Frontier Nursing in Appalachia: History,
Organization and the Changing Culture of Care

Edie West

Frontier Nursing in Appalachia: History, Organization and the Changing Culture of Care

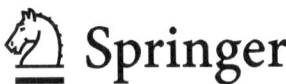 Springer

Edie West
Indiana University of Pennsylvania
Indiana, PA
USA

ISBN 978-3-030-20026-8   ISBN 978-3-030-20027-5   (eBook)
https://doi.org/10.1007/978-3-030-20027-5

This Springer imprint is published by the registered company Springer Nature Switzerland AG
The registered company address is: Gewerbestrasse 11, 6330 Cham, Switzerland

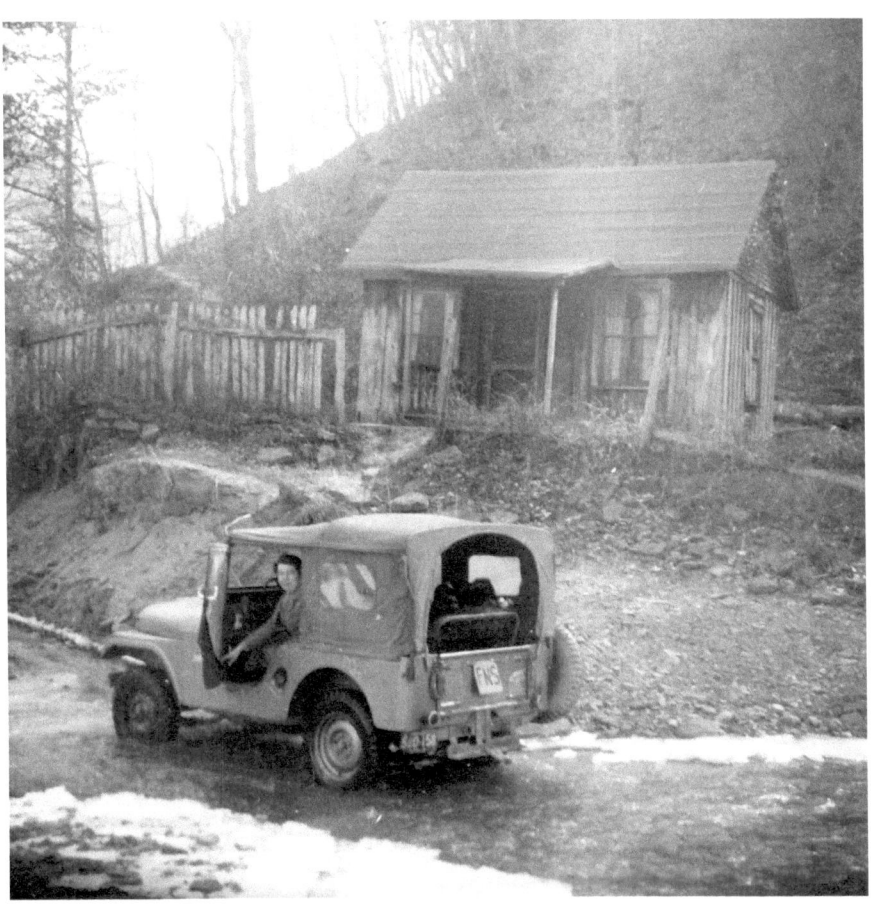

Former British Frontier Nursing Service Nurse Maggie Willson on an Appalachian home visit (circa 1960s)

Illustrations

Photographs

1. Former British Frontier Nursing Service Nurse Maggie Willson on an Appalachian home visit (circa 1960s), Book Cover.
2. Judy Halse posing for FNS *Bulletin* (1960).
3. Mary Breckinridge with "Third Generation" FNS 'Baby' outside of her home and administrative offices, 'The Big House' (Circa 1960s).
4. 'Big House' interior, then and now, with Molly Lee at Thanksgiving Dinner in 'then' photo (circa 1960s).
5. Former British FNS Nurse Maggie Willson (standing) with (left to right): Helen Browne, FNS Founder, Mary Breckinridge and her Cousin, Marvin Breckinridge.
6. Former British FNS Nurse, Maggie Willson with 'Baby in her Saddlebag' promotional photograph.
7. Author, Dr. Edie West, with former British FNS Nurses Judy Halse and Maggie Willson, then and now.
8. Former British FNS Nurse, Molly Lee, with Appalachian mother and twins she delivered.
9. Former British FNS Nurses: Molly Lee & Betty "Hilly" Hillman… then and now.
10. Former British FNS Nurse, Betty "Hilly" Hillman on an Appalachian home visit.
11. FNS Nurse Betty Lester (on white horse), FNS Founder, Mary Breckinridge, former FNS Nurse Molly Lee (far right) and one other FNS Nurse on horseback preparing to ride on "Mary Breckinridge Day."
12. Unidentified FNS Nurse, her dog and jeep (circa 1960s).
13. Former American FNS Nurse and one of the first graduates of the Frontier Graduate School of Midwifery, Doris E. Reid and her dog on horseback.

Maps

Preface

Mary Breckinridge established the Frontier Nursing Service (FNS) in a poor, rural, underdeveloped area of the Appalachian Mountains of Eastern Kentucky in 1925 and, in so doing, marked the first effort to professionalize midwifery in the United States. Since its inception in 1925, the FNS has survived many challenges and still exists today. This historical analysis of the FNS's 'early years' (1925–1970) yields valuable insights not only on how such a remarkable feat was achieved but also on how these insights could benefit nurses today. The contemporary nursing profession is struggling with many of the same internal and external environmental forces that challenged those 'early nurses'.

The FNS's culture is explored, and its formation as a community-/people-focused organization at a time in history when the nation was moving towards a corporate-/consumer-focused society is examined. The political implications for the FNS and its founder as the service negotiated its place in both Appalachian and wider societies, the lack of clarity and disruptions that developed within the organization with regard to its move from a decentralized to centralized power structure and resultant relational transformation within its community and its work environment, nurse-physician relationships, educational environments, nurse recruitment and retention practices and public image are then examined. The oral history narratives of FNS nurses and non-FNS nurses currently in practice as well as nurse and non-nurse FNS staff and community members have been employed in the study to build as complete a picture as possible of the FNS, the nurses who worked within it and the culture of nursing.

Critical threads that emerged in relation to nursing's chronic recurrent recruitment problems include retention, work environment and public image. These 'crisis issues' are woven throughout the wider socioeconomic, political and health-care agenda of the US national culture. This cultural change has gradually intruded into the Eastern Appalachia and is still reflected in the narratives of nurses in practice today as reported here. A more comprehensive, albeit complex, set of insights to nursing's ongoing crisis issues includes consideration that the profession has inherited a culture that has proven to be self-defeating as it has perpetuated many of the corporate cultural traits that can be seen to be incongruent with its professional identity and goals. The continual crisis issues commonly cited as causes of 'nursing shortages' are not created solely by those barriers which exist external to the profession, such as a lack of political power, funding, or even the institutionalization of health care. They are also being perpetuated by the profession's inability to deal with the barriers inside the existing culture.

The question emerging from this analysis of the FNS which needs to be posed to the profession as a whole is as follows: 'Has the embracing of institutional identity (viz., the business and medical models) within the nursing profession, its higher education and practice settings impeded the discipline's ability to impact more successfully for sustained, positive change within these environments?' In order for sustained positive change to occur, nurses must be willing to unveil those barriers within the profession itself that deal with the very basic question of professional identity. This historical analysis supported by the oral history testimony offers some insights into how this question might be further explored.

Indiana, PA, USA   Edie West

Acknowledgements

I must thank first and foremost my Lord and Saviour, Jesus Christ, without whom, I can do nothing, and former American FNS nurse, Miss Doris Reid (1918–2004), whose life and work inspired me to do this research and write this book. A heartfelt thank you also goes out to the British and American FNS nurses who shared so much more than their expertise, wisdom and incredible life experiences with me. They also opened their hearts, hands and homes to a total stranger in need, reminding this researcher of all that is great and good about nurses. I want to thank all the nurses who participated in this study and gave of themselves through honest reflection for the ultimate benefit and advancement of their chosen profession.

A special thank you goes out to Dr. Ron Iphofen, Dr. Will Griffith and Mrs. Katherine Williams for all of their insights, guidance and support and to the archival staff at the University of Kentucky in Lexington and the 'Oral History Project' staffers there who graciously assisted me in the transcription of the FNS oral history audio tapes. I also wish to express my appreciation to the FNS, especially to Barb Gibson, who helped me find former FNS staff and offered me hospitality and access to the memorabilia, photographs and archival materials located in Wendover, Kentucky.

I also gratefully acknowledge my family, friends and colleagues who let me vent, spurred me on and kept me sane over the 4 years it took to complete this work and most especially to my parents, Ken and Virginia West (my prayer warriors), who made 'no writing Sunday' a special place of refreshment weekly.

Finally, this book is dedicated to the memory of my big brother, Wayne Jacob West (1954–2018), my webmaster, audio-visual department and tech support guy all rolled into one, an incredibly smart, funny, big-hearted, generous man to all who knew him. I never could have completed this work without him. I miss you daily, my brother, and long for the day when we will be together again.

Contents

Chapter 1
Background and Introduction

1.1 Modern Problem, Historical Perspective and the Frontier Nursing Service

1.1.1 Modern Problem

Contemporary nursing undoubtedly compares favourably with other professions if one judges by the standards of public service, idealism and professional solidarity. Yet entire volumes have been written on the medical profession's contributions to the miracles of surgery or the triumphs over infectious diseases, whereas hardly a word has been written on the nurse's contributions towards this progress [1]. Though it could be argued that much has been written about nursing since Dock made this statement in 1932, if the passing reference made by Drake (2001) in *The History of Appalachia,* which referred to the Frontier Nursing Service as a "mission" while simultaneously lauding Lexington's "prominent physician's" is any indication of what is being written, then one could question the value placed upon nurses and nursing by the general public [2]. Furthermore, the discipline has historically been modest, self-effacing and not fully cognizant of the role their profession has played in the modern warfare against disease [3]. The need for professional nurses to honor their own work, attain recognition from physicians and the general public and rid themselves once and for all of this notion that they are compelled to work under the constant eye of physicians and automatically carry out their orders is certainly not new. However, it is a need that has yet to be fully satisfied.

Unfortunately, like other predominantly female professions, nursing remains under-valued. While the public indicates high trust of nurses, there is a lack of understanding about what nurses do. Nurses today are still burdened by the image of "handmaiden" and this lowered status has implications for the value of nursing to society [4]. Indeed, this image has been a major contributor to the nursing shortages over the years. Though it is not possible to isolate a single causative factor as the problem is complex and interrelated and there is no simple description on the status

© Springer Nature Switzerland AG 2019   1
E. West, *Frontier Nursing in Appalachia: History, Organization and the Changing Culture of Care*, https://doi.org/10.1007/978-3-030-20027-5_1

of the most recent nursing shortages in the literature, there is agreement that the problem is having a negative impact on the current nursing practice environment. The profession's inability to recruit enough nurses to meet the demand, particularly in an aging population, into environments that are not wholly conducive to keeping them in practice remains a problem that is global in scope [5]. Most experts also agree that for sustained change and assurance of an adequate supply of nurses, solutions must be developed in areas of education, health care delivery systems, policy, regulation and image [6].

1.1.2 Historical Perspective

Society created the need for nursing, and also led nursing to develop over the years in order to meet its ever-changing needs. Social change occurs as a result of economic, religious, demographic and cultural climate shifts, or any combination of them, over time. Other forces for change within any given culture are scientific revolutions, wars, political powers, and mass media [7]. The relationship between these various catalysts for change is a complex one. They can hardly be considered mutually exclusive and can be extremely far reaching in their impact. Such change, both external and internal to any cultural entity produces new demands for, among other things, improved health care.

An historical approach to contemporary nursing issues can provide us with the same intellectual and political tools that our predecessors applied to shape nursing values and beliefs to the social context of their time. Indeed, history shows us how our predecessors struggled with problems almost exactly like those we face today. It also reveals methods, not wholly unlike our own, which could yield similarly remarkable results. History discourages by its habit of repetition and discloses the human race's tenacity for outmoded ideas and methods. It also encourages, by bringing to light progress made, and the role earnestness and persistence played in its advance [8]. If we consider the long history of nursing as a whole, we see how uneven and halting progress has been, rising by slow stages for many centuries only to decline again up to the threshold of modern times [9]. The contribution of Florence Nightingale in the latter half of the nineteenth century was to create a profession based upon sanitary knowledge and scientific medical discoveries; secular in the full sense but humanitarian, independent and self-supporting. It is still this emphasis on expert skill and knowledge which distinguishes the modern professional nurse from the older idea of the voluntary religious or personal service nurse, or that of the manual labourer. Nursing then had the distinct advantage of being the only profession that offered serious, solid, courageous women a career that promised prestige, adventure and the opportunity to become a constructive reformer. However, nursing's progress in the twentieth century tended to be governed by the laws of industry (supply and demand) fuelled to a large degree by two World Wars. The feminist movement also first helped and then hindered the profession by opening many career fields to women that were not possible several decades before [10].

1.1.3   The Frontier Nursing Service

Intentional communities consist of groups of people who have committed to live together to pursue some ideology, whether spiritual, economic, environmental and/or social [11]. The Frontier Nursing Service (FNS) was one such community that began its health care service with remarkably similar beliefs and values as that of its chosen service community in the Service's early years. Mary Breckinridge established the FNS in a poor, rural, underdeveloped area of the Appalachian Mountains of Eastern Kentucky in 1925 and in so doing, marked the first effort to professionalize midwifery in the US [12]. She based her organization on an established scheme that existed on the Inner and Outer Hebrides Islands of the British Isles, which was very similar to the terrain of Eastern Kentucky, called the Highlands and Islands Medical and Nursing Service [13]. Using the Highlands concept Breckinridge expected her nurses to serve as public health and district nurses in addition to being nurse-midwives. Her organization was originally known as the Kentucky Committee for Mothers and Babies and later named the Frontier Nursing Service. She founded her organization on these two major goals: improving the health of children and pioneering a system of rural healthcare that could serve as a model for healthcare systems serving the most remote regions of the world. She chose Eastern Kentucky for her demonstration project, an area with few roads and no physicians. She felt that if the work she had in mind could be done there, it could be duplicated anywhere. Of the area she had chosen, and her ideas about rural health care, Breckinridge wrote:

> In 1925 the territory in the Kentucky Mountains, where the service began its field of operations, was a vast forested area inhabited by some 10,000 people. There was no motor road within sixty miles in any direction. Horseback and mule team were the only modes of travel; brought-on supplies came from distant railroad points and took from two to five days to haul in [14].

In the summer of 1923, travelling on horseback, Breckinridge initiated a research study of the health needs of the people of Leslie, Clay, Perry and Harlan counties. She rode over seven hundred miles interviewing families and the 'granny' midwives. She found that women lacked prenatal care and gave birth to an average of nine children, primarily attended by self-taught midwives. She saw high rates of maternal mortality and came to believe that children's health care must begin before birth with care of the mother and follow that care throughout childhood while including care for the entire family. The FNS became the first organization in America to use nurses qualified as midwives.

In the organization's 'early years,' nurses who had equestrian experience had to be recruited from Great Britain as there were no midwifery schools in the United States. The majority of these nurses were British though Breckinridge also educated interested American nurses with equestrian experience by sending them to Great Britain for midwifery training. Breckinridge paid full scholarships that included housing, food and transportation, which at the time meant a round-trip journey by ship for her American nurses to go abroad for the required 6 months of training. She also paid the fare of interested British nurses to come to Kentucky. These nurses contracted to work for the FNS for a period of 2 years. They could leave before then if they chose, however the Service would not pay for the return trip if they opted to leave before their contracted length of stay. There were few who chose to leave before the contracted length of stay but those that did were able to return on the pay they received as the FNS provided free room, board and transportation for all of its employees. These nurses' practice environment necessitated fording raging rivers on horseback through some of the roughest, wildest areas of Appalachia, delivering babies, providing district and public health nursing in rustic cabins, many without running water or electricity. Essentially, they provided care to people who considered their fellow Americans 'foreign' [15].

Breckinridge, the daughter of a wealthy and prominent Southern family, initially financed the Service through her personal funds. No state or federal agency was either able or willing to help with her project in its infancy though later these agencies took over the bulk of the Service's operations once it had become a trusted, established component of the local community. When her personal funds were exhausted, she garnered support through her family connections and friends. Breckinridge spent much of her time outside the mountains in the early years, developing the base of financial support that survived the depression and enabled the FNS to carry on in the ensuing years. She organized support committees of philanthropic individuals in many large cities, which included Boston, Chicago, Cincinnati, Cleveland, Detroit, Louisville, New York, Philadelphia, Pittsburgh, Providence, Rochester and Washington DC.

It was through the loyal work of these members the FNS survived through the stock market crash of 1929, the depression, numerous droughts, floods and the advent of World War Two. In 1939 Breckinridge faced major recruitment and retention problems, as the majority of her nurses returned to England to serve their country in World War Two. She was compelled to start the first midwifery school in the US in order to keep the FNS's doors open. It is interesting to note, that many of those British nurses chose to return to the FNS after the war and some of them are buried there. Despite these difficulties, between 1925 and 1930 the FNS grew rapidly. The first clinic was opened in Hyden, Kentucky in 1925 with the help of two nurses. By Christmas of that year Breckinridge had built the log house at Wendover, Kentucky that was to be her home for 40 years and which was the beginning of the complex, which has served for more than 80 years as the administrative headquarters of the FNS. The Hyden Hospital and Health Centre was completed in 1928 and in response to the demand from local citizens for accessible nursing care, nine outpost nursing centres were built in Leslie County and the Red Bird River section of Clay County [12].

The Service began as a decentralized health care system with a hospital and six out-post nursing clinics located within a five-mile ride on horseback to its service community. The region served by the FNS was divided into nine districts. These centres were staffed by nurse-midwives, who held clinics, made rounds on horseback, provided home care, and attended home births. They served an average of 250 families per outpost, held immunization clinics at one room schools and provided advice regarding sanitization of wells and outhouses. They also made arrangements for high-risk patients to be seen at Hyden Hospital. The hospital provided nurses and a physician who could perform surgeries. They also had visiting doctors who would hold specialty clinics such as gynecology, eye, ears, nose, throat and ortho-pedics. A system of referrals was developed to ensure that FNS patients could get specialist care beyond the mountains which could not be provided by the Service's own professional staff, a system that continues today [14].

A major challenge of providing care in this region was communication, both physical as well as cultural. In the Service's 'early years' nothing came into the hills except mail and that only once a day. Later, an unreliable phone service arrived. To cope with this problem, meet the supply needs of the outpost clinics and help with all the work that had to be accomplished each day by the nursing staff, Breckinridge started a volunteer service and called the participants 'Couriers.' The Couriers were initially recruited from Breckinridge's many family and friends. Most were young women seeking adventure and an opportunity for public service. Couriers spent much of their days in the saddle carrying news and supplies between the many clin-ics and the hospital. They guided visitors, transported patients and assisted the nurses when necessary. They also had the charge to care for all of the horses and later the jeeps used by the Service [14].

The health care system established by Breckinridge worked so well that there was an immediate decrease in infant and maternal mortality. The FNS kept precise statistics and evaluated the Services' progress after every 1000 births. These statis-tics were tabulated by the Metropolitan Life Insurance Company. The report on the first 1000 births stated that the study showed conclusively what had in fact been shown before, that the type of service rendered by the FNS safeguarded the life of mother and infant. If such service was available to the women of the country gener-ally, there would be a saving of 10,000 mothers' lives per year in the US; there would be 30,000 less still births and 30,000 more children alive at the end of the first month of life. The study demonstrated the need to train a large body of nurse-midwives, competent to carry out the routines that had been established both in the FNS and in other places where good obstetrical care was available.[1]

In the late 1960s, the FNS recognized that as health care options became more complex, a broader based education was necessary for nurses to be able to provide comprehensive primary care to all family members. At this time, the Frontier School developed the first certificate program to prepare family nurse practitioners (FNP). In 1970, the name of the School was changed to the Frontier School of Midwifery and Family Nursing (FSMFN) to reflect the addition of the FNP program. In 1975, the Service completed and opened the modern, 40-bed Mary Breckinridge Hospital and Health Center. This hospital has served the health care needs of the people of Leslie County for the past 30 years and continues its operation today as a critical access hospital. Over the ensuing years, there were many changes in the Southeastern

---

[1] Reprint from the FNS Quarterly Bulletin, winter 1935 (No. 3). University of Kentucky, Lexington. 85M1: FNS, Box 25, Fol. 2. 'Organization & Supervision of the Filed Work of the FNS'.

Kentucky region. The opening of roads brought an end to the era of nurse on horse-back. Today the Service operates five federally designated rural health clinics, a critical access hospital, and a home health service. The Frontier School of Midwifery and Family Nursing is the largest school of midwifery in the US. The School also offers programs for aspiring family nurse practitioners and women health care nurse practitioners. Programs are also offered to students in remote and rural areas through distance education. Wendover continues as the administrative centre of the service. The original log cabin fondly called 'the Big House' that was Mary Breckinridge's home for over 40 years was honored as a National Historic Landmark in 1991 and became a Bed and Breakfast in 2001. The Courier program today is an internship program. Students come and shadow nurse-midwives, nurse practitioners, physicians and help with the many day-to-day tasks of operating the Service. The Service developed by Breckinridge has provided care to the people of Eastern Kentucky for over 80 years and has graduated over 17,000 nurse-midwives and nurse practitioners who serve all over the world.

The FNS celebrated 75 years of service in the year 2000 and has evolved over the years. The FNS today owns and operates Mary Breckinridge Healthcare in Hyden, Kentucky, four rural clinics (Beech Fork Clinic, Community Health Clinic, Kate Ireland Healthcare and the Dr. Anne Wasson Clinic). The Frontier School of Midwifery and Family Nursing consist of a master's Science in Nursing education program with specialties in Nurse-Midwifery and Family Nurse Practitioner. The fact that Breckinridge's organization is not only viable but still thriving over 80 years later is a testament to the effort, skill and determination of both its founder and her nurses, and to the value placed on them by the community they served.

Though many have come to the FNS to study Breckinridge's organizational model over the years in order to duplicate it in rural areas all over the globe and some research has been done at the Service on nurse midwifery and even analysis from a social or ethnographic perspective, no one has ever examined the FNS from a cultural and historical perspective. The major crisis issues (recruitment, retention, work environment and public image) that this organization faced are common to nursing and are issues that still have a negative impact on the profession today. Analysis from a cultural perspective is lacking in the prevailing literature and as a result, the response or proffered solutions to these issues have tended to be simplistic or linear analytic responses to extremely complex socio-cultural and economic problems when looked at holistically.

1.2   Methodological Discussion

Historical research in nursing is a relatively new method of inquiry and qualitative research has particularly developed in nursing in the last 25 years in the UK and US. The profession's thrust to date has been on quantitative research, which deals more with nursing 'science' than 'art.' The intrinsic and extrinsic value of historical research in nursing was first published in 1965 in a landmark article entitled 'The

Case for Historical Research.' Up to that time there were very few research studies being done in nursing history [16]. The American Nurses Association in 1965 formally recognized historical research as a direct result of Newton's article. Since that time, the need for historical research in order to facilitate a clearer understanding of nursing's ongoing challenges and to provide for a more successful approach to current professional problems has been supported in more recent publications [17]. Historical nursing research is also developing rapidly in a number of academic institutions in the United Kingdom, elsewhere in Europe, the United States and Australia.

This study of the FNS proved to be challenging in regard to theoretical and methodological analysis. The research conducted for this thesis comprised both an historical analysis of the FNS together with an assessment of oral history interviews with a sample of nurse and non-nurse participants. By its very nature this research has necessitated a much more eclectic approach in regard to both theory and methodology, and the available literature advocates the use of a range of resources and tools in compiling historical data for use in nursing research [18]. The oral history interviews of British and American FNS nurses, FNS staff and local community members served to enhance the depth and richness of this work and are presented throughout the study to offer authentic insights into the personal experiences of professionals imbedded in a novel cultural experience in which the practice of their profession was sustained by organizational and community processes that were not existent elsewhere in the US in the Service's early years. In addition, the oral histories of North American nurses currently in practice exemplify the similar and disparate cultural experiences of nurses in regard to professional recruitment, retention, work environment and image issues. The goal of this study was to seek the main theme or themes to be illuminated by an analysis of conventional historical data and of oral history data generated by the nurses via taped interviews and surveys.

Twelve former FNS nurses (five British and seven American) were interviewed or surveyed. Of these twelve, all twelve were surveyed and nine also agreed to be interviewed. An advert was placed in the FNS's *Quarterly Bulletin* asking former FNS nurses interested in participating in the study to contact the researcher. A website was created to solicit the participation of nurses in practice and an advert placed in *RN* and *AJN* magazines asking nurses interested in participating in the survey to go to the website. Twenty non-FNS nurses in practice participated by submitting the completed survey on-line. The interviews followed the principles, standards and evaluation guidelines set forth by the Oral History Association and were analysed from a hermeneutic perspective; that is a final interpretation of the data was reached only after careful analysis between texts, and then testing all or part of these interpretations against the global meaning of the texts, with proper attention also being given to presuppositions [19]. The survey questions were open-ended and required nurses to either write or type responses to them in 'free-text' style. Interviews and surveys were elicited over a 4-year period from 2003 to 2007 (Appendix A).

The Oral history narratives of FNS nurses (coded FNS 01-12) and non-FNS nurses currently in practice (coded SWN 01-20), as well as nurse and non-nurse FNS staff and community members retrieved from the University of Kentucky's Oral History Project (coded Interview # 1978–1982) were used in the study to build as complete a picture as possible of the FNS, nurses and the discipline of nursing, within an historical context. The emerging themes were then quantified. To further ensure that the research findings accurately reflected people's perceptions, whatever they may be, and to increase the researchers understanding of the probability that the findings would be seen as credible and worthy of consideration by others, corroboration was sought between the nurse narratives and the primary and secondary sources (i.e., archival information, newspapers, journals, books and internet sources). Internal criticism of the historical data focused on authentication of the generator of the data being analysed as well as on whether witnesses agreed with one another. External criticism to determine if the evidence was authentic and genuine as well as if valid sources which could be admissible as evidence were being used was also crucial to the study. The interviews offered a clear advantage in fostering a fuller understanding of the individual nurse's private yet crucial areas of family and personal relationships, and experiences which prompted career decisions. An individual life and the role it played in the larger community are best understood through in depth oral history interviews [20]. Despite the inevitable loss of certain information and the undoubted subjectivity on the interviewee's recollections, the process gives voice to those working and middle-class nurses who did not choose to write autobiographies, as did the FNS's celebrated founder, Mary Breckinridge. Streubert and Carpenter's (2011) guidelines for historical analysis were also been employed in order to rigorously assess the generation of data, treatment of data (which encompasses the assessment of primary and secondary sources), analysis of data (which refers to the analysis of organization, theoretical framework, bias and ethical considerations), and finally the study's significance to nursing. The researcher's interpretations of the findings were also analysed to determine if the findings were sufficiently and dispassionately explored [21].

Historical knowledge arises from the extensive study of individuals within societies. Historical sources encompass every form of human evidence and are based squarely on what the historian can read in documents or hear from informants [22]. Idealist school historians are most concerned with getting inside an event and understanding the thoughts of individuals within a specific time, place and situation and as this framework represented more closely the values of qualitative research it seemed to suit the study's aims. Yet most historians question whether there exists any one way of explaining change. Therefore, elements of a grounded theory approach also seemed to fit the exploration of nursing recruitment, retention, practice environment and image issues at the FNS; whereas understanding phenomena from the nurse and non-nurse subjects' own perspectives suggested a phenomenological approach to the interview data. Add to this the fact that a majority of the FNS's 'early years' nurses were imported from Great Britain, while the Appalachian Mountain culture of Eastern Kentucky was their field of practice and an argument can also be made for an ethnographic approach to the study [23]. In sum, the breadth of this study made it difficult to identify a single theory or methodology that would have adequately encompassed the analytical requirements of the topic.

1.2.1 Scientific Method in Human Cultures

Though there is no standard definition of culture, most alternatives incorporate the work of Franz Boas, one of the pioneers of modern anthropology who was famed for applying the scientific method to the study of human cultures and societies, a field which was previously based on the formulation of grand theories around anecdotal knowledge. Boas believed in historical and cultural relativism, which points out that the differences between people, were the result of historical, social and geographic conditions and that all populations had a complete and equally developed culture. For the purpose of this study, Boas' approach was adopted whereby culture was defined as 'the system of shared beliefs, values, customs, behaviours and artefacts that the members of a society use to cope with their world and with one another, and that are transmitted from generation to generation through learning' [24]. Moreover, with the evolution of institutions within cultures come more rigidity and resistance to these natural impulses. Indeed, these organizations and institutions themselves can be viewed as cultures within cultures [25].

1.2.2 Environmental and Organizational Cultures

Though most organizations are established to achieve economic or political objectives, the FNS was not. It did, however, out of necessity require economic success and needed to be politically connected in order to achieve its altruistic goals. It is therefore essential that the study of this organization include structural, material, economic and environmental factors as well. The most rapid cultural changes within a given society occur in times of crisis and these changes also affect health care parameters within society. Therefore, the organizational culture of the FNS, a unique health care organization, located within the equally unique sub-culture of Eastern Appalachia at a time of unprecedented change in the US's overall socio-economic history presents some challenges regarding what perspective to take when examining it. The organization does not fit any one of the three reigning social scientific perspectives on the nature of change in organizational cultures, which are integration, differentiation and fragmentation [26].

The integration perspective interprets all cultural manifestations as consistently reinforcing the same themes. All members of the organization are said to share in an organization-wide consensus and culture is described as a realm where all is clear, and ambiguity is excluded. The differentiation perspective describes cultural manifestations as sometimes inconsistent and sees consensus only within the boundaries of subcultures, which often conflict with each other. Ambiguity is characterized so that it does not intrude on the clarity which exists within these subcultural boundaries. However, the fragmentation view of culture most fits the overall objectives of this study, namely, to bring the sources of ambiguity (i.e., where a culture or subculture begins or ends, as these boundaries are permeable and fluctuating) to the foreground of a cultural description. It builds on the complexities introduced by the nexus approach to understanding culture, which states that an organization is a microcosm of the surrounding culture. Many external societal influences will therefore permeate the organization's periphery and be enacted within it. It builds on the complexities introduced by the *nexus approach* to understanding culture.

The nexus approach argues that in many ways, an organization is a microcosm of the surrounding culture. Many external societal influences will therefore permeate the organization's periphery and be enacted within it. This premise of 'feeder cultures' suggests a better resolution to the uniqueness dilemma presented when looking at organizations, which quite often contain very diverse environments from one another as a result of the variance that also exists in the surrounding culture in which they subsist. Acknowledgement of 'feeder culture' influences permits a redefinition of organizational culture that sees an organization as 'a nexus where a variety of cultural influences come together within a boundary.' Some of the cultural elements within that boundary will be truly distinctive to the organization. Other elements, some of which may well be erroneously believed to be unique, will reflect cultural influences external to the organization. This premise of 'feeder cultures' suggests a better resolution to the uniqueness dilemma presented when looking at the FNS, which contained very diverse environments both within as well as without the organization. In addition, the fragmentation approach views culture as a loosely structured and incompletely shared system that emerges dynamically as cultural members experience each other's events and the organisation's contextual features and for the purposes of this study, this analytical approach was adopted [27]. Many fragmentation studies emphasize environmental sources of change and acknowledge that power is not localized solely at the top of a hierarchy or even at the sub-cultural level of analysis but rather is broadly diffused in the environment. In the FNS's long history it served as a 'feeder' as well as a 'fed' culture by the national and international environments it relied heavily on for funding and health care providers from outside of the Appalachian region and the local community, which provided the purpose for its very existence [28]. Much of the turmoil experienced by the organization in its latter years stemmed from the power shift that accompanied a move from a decentralized to a more centralized organizational structure within this environment. Fragmentation is the approach that most acknowledges the environmental changes in feeder cultures, a reality that has profoundly changed not only Appalachia and the FNS over the years but also the discipline of nursing as culture as well. This perspective acknowledges the integration perspectives search for consistency and the differentiation perspective's search for inconsistency within organizational cultures but goes further, deeper, on to complexity and if there is one word that can best describe the FNS, Appalachia and the discipline of nursing most succinctly, it is 'complexity.'

Nurse-Midwife and FNS founder, Mary Breckinridge believed in the concept of power being broadly diffused. She strongly believed that even after birth a young child is not an isolated individual. His care not only means the care of his mother before, during and after his birth, but the care of his whole family as well. She felt that bedside nursing of the sick in their homes was as essential in rural areas as in the Visiting Nurse Associations to be found in cities. This approach to health care meant including the whole family and community, because the young child was part of both. She thought that health teaching must also be on a family basis and in the homes. Breckinridge understood that culture does not imply a 'uniformity' of values but rather a shared recognition of relevant issues, which for her focused on the people of a particular rural community in the US and her organization's responsibility to care for these people's well being in the promotion of health as well as in the care of the sick [27]. It should be noted that the concept of community wellness in addition to the treatment of the sick was an idea that was in a state of transition in 1925, when the service was founded. Breckinridge's introduction of midwifery to the US and linking it with public health and district nursing to provide a generalized community-focused, health and wellness approach to health care was not a new concept. However, she was establishing it at a time when the rest of the nation was moving toward the business model of specialized, technology-driven care of the sick and the more institutionalized delivery of care system that this focus necessitated [12].

Breckinridge had this to say about the question when she wrote the following entitled 'A Few Notes On Nursing By An Old Nurse' in her organization's Quarterly Bulletin's Spring 1948 issue:

> The tendency today is toward standardization in certain fixed patterns—One need not lack standards in avoiding standardization, just as one need not lack unity in avoiding uniformity. There should be no falling below a certain standard for nursing schools, but above which the sky should be the limit. Experimentation should continue and be encouraged. Nursing owes its growth to avoid rigidity.[2]

The FNS in its early years was more of a microcosm of the surrounding Eastern Appalachian culture. In the Service's latter years, it reluctantly served as a 'feeder' culture to the Eastern Appalachian region of the corporate culture that existed outside of the hills. As a philanthropic organization, it relied heavily on 'feeder cultures,' which consisted almost entirely of people and organizations that existed outside of Appalachia for personnel, finances and supplies. Though the FNS had always made a concerted effort to include the local people and their cultural norms when making decisions regarding the services they provided, eventually a schism developed between the organization and the local population, as well as within its organizational ranks, as it began to look and function in much the same way as health organizations outside of the region. Adjustments in care provision and practices that the FNS had to make in order to survive were forced upon them by its 'feeder culture' and eventually this affected its ability to meet the needs of the people in a manner that was culturally congruent and acceptable to them. The FNS, in its latter years became a conduit for the propagation of the type and manner of care

---

[2] FNS Quarterly Bulletin 1948. 85M1: FNS, Box 25, Fol. 21. 'A Few Notes on Nursing by an Old Nurse' by Mary Breckinridge, Reprint from the FNS Quarterly Bulletin, spring 1948 (No. 4). University of Kentucky in Lexington, USA

being done outside of the region. This, coupled with improved access into the region via roads, resulted in the area becoming less and less remote to an ever-encroaching culture that was in many ways alien and to which the people were unwilling to fully assimilate.

Ironically, in the FNS's latter years it was a trait from both of these competing disparate cultures that helped the organization survive. The local people had developed rapport with the FNS founder and her nurses. Therefore, even in the face of rapid and often troubling changes in the organization's provision of care, the people, for the most part, remained loyal to the organization [29]. Consequently, the national health care (medical/business) model of 'corporate America' that eventually eclipsed the Service in the 1960s and 1970s, capitalized on this loyalty by using the FNS's history, positive image, stories and myths to market it as a valuable commodity to the community despite its agenda shift from Breckinridge's custom-made, community health and wellness focused, people-oriented approach to the national, mass-produced, medical/business model, industry-focused approach in the provision of health care [30]. This culture shift forever changed the relationship between nurses and other health care personnel within the organization as well as the organization's relationship with the community it served.

An Analysis of the FNS and surrounding region, which simultaneously underwent these changes and made the choices necessary for survival, will help us to validate the reliability of those choices. A re-thinking of the FNS's past, including a re-examination of the ideas of its founder, nurses and community, which helped to shape the organization, can authenticate those issues previously identified within the literature as primary causes for nursing's continual recruitment, retention, work environment and image woes. Further, when compared with the ideas of nurses presently in practice today, other possible causes can then be identified that have either not previously been investigated or perhaps have been deemed less relevant. For instance, the impact that organizational culture such as governmental agencies, health care practice settings, educational institutions and professional nursing organizations as well as the wider local, national and popular cultures have had upon these crisis issues.

The FNS's culture from a local and national perspective is explored and its formation as a community-people focused organization at a time in history when the nation was moving toward a corporate-consumer focused society is examined in Chap. 2. The political implications for the FNS and its founder as the Service negotiated its place in both Appalachian and wider-society frames (Chap. 3) while the lack of clarity and disruptions that developed within the organization with regard to its move from a decentralized to centralized power structure and resultant relational transformation within its community is presented in (Chap. 4). The remaining chapters reflect the main themes illuminated by the historical and oral history data. They are; environment (Chap. 5), nurse-physician relationship (Chap. 6), educational environment (Chap. 7), nurse recruitment and retention practices (Chap. 8) and public image (Chap. 9).

Many of the institutional and organizational cultures that were being introduced by the local, state and federal governments into Appalachia in the 1960s had differing objectives and agendas for the Service as well as the community. All of the subsequent chapters examine the national culture that impacted Eastern Appalachia and more specifically the organizational culture of the FNS, which had ties to both of these cultures and beyond [31]. The critical threads which emerged in relation to nursing's chronic recruitment, retention, work environment and image issues are woven throughout the wider socio-economic, political and health care agendas of America's national culture, which eventually gained access into Eastern Appalachia and are still reflected in the oral history narratives of nurses in practice today [31]. Through an exploration of the common ground between these cultures, the motivations of the FNS and new governmental and non-governmental agencies and industrial concerns within the region as well as the divergences between them and especially through a re-examination of the compulsions of the FNS, a more comprehensive, albeit complex, set of insights to nursing's ongoing crisis issues is unveiled. The historical impact of these crisis issues on 'professional identity', the discipline's proclivity to be negatively influenced by the culture which breeds them and its ability to influence for sustained positive change within them is then proffered in the concluding chapter.

References

1. Dock L. A short history of nursing. London: Putnam's Sons; 1932. p. 1.
2. Drake R. History of Appalachia. Kentucky: University Press of Kentucky; 2003. p. xiv.
3. Buresch B, Gordon S. From silence to voice: what nurses know and must communicate to the public. Ottawa: Canadian Nurses Association; 2000. p. xv.
4. Snavely T. A brief economic analysis of the looming nursing shortage in the United States. Nurs Econ. 2016;34(2):98–100.
5. American Association of Colleges of Nurses. About the nursing shortage. 2019. https://www.aacnnursing.org/News-Information/Nursing-Shortage-Resources/About. Accessed 1 Jan 2019.
6. Buchan M, O'May F, Gilles D. Nursing workforce policy and the economic crisis: a global overview. J Nurs Scholarsh. 2013;. https://doi.org/10.1111/jnu.12028
7. Baly M. Nursing and social change. 3rd ed. London: Routledge; 1995. p. 56.
8. Goodnow N. Outlines of nursing history. New York: Saunders; 1921. p. 11.
9. Dock. A short history of nursing. London: Putnam's Sons; 1932. p. 117.
10. Bullough V. Emergence of modern nursing. London: Croom Helm; 1979.
11. Abramson R, Haskell J. Encyclopaedia of Appalachia. Knoxville: University of Tennessee Press; 2006. p. 151.
12. Breckinridge M. Wide neighborhoods: a story of the Frontier Nursing Service. Lexington: The University Press of Kentucky; 1952.
13. Dodge B. The story of nursing. Boston: Little, Brown & Company; 1965.
14. Frontier Nursing Service, Inc. History information. FNS website. 1925–2008. http://www.frontiernursing.org/. Accessed 10 May 2007.
15. Gardner C. Cleaver Country: Kentucky mountain trails. New York: Fleming H. Revell; 1931.
16. Newton ME. The case for historical research. Nur Res. 1965;14(1):20–6.
17. Fasoli D. The culture of nursing engagement: a historical perspective. Nurs Adm Q. 2010;34(1):18–29. https://doi.org/10.1097/NAQ.0b013e3181c95e7a.
18. Lewis S. Qualitative inquiry and research design: choosing among five approaches. Health Promot Pract. 2015;16(4). https://doi.org/10.1177/1524839915580941

19. Oral History Association. OHA principles and best practice. 2019. http://www.oralhistory. org/. Accessed 1 Jan 2019.
20. Abrams L. Oral history theory. 2nd ed. London: Routledge; 2016. p. 250.
21. Streubert H, Carpenter D. Qualitative research in nursing: advancing the humanistic imperative. 5th ed. New York: Lippincott, Williams and Wilkins; 2011.
22. Tosh J. The pursuit of history aims, methods and new directions in the study of history. 6th ed. London: Routledge; 2015. p. 198.
23. Smith J. Qualitative psychology: a practical guide to research methods. 3rd ed. New York: Sage; 2015.
24. Bates D, Plog F. Cultural anthropology. 3rd ed. Berkshire: McGraw-Hill College; 1990.
25. Ryan R, Deci E. On assimilating identities to the self: a self-determination theory perspective on internalization and integrity within cultures. In: Leary MR, Tangney JP, editors. Handbook of self and identity. New York: Guilford; 2003. p. 253–72.
26. Martin J. Cultures in organizations: three perspectives. Oxford: Oxford University Press; 1992. p. 42.
27. Martin J. Cultures in organizations: three perspectives. Oxford: Oxford University Press; 1992. p. 159.
28. Martin J. Cultures in organizations: three perspectives. Oxford: Oxford University Press; 1992. p. 150.
29. Puckett A. Seldom ask, never tell: labour & discourse in Appalachia. New York: Oxford University Press; 2002. p. 31.
30. Schultz M, Hatch MJ, Larson MH. The expressive organization: linking identity, reputation and the corporate brand. Oxford: Oxford University Press; 2000. p. 13.
31. West E. British and American Frontier Nursing Service (FNS) nurses (1950-1960s): oral history narratives on nursing. J Oral Hist Soc. 2007;2:35.

Chapter 2
Rights and Claims: Culture and Communication in Appalachia

2.1 Rights and Claims: Communicative Repertoire in Appalachia

The isolation created by the geographical location of Appalachian peoples has fostered self-reliance, dependence on family and kin, and distrust of outsiders often referred to as cooperative independence [1]. Because of the long history of isolation as well as outside exploitation of these peoples, they tend to be distrustful of outsiders and outside organizations [2]. Obtaining the trust of Appalachian people requires that one become a part of their culture, engaging in the community's activities. Appalachian culture is person oriented rather than task oriented, and person's identity is dependent on their community and kinship ties.

To engage in the most basic request communication for socio-economic transactions in Appalachia, a resident must have a right to both make the request and to ask for whatever object the request entailed. In addition, these rights were not granted on the basis of education, professional qualifications, law, statute or perceived social class but were predicated on what actions are appropriate within gender, age, religious status categories, or other kinds of *people* criteria. Individuals within this culture engaged in labor, economic exchanges and dialogue according to these rights. If no kinship relationship existed, then in order to belong one needed to acquire a fictive kin categorization, only then could one have a status in the community from which to interact [3].

In 1923, prior to founding her Frontier Nursing Service (FNS) in 1925, Breckinridge toured the mountains of Leslie County on horseback, visiting all the local "Granny" midwives she could find. She made contact with the 'Granny Women' first and foremost to forge *relationship with* them before offering assistance *for* them. She also introduced herself to the local people. One 'early nurse' explained that they were not immediately 'liked' by everyone, 'If you were riding up a creek and saw a door shut, you didn't go in. You knew they didn't want you' [4]. In speaking of the start of her organization Breckinridge stated that the FNS was

© Springer Nature Switzerland AG 2019   15
E. West, *Frontier Nursing in Appalachia: History, Organization and the Changing Culture of Care*, https://doi.org/10.1007/978-3-030-20027-5_2

not called upon by the locals for quite some time after her arrival in the hills until one day a 'Granny Woman' had an emergency labor situation in which the pregnant woman had received no prenatal care. She called upon the FNS Nurse-Midwife when the situation became dire and thought hopeless. The nurse saved both mother and child. Breckinridge later wrote that it was equally possible that the nurse could have lost them both in this situation and that if she had failed to deliver both mother and child safely, it might have been the end of the FNS before it ever began. As it was, once word of her success spread, FNS nurses were called upon more by both the 'Granny Women' and individual families within the community [5]. Though it is certainly true that the FNS Nurse-Midwives did eventually replace the lay mid-wives it is equally true that it was the choice of the individual family who they wanted to see and if they chose the 'Granny Midwife' it was accepted by the FNS as, 'Whoever they wanted they had'.[1]

Breckinridge would have been labelled aristocrat, progressive and suffragette by the culture from whence she sprang. However, she was initially considered a 'fotched-on woman' as was all her early nurses by those belonging to the culture in which she chose to live and work for most of her adult life [6]. This term, used prin-cipally in Eastern Kentucky is the obsolete past tense of an old English verb, 'to fetch' and means 'brought from a distance.' Literally, it was used to describe women who were so diverse in background, personality, perspective, mission and method that few generalizations about them withstand scrutiny except that they all came from outside of the Eastern Appalachian region of the US. Popular historical accounts of these women tend to depict them as 'virtuous, high-principled, Christian, altruistic servants and bringers of the blessings of modernity to mountain people' [7]. Other accounts of these women characterize them as distrusted 'furriners' (for-eigners) and the most recent accounts by scholars both inside Appalachia and with-out have argued that these women, including Mary Breckinridge, served as either unwitting or intentional legitimizing agents of an advancing industrial capitalism that entailed high social and cultural costs for mountain environments, communities and people [8]. Nurses who know anything of Mary Breckinridge at all generally view her as a Nurse-Midwife and health reformer who had the distinction of being one of the few nurse entrepreneurs to have succeeded in founding and managing an organization devoted entirely to nursing, the provision of nursing and medical care (in that order) and in bringing Midwifery to the US despite opposition from many in the medical profession and others in positions of power who did not support these concepts [9]. The 'saintly' image was one Breckinridge purportedly loathed and did her best to countermand while she was living though much has been done to per-petuate it as well as the image of 'capitalist colonizer' since her demise.[2]

---

[1]Interview #82OH12FNS155 1982. Betty Lester, former longtime FNS nurse (English): 2nd inter-view on 27 July 1978. Interviewer: Dale Deaton, FNS Oral History Project Interviews # 1978–1982.

[2]Interview #82OH15FNS158 1982. Lydia Thompson, Prominent Committee Member outside of the FNS, interviewed: unknown. Interviewer: Dale Deaton, FNS Oral History Project Interviews # 1978–1982.

The FNS, in its early years provided a service that was congruent within the existing Appalachian culture. Once the local population began to utilize the Service a fictive kin categorization was established that created a status within the community from which the FNS could communicate. The Service needed this status as it had none of the kinship ties necessary to interact with the local community otherwise. This new category recognized the nurses as belonging to the culture. Once introduced by one already in the community as 'the gal who delivered my baby' direct greeting and exchanges could then occur with other community members. These relational experiences were necessary in order for communication and socioeconomic activity to occur [3]. These belonging networks also provided benefits to their members. For FNS nurses and the people they served these benefits were decidedly relational and thus also reciprocal.

One FNS nurse said that the people came to us by choice and as a rule once they had a baby with us, they 'came back for more'.[3] When asked why she thought this occurred, she responded with one word, 'attention.' When asked to elaborate on this, she stated that some of the young girls were afraid to 'have a man' and that the nurses answered their questions and were available to 'just talk' if they needed them. She also noted that physician attended deliveries required more pain medication for these women, whereas the nurses used much less. She attributed this to the fact that the midwife was more than just present *for* the delivery but was 'there *with* them' every step of the way, and that this made all the difference not only to the patient in ways of optimal care delivery but also to the nurse in ways of reward or feelings of making a difference. This took care beyond provision of a service to the patient for which the giver of care was compensated monetarily. It also encompassed 'relational' benefits that not only gave the nurse job satisfaction but also improved the actual care of the client as well as kept the costs of said care lower.

The prevailing objection for continuing community based or public health nursing in the wake of institutionalization and specialization in the health care system to people in isolated areas was that such services would never be able to carry the full cost for these services themselves. Breckinridge conceded that this was quite true. She also said that it was equally true of "every nursing service and every public institution and of a large fraction of public schools in the entire US. It is equally true of all hospitals, except very expensive private ones for a few very wealthy people none making use of hospital or district nursing services in large cities pay anything but a small part of the cost of their maintenance. Private endowments and gifts of those more fortunately situatcd have to meet the bulk of the expense if such services and hospitals are to exist at all".[4] Another prevailing ideology of the day was that rural work must be more expensive than city work

---

[3] Interview #78OH148FNS08 1978. Martha Lady, FNS Midwifery School Graduate of 1960 interviewed 4 Aug 1978, Interviewer: Johathan Fried, FNS Oral History Project Interviews # 1978–1982.

[4] FNS Quarterly Bulletin 1928. 5M1: FNS, Box 25, Fol. 1. 'Statement of Costs of FNS during Fiscal Year, 1 May 1926–1927, by Ella Woodyard, PhD', Reprinted from the FNS Quarterly Bulletin, February 1928. University of Kentucky in Lexington, USA.

due to the added travel costs. Yet, this was not the case for the FNS. Nurses at the FNS were on horseback, not cars, which required no fuel and much less mainte-nance, and travel time was kept to a minimum by a plan of decentralization whereby nurses lived in centers in the heart of the districts they served and rarely more than five miles from the farthest patient. Indeed, this paradigm worked in favor of this organization being accepted by the people as it set the entire opera-tion up as being culturally egalitarian. The nurses went to the people to deliver care but only after they were asked to do so by them, and they lived amongst them as equals. Each nursing center covered a five-mile radius or 78 square miles (see Footnote 4). This decentralized plan included an expressed intent by the FNS to keep patient care from becoming too 'specialized' as well. Specialization would undoubtedly have increased operational costs as well as fragmented the care of individuals, families and communities. In addition, it would have gone against the culture's collectivistic family/*people*-oriented culture as well as the community's ethic of neutrality, that is the avoidance of assertiveness, interference or domi-nance over the lives of others [10].

2.2 National Versus Eastern Appalachian Culture

While communities can be well understood through their families and kin groups their economic and cultural personalities are also shaped by recurrent pulses of immigration, by the evolution of technology and by the landscape and natural envi-ronment. Before the industrial transition (1880–1920) that witnessed the Appalachian region becoming the main fuel source and a principal foundry of the American Industrial Revolution, Appalachians had largely depended upon agriculture and local enterprises such as logging and salt production. Family and kinship have formed the backbone of rural and small-town American life since colonial times but in few places, does the family remain as essential a component of culture and soci-ety as in Appalachia. Scholars and residents of Appalachia have come to see the entrenched social, political and personal influence of family *relationships* [italics added] as the dominant thread in the areas cultural framework, as well as a feature that distinguishes Appalachia from much of the US [11].

The nuclear family is the fundamental unit of social organization in America but rather than being independent, as is the norm for nuclear families in the larger US culture, in Appalachia nuclear families frequently are connected to a larger social organization that includes the parents and siblings of the nuclear family's parents. These family-group households also tend to reside geographically closer to one another than in other parts of the US, a characteristic not uncommon for poorer rural communities. These families generally followed traditional gender roles, which have been historically patriarchal with men controlling income use and making decisions, serving as heads of households, directing production and owning land; while women act as loving nurturers to their husbands and children [12]. Though traditionally speaking, Appalachian culture is patriarchal, the exception to this rule is if the woman makes more money than the male. Decision-making tends to be either egalitarian or matriarchal [13]. Many areas engaged in farming until the late nineteenth and early twentieth century, although parts of the region had been industrialized. On the farm, the husband and wife worked as a team because the labour of both was needed to support the family. This routine work was divided spatially, where mothers and daughters were primarily responsible for work done in the yard and house, and fathers and sons were responsible for chores beyond the house and crop production. The entire conjugal family, which often consisted of extended kin and neighbours worked together. Children shared in the family work and learned culturally appropriate gender behaviours by modelling their parents. Hence, traditional expectations with regard to gender roles were incorporated into the child's sense of identity. These mixed-sex teams commonly hoed corn together.

There were few of the job taboos for women in the hills that existed for them in other parts of the US, and little stigma attached to doing what was traditionally viewed as 'men's work,' particularly in childhood. However, women were routinely deployed in men's field activities but men rarely did housework and the phrase used by Appalachian men to characterize the fieldwork done by their women was 'helping out.' This has been interpreted by researchers to signify the 'diminished significance of the female contribution' that has been used to 'maintain the centrality of males' [14]. However, from a cultural perspective the language used by researchers from without Appalachia to interpret this phrase is as significant as the language used by the Appalachians to describe the work done by their women. The term 'helping' here to describe the work being done is interpreted as an activity of 'diminished significance' to that of the work being done by the men, even though the work that was being done is identical. Beyond the designated role assignment or even gender considerations, 'helping' is clearly a cultural value that is deemed of less worth by society. This value assignation has proven to be problematic to the discipline of nursing in its struggle for professional status as the work continues to be viewed as either 'helping' the doctor or the sick.

With few exceptions research indicated that items or services Appalachian women had control over fell into the following domains: the bearing, caring and rearing of children, domestic spaces and activities, food preparation and related activities, healing and caring for the sick, literacy activities and spiritual or moral matters involving church activities or the evaluation of people's behavior. All of these items and services tended to focus on activities *for* people. Men tended to have authority and control over matters related to money, machinery, politics, land transactions and outdoor activities though these patterns changed as more women found jobs outside of the home in which they worked together with men. All of these domains are clearly more concerned with the activities *of* people. This state of affairs was not much different for women outside of Appalachia as families were constructed upon patriarchal social relations that were common throughout the nation, even more so in rural America and the intrinsic value placed upon these relations were not equal in either culture [15]. Though certainly not equal, in Appalachia 'helping out' was definitely of higher social value than in the rest of the nation as within this culture it implied 'loyalty' on the part of the one doing the 'helping' that often required personal sacrifice and for which no monetary payment was expected. This cultural trait was done by both males and females in Appalachia. The only difference being that the males were expected to provide this service toward benefactors who took care of them and their families within the sphere that they had control over, namely to their wage providing employers. Females provided this service within the sphere that they had control of within the culture, specifically family and local community endeavours [16].

Rural America, principally farmers, who never did reap any of the wealth of the 'prosperity years' were the worst hit during the Great Depression of the 1930s and had added to their suffering seeing their overworked land reduced to a bowl of dust via some of the worst droughts in the history of the American mid-West. In the Appalachia's the depression's effects were minimal when compared to other regions of the US. Those with families who were subsistence farmers bartering for locally produced goods in either goods or services needed little money to maintain living standards, which were not all that high to begin with. Many of the Mountain people found the drought of 1930–1931 a worse ordeal than the Great Depression [17]. The Appalachian coal miners who were full time wage earners were the hardest hit by the depression and some subsistence farming on the side cushioned what they suffered from partial or total unemployment while the 'new deal' works programs mixed benefit with harm for the Appalachia people. 'New deal' money injections harmed textile and coal industries but helped save the land by making many people less dependent on farming the already overworked land. Appalachia let much of its topsoil wash away in the 1930s and 'new deal' agencies intervened by initiating financial incentives for soil conservation. The greatest immediate and daily benefit to those living in the Appalachia's of all of Roosevelt's 'works projects' were road improvements [18].

The economy of Appalachia, which was once insular and self-supporting over the course of a century and a half, became inexorably dependent on business trends in the rest of the nation and the world. The problem was that the people kept-up their end of the bargain, while industry either chose not to, or found that they were not able to do so. The rise of industries connected with extrication and distribution of coal, iron, timber and commercial agriculture products in the late nineteenth century presented those goods to the world beyond, causing national and international boom–and-bust cycles to resonate increasingly in Appalachia. By the coming of the twentieth century, the arrival of cash wages had lured many Appalachian residents away from their traditional subsistence-based economy into mines, mills and logging camps. From 1900 to 1930 the number of the region's wage earners increased by 75%, 15 times the increase in its number of farmers [19]. Central Appalachia (including Eastern Kentucky, West Virginia, southwest Virginia, and northeast Tennessee) remained the area with the weakest economy in the region throughout the final decades of the twentieth century [20].

Between the years 1950 and 1970, 65% of men aged 15–34 left the region for industrial cities, often choosing to join kith and kin already established on the outside, hence maintaining the kinship ties essential to cultural identity [21]. As the region moved from a predominantly agrarian society and family-planning became more readily available, family size declined throughout the early twentieth century. However, compared with other rural American regions the level of fertility in central and southern Appalachia remained high. The combination of population increases, family farm subdivision, cultivation of increasingly marginal steep land and alternative uses of land such as coal mining and timber harvesting resulted in economic decline [22]. The problem was that the incoming system of a solely money-based economy was at odds with the values, which were intimately connected to the idea of volunteer reciprocity ingrained in the Appalachian culture's existing system of subsistence-barter-and-borrow economy. The focus of the existing system was on the relationships between the people involved with work rather than the object of the work [23]. This people orientation' of the Mountaineer could prove aggravating to employers as they would often not show up for work if they could not get the needed time off to attend a second cousin's funeral. They would risk being fired rather than risk being ill thought of by the community back home. Yet the same cultural trait could also be viewed as a valuable commodity as Mountaineers saw employers as entering into 'relationship' by providing employment and were willing to come out day or night to help while spurning offers of pay [24]. They were loyal, willing and rendered good service because 'work' was viewed culturally as something more personal than even a binding contract between employer and employee; it was a kinship connection designed for the purpose of mutual benefit. In Appalachia, if one is in the lesser value position in terms of access to power and resources, one may need or want to make a request of another who controls these resources. In return, the one in the higher value position will want and need the requester to validate his continued control over these resources. This inherent access and control gives this person the right to 'take care of' others. Indeed, it is considered his 'place' to do so [25]. Once a transaction is successful in this socio-economic communicative repertoire, both participants benefiting from the transaction will be indebted to one another. The recipient to the benefactor in ways that create loyalty, gratitude or political fidelity and the benefactor is obligated to continue to provide future commodities or services which he or she has control of as long as the beneficiary recognizes this fidelity through such actions as political support or continued business. Hence, the departure of industries that provided the work needed for family survival when Appalachians were no longer in a position to subsist without them, particularly after they were told that their loyalty to these companies would ensure it, was perceived by the culture as a 'reneging' of an obligation on the part of the benefactor, and when unemployment (welfare) was offered to the people instead of work, these people took it without qualm, viewing it as compensation by one 'outsider' for the failure of another to meet its obligation to the community. This was a cultural trait that was foreign to most Americans and offended the work ethic sensibilities of many of them. Work outside of this culture was viewed much less personally, as a business endeavour, an object pursued for esteem, advancement and/or to provide more or better material possessions for oneself and one's immediate family; whereas work in Appalachia was done for family survival and moreover, was a community endeavour [26].

The Appalachian peoples have been accused of being suspicious of outsiders, resistant to any interference and vigorous resisters of any form of governmental intrusion, especially that which could be perceived as charity [27]. Initially, this trait was due to a communist movement in Europe that occurred during the industrial revolution. When American union strikes against manufacturers led to a bombing outrage in the US, a communist scare ensued, which led to the arrest and expulsion of many communist and socialist sympathizers, many of whom were not part of the violence [28]. This event in US history created an aversion toward any political ideology that negated individual liberties by most Americans and was viewed by the existing Appalachian subculture to also include any outside domination by the US Government. Later, this aversion toward outside interference by Appalachians was based upon more recent, bitter experience with outsiders as by the end of the 1950s Appalachia was in economic and social distress; marked by government intervention, corporate exploitation and environmental debacles.

Appalachia had become a rude name, implying not only poverty but also most of the blame for the descent into that condition within a predominantly prosperous nation.

By 1960 many explanations were being put forth for Appalachia's problems, among them were environmental degradation; soil erosion; well-intentioned policies that were limited in scope, paternalistic and set into motion by the government; economic, social and political displacement and disenfranchisement of the people; and there were even a few explanations that blamed the poor human qualities of the people for their own problems. Different interpretations clashed, but all groups identifying the problems in these various ways suffered from a lack of ability to do much about them. It was at this time that the Federal government, more specifically the Appalachian Regional Commission (ARC), defined, and has since redefined, the Appalachia region as encompassing what is now a grand total of 420 counties in portions of thirteen states (Illustrations Map 14). With economic need as the criterion, lawmakers fashioned an Appalachia composed of upland counties, including the whole of West Virginia and areas more or less adjacent with the mountains in Alabama, Georgia, Kentucky, Maryland, Mississippi, New York, Ohio, Pennsylvania, Tennessee, Virginia and the Carolinas [29]. From its inception and thereafter, the federal map reflected the constraints of not only economic need, geography and culture but also congressional politics.

In 1925 the Frontier Nursing Service (FNS) was founded in Leslie County, Kentucky. The organization opened its first clinic in the neighboring county of Hyden, Kentucky that same year, followed by the Hyden Hospital and Health Center in 1928 and a total of nine outpost nursing centers in Leslie County, and the Red Bird River section of Clay County, Kentucky. These counties are still listed as "distressed" by the Appalachia Regional Commission today. This means that these counties have at least twice the national poverty rate and have a per capita market income 67% of the national average or a 3-year average unemployment rate that is twice the national average [30]. In addition, demographically though there are counties with more diversity in the Appalachia region, 98% of the population in the county that the FNS serviced was white and of English and Scotch-Irish descent. Breckinridge, as well as many of the other former FNS Nurses who penned their experiences in Leslie County describe a form of Elizabethan English historically indicative of Appalachia that is still spoken in some communities there today [5]. This is a dialect that famously uses different vocabulary and meanings, some of which may be archaic, such as *"britches"* (trousers), *"poke"* (bag), *"sallet"* (salad, as in a poke-sallet, of pokeweed rather than bags!), *"afeared"* (afraid), *"fixin"* (getting ready, as in "I'm fixin to do something"), *"allow"* (suppose, as in "I'll allow as how I'll go over yander for a leetle spell"). But words are the least of it. Appalachian accents also differ markedly from the standard, such as in words ending in "oh" sounds, such as *"holler"* (hollow), *"winder"* (window), *"tater"* (potato), or "ah" ending words, such as *"sody-pop"* (soda-pop). It's one of the ways Appalachian communities show solidarity and belonging. It also demonstrates how important and deeply ingrained within the culture collectivism runs [31].

Economically, the most common employment sectors for those who live in Leslie County, KY were, and remain mining, quarrying, oil and gas extraction. Though in large part due to the work of the FNS in the mid-twentieth century in Eastern Kentucky, today healthcare, social assistance and educational services are also major employers in this area [32]. Surface and underground coal mining has created many environmental as well as health problems for this population. Environmental issues include destruction of large areas of land, demolition of landscape and natural habitat, lack of surface subsidence, abandoned shafts, extensive surface spoil heaps, mine explosions, collapses and flooding. Aside from the obvious physical danger associated with mining, the corresponding long-term health issues created from a lifetime of toil in a mine can be equally life-endangering. They include lung ailments related to coal dust, silica dust, diesel particulate matter, welding fumes and asbestos. Also, hearing loss associated with noise, skin disorders, and poisoning associated with exposure to lead and other minerals [33]. These ailments were treated by the nurses at clinics along with "worms" (tapeworms) in children drinking out-house contaminated water, and trachoma—a contagious bacterial infection of the eye that could cause blindness, as well as a vast variety of gynecologic, obstetric, orthopedic and pediatric diseases/disorders in their unique role of Public Health-Nurse-Midwives [34]. However, the main focus of the FNS in its early years was meeting the pre and post-natal needs of women and children in their homes.

Of all of America's distinctive regions, Appalachia has perhaps the most complex history, for as much as it is a geographical entity; it has become a cultural concept constantly evolving even as its borders and geographical boundaries are drawn and redrawn. In 2010, further additions brought the total number of 'Appalachian' counties. Over the years, the region's maps have changed to suit distinct and varying political and historical frameworks and to serve countless purposes. While all of the various efforts to define the region acknowledge the importance of the Appalachian Mountains, none of them adopt its physiographic or topographic boundaries as the sole determinant of its regional classification. In the case of other identifiable regions of the country, state or county lines help with geographical definitions but in the instance of Appalachia, these boundaries are of no use in defining either the geographic or cultural outlines of the region. Thus, the limits of Appalachia are a subject of chronic rumination; though in every conception the region stretches from the Deep South far beyond the Mason-Dixon Line into the

North, assuring that both its political and cultural histories are as complex as its landscape [35]. What prompts outsiders to find Appalachian culture most singular is the relational 'grounding' that permeates all other aspects of cultural identity. The language, economics and politics of the region are all rooted in kith and kin-focused and distinctly people-oriented system of communication. Requests in much of the region are indirect rather than direct as residents of close-knit communities assume they know each other well enough to provide wants and needs without being asked [36]. Direct requests usually required the requestor to be in a close relationship with the one from whom he or she has made the request.

A complex local economy with a power structure of 'rights,' 'place' and 'claims' were embedded within the existing community 'belonging' networks. However, many of the goods and services that required cash money depended on other patterns of organized requesting practices to develop within the existing socioeconomic communicative repertoire in Appalachia. Therefore, residents designated two other patterns, 'takin' care of' and 'tradin.' Those Appalachian wage-earners receiving benefits from 'takin' care of' benefactors (wage generating businesses) were obligated to provide loyalty through 'helpin' out' services to these benefactors, sometimes at great personal sacrifice. In this way, relationships were forged between 'takin' care of' constituencies that came into the region and the existing belonging networks and they often overlapped [37].

2.3 National Versus Frontier Nursing Culture

Breckinridge ostensibly requested time away from the service only once (in 1935) in all of her tenure at the organization's helm, from its inception in 1925 until her resignation as 'Volunteer' Director in 1962 at the age of 81. The reason given to her executive board for the request was her health. It is interesting to note that discussion also ensued at this same executive board meeting regarding the sale of Breckinridge's Russian Imperial China, once owned by Peter the Great, to help with the organizations dwindling finances during the height of the depression.[5] In order to understand how the FNS formed its unique cultural identity as an organization one must also comprehend the cultural identity of its founder, since she exerted such a strong influence on its culture while she lived [38].

> The organization was her, her personality… the way we are living now and the way things are now—her kind of organization are not going to exist—there is too much government.[6]

---

[5]FNS Summary of Executive Committee Meetings 1925–1935. 85M1: FNS, Box 2, Fol. 1. Includes resolution made on 10 March 1928 to invite the Dr. and Mrs. MacKenzie to the FNS and Breckinridge's request for time off due to 'exhaustion', 14 November 1930. University of Kentucky in Lexington, USA.

[6]Interview#82OH34FNS177, 1982. Mary Stewart, former FNS Courier, Interviewed 15 January 1980. Interviewer(s): Marion Barrett and NancyAlbertson, FNS Oral History Project Interviews # 1978–1982.

The decades in which Breckinridge lived, both before and after the First World War, were ones of immense and rapid change that was unparalleled since the country's founding. The US was in a state of accelerated change from a system centred on agriculture to industry [39]. By 1900 as a direct result of this rapid expansion America had become a divided country of an industrial aristocracy and of immigrants living in tenements. Indeed, many of these issues were shared by virtually all of the Western world's existing and emerging industrial powers.

The year's 1900–1917 brought about a need to confront the changes brought on by modernization. People began to seek public solutions to social problems and a social gospel was born in which charity work became paramount to fixing the social ills of the day [40]. Also, at this time the women's movement, whose European political birth began in earnest in the late 1890s, re-emerged as the suffrage movement in the mid-1900s [41]. It reflected women's involvement in social work and local service between those years and it spread across Europe and into the US as it gained momentum. Women were determined to bring about a more just and humane society, and relieve the suffering of women and children brought in the wake of an industrial aristocracy which impoverished and brutalized men, women and children, abandoning them in a time of crisis to public charity. Women, who were now making a more coordinated social and political impact than ever before, began making changes by forging political alliances, organizing, pressing for legislative changes and ultimately running for public office themselves [42]. Women's pressure groups at this time all sought not only to improve the economic conditions of women and children or merely to secure the right to vote, but also pressed for better health care for women and children. Suffrage reformers campaigned for child benefit and better maternity services and governments quickly recognized that the productive power of the economy and military strength of the nation depended on a large, able-bodied (mostly male) work force. Future work forces and armed forces depended on a good supply of healthy babies and children. So, childbirth was to be protected, supervised, measured and fed. Thus, a public health focus on preventative health care arose [43]. The focus was on the prevailing threat of poor health to the overall population as well as the individual.

At the beginning of the twentieth century nursing also had a decidedly public health focus and as such dealt with society as patient [44]. Nursing advances at this time went part and parcel along with those of the progressive era and included taking physical, social, mental health and teaching out into community neighbourhoods, homes and schools. The major social and medical changes in the second half of the century facilitated the development of nursing as a respected, paid occupation for women, one of the few. Yet nursing, as well as any other paid public work available for women at this time, was strictly controlled by the culture which existed both outside and inside the institutional setting, which was decidedly male-dominated and one in which women worked within a hierarchy whereby there were one set of rules for women and another, less punitive, for their male counterparts [45].

The field of public health work for nurses at the turn of the century swelled in America and with it the support of professional, private and governmental organizations within the communities that these nurses served. The community-based provision of care model, with its generalized approach to meeting the health needs of people, wellness and prevention focus and more localized power structures and distribution methods had helped American nurses to win a legislative place in each state of the union, where 'progressive' nurse leaders pressed relentlessly, in the face of the medical community's growing opposition, for a higher standard of education for nurses and the necessary funds to achieve this goal. In contrast, Britain had at this time a growing demand for hospital care, a deepening financial crisis for hospitals and new and different employment opportunities becoming available for women. The resulting crises ultimately lead to the post-World War Two creation of the National Health Service (NHS) that exists today [46].

It was into this era of industrialization; rising feminism and 'progressive' politics that FNS founder Mary Breckinridge was born in 1881. Breckinridge was the daughter of a wealthy, privileged and prominent Southern family. In her youth, the social role for women created a dilemma for her. She, like many women of her day, complained of feeling 'idle' and she stated in her autobiography that she 'chafed' at the complete lack of purpose in the things she was allowed to do. Several times she suggested to her mother that it would be nice to do something useful, but wrote that she never 'got anywhere with such an idea' [47]. She explained, that her mother was broadminded and advocated women's suffrage when it was frowned on but that she also believed, like nearly everybody then, that the only place for a woman was in her father's house while she was single, and her husband's if she is married [48]. Though Breckinridge certainly subscribed to many of the prevailing Victorian ideas regarding nursing as 'vocation,' she also advocated nursing as a profession, which was autonomous and one requiring advanced education. Her personal circumstances at aged 28 changed her views regarding education from those she held at age seventeen, when after completing finishing school and deciding not to go on to college she wrote that as much as she loved study, she loved adventure more, so that the temptation college held for her lay solely in providing an open wedge for larger liberties. She later came to believe that education came not only from formal sources but also from relationships and personal interaction with people. This formed the philosophical foundation upon which nursing education and practice environments were built at the FNS both for its founder and her nurses.

Breckinridge had a son who died at age four and a daughter who died at birth. She later wrote that the generation to which she belonged thought it in poor taste to discuss 'a broken marriage' and that hers was broken after her children were dead [49]. She readily admits in her autobiography that if circumstances had been different in her life, there may have never been a FNS. It was the character of the individual woman, her personal tragedies and life experiences that coalesced to change the trajectory of her future life and chosen work. A chosen work that was decidedly more available to a woman of her breeding, financial privilege and social prominence, yet still one viewed as not altogether seemly for a woman of her class.

In 1918, after the First World War had ended, Breckinridge volunteered to work with the American Committee for Devastated France where for the first time she saw the value of formally trained midwives in France and also identified the need for the then unheard-of health practice of prenatal and postnatal care for families.

She returned to the US in 1921 with an idea on how to provide health care to the people of rural America. Because her family's roots were in Kentucky, she had a concern for the health of the mountain people.

To further prepare herself to carry out her plans, she took some courses in the latest developments in public health at Teachers' College of Columbia University in New York in order 'to learn about American methods' [50].

In the 1920s, the decade Breckinridge began her Service, the nation was fraught with a sense of struggle to make sense of the First World War, and perhaps in a wider context, America's place in it and the world. The national feeling was one of loss with regard to the personal, moral and spiritual values that had prevailed at the start of the twentieth century. A new America was emerging and, at the same time, dramatic advances in science, technology, urban growth, acceleration of educational levels and an increase in socio-economic mobility created a sense of rebellion against the Victorian idea of decency [51]. Yet, Breckinridge could hardly be characterized as the epitome of the 'new American woman' who emerged from the First World War strongly influenced by the changing culture and technological innovations of the era. In 1925, the year that she established her nursing service in the Eastern Appalachian Mountains of Kentucky, Breckinridge was 44 years of age and had experienced not only the death of her two children and first husband but also the divorce of her second husband. In addition, in the American South where Breckinridge's people had both the wealth and breeding that dictated the powerful, privileged roles they held in society, females had been conditioned to speak not of their rights but of their responsibilities. Women expanded their ascribed sphere into community service and care of dependents. This was considered 'domestic politics' not fully a part of what was considered 'men's politics' or even 'women's politics 'of the time.' Also, well into the Twentieth Century the persistence of a high birth rate in some sections of the Southern Highlands severely curtailed both the cultural changes occurring elsewhere in the US and the resulting options available for women at this time (see Footnote 2). From a cultural perspective, the value disparity which existed between rural and urban environments in regard to the intrinsic worth that was placed upon those cultural traits being ascribed to gender within patriarchal societies created the need for women to suppress their own gender consciousness at the same time as attempting to suppress effectively gender consciousness among men [52]. Suffragette's at home and abroad called the rearing of the child 'crop' the most vital to the nation of all its 'industries, being that which alone give to other industry any meaning or importance'.[7]

The interwar years ushered in a seemingly unending onslaught of biomedical technology which created the need for laboratory and radiographic departments in order to properly diagnose and treat illnesses, and physicians had to concede that they could no longer meet their patients' needs without the outside assistance of commercial medicine. Yet, even with the appearance of an 18-bed hospital (institu-

[7]Interview #78OH148FNS08 1978. Martha Lady, FNS Midwifery School Graduate of 1960, Interviewed 4 August 1978, Interviewer: Johathan Fried, FNS Oral History Project Interviews # 1978–1982.

tion) into the hills, this model of decentralization and general care was the norm at the FNS.[8] When additions fuelled by advances made in the biomedical and physical sciences began infiltrating the hills as well, nurses provided what came to be a unique, universal type of patient care as evidenced by the statements made by former FNS Nurses regarding their job descriptions, which included doing haemoglobins, typing and cross matching blood, taking X-rays and running clinics in addition to fulfilling the more traditional nursing role of home visitor in rural settings.[9]

One former British FNS Nurse describes the 'best job she ever had' as something coined by the FNS as a 'triple worker,' which was, 'a district nurse, district midwife and health visitor all rolled into one.' The care was individual, family and community focused. The scope of nursing practice was from cradle to grave.[10] In other words, the prevailing philosophy of both the organization as well as the nurse's practice environment was one of comprehensive care. There was a connectedness with, among and for people and the nurses.

They gave a great deal but received a great deal back, not only from the organization, but from their patients as well. This particular nurse saw many of the changes that occurred at the FNS and summarized it thus:

> There is something that those of us who were down at the FNS got that you don't get anymore, I don't think. It's this... I think when we were down there it was a sort of pioneering spirit, you know, doing things on the rough. There was just a little bit of adventure-type to it and there was a sort of sense of... sense of working together, being united in this thing. And I think everybody kind of goes his own way now.... You were dependent upon other people to a certain extent (at FNS) and yet you were independent. But you saw other people they had a special value to them. They were important to you.[11]

Breckinridge realized that her organization's success in Appalachia hinged upon its ability to develop 'relationship' with the local community. In addition, in order for her organization to grow it also had to maintain the relationship network it had already formed outside of Appalachia for its financial assistance. Finally, for the service to be sustained and strengthened solid relations had to be forged within her organization between its personnel and the community they served. The provision of health care by the FNS in the Eastern Appalachian culture was difficult to achieve but it was particularly difficult to accomplish in a culture where 'rights,' 'place' and 'claims' relationships were so necessary and so very complex.

---

[8]FNS Quarterly Bulletin 1928, 85M1: FNS, Box 25, Fol. 1. 'Statement of Costs of FNS during Fiscal Year, 1 May 1926–1927, by Ella Woodyard, PhD', Reprinted from the FNS Quarterly Bulletin, February 1928. University of Kentucky in Lexington, USA.

[9]FNS Quarterly Bulletin 1935, 85M1: FNS, Box 25, Fol. 2. 'Organization & Supervision of the Filed Work of the FNS', Reprint from the FNS Quarterly Bulletin, winter 1935 (No. 3). University of Kentucky in Lexington, USA.

[10]Judy Haralson-Rafson, American former FNS Nurse (1971–1976; 1971 Graduate of FNS Family Nurse Practitioner Program), Date surveyed: 31/07/2003. Date interviewed: 12/05/2006. Interviewer: Edith A. West.

[11]Margaret (Maggie) Willson, British former FNS Nurse-Midwife (1955–1967), Date surveyed: 10/08/2003. Date interviewed:09/04/2005. Interviewer: Edith A. West.

Though nationally, women began taking jobs outside of the home more after 1928 at which time there were five times as many women employed outside of the home than in 1918; marriage, family and homemaking were still a woman's first priority. The numbers of working women outside of the home rose from fourteen to 19 million and by the end of the Second World War 36% of these women were in employment outside of the home.[12] Marriage and family maintained a high priority with women in the 1940s and 42% of 18–24-year-old women were married. A Gallup poll taken in 1936 found that 82% of respondents were opposed to married women in the labour force. *Fortune* magazine's survey the same year found that 85% of men and 79% of women believed married women should not work outside their home [53]. Yet women were brought back into the work force *en masse* once again out of necessity at the start of World War Two. The historic patterns of women *'helping out'* begun in World War One, that is having women serve *with* rather than *in* all branches of the armed services, resumed while public opinion continued to be ambivalent about how far from the traditional roles of women society was prepared to deviate even in a time of world war. Those women who expected to remain in the labour force after the war were disappointed by the reversion to policies which barred married women from working and limited the hours or conditions under which any woman could work and the resumption of official and non-official 'male' and 'female' job categories in the post-war years [54].

From a cultural perspective, when the use of language is considered to describe any form of 'domestic service' by women who were leaving it for war work, it becomes evident just how little value was placed upon it by society. Recurring descriptors to depict it are 'drudge' and the work was often equated by the women with feelings of being confined 'within' a cage.' One woman referred to herself as a 'cabbage' when describing her 15 years as a 'housewife' prior to her doing part-time war work. When one considers that the work these women were often leaving home to do was factory work, which could be just as menial and monotonous as domestic service or homemaking, the true depth of disparity between the value societies attributed to each becomes painfully apparent. Indeed, men returning from both World Wars would not take the jobs that were considered 'domestic service' work, expecting women to go back to them (or go home) and became incensed when they did not [55].

The division of labour began to shift for Appalachian women also during war time. However, Appalachian mothers and daughters continued to work within the family while they took on management of the farm in the absence of their male kin who began to work for wages in factories outside of the region. Appalachian women were not permitted by company policy to work as loggers, coal miners or in any of the mills that served as sole wage providers within the region [56]. The work of both men and women was crucial to the economic survival of the family, yet Appalachian women have generally been overlooked by larger society, which tends to maintain

[12] Interview #78OH148FNS08 1978. Martha Lady.

more traditional views regarding the ascription of value to gender roles and wage versus 'volunteer' work. The industrial boom initiated by the Second World War also created opportunities for those Appalachian men willing to leave the hills in the hope of finding public works jobs like the rest of the country. What no one could foresee was how much economic and cultural harm the move to total dependence upon industry would eventually create when those businesses abandoned the region using the same roads it helped to create to enter the area.

The FNS lost the bulk of its staff when British nurses in 1939 chose to return home to join the war effort. Unable to replace the nurses or train American nurses in Great Britain due to the war, Breckinridge opened the FNS Graduate School for Midwifery, something she planned on doing in the future but Hitler expedited with his invasion of Poland. She strategically also began giving 6-month training in district nursing to senior Cadet nurses from Johns Hopkins Hospital in Baltimore and the Henry Ford Hospital in Detroit who were in the federal government program to help the American war effort while simultaneously staffing her Service in her British nurses' absence [57]. Breckinridge also made an appeal at this time to 'remember women as well as men at this time of war. In the last three score years and ten, 51,210 men have been killed in war while several hundred thousand young women have died in childbirth,' fearing that the philanthropic support the service relied upon would drop off.[13]

Though war time certainly tightened her resources, Breckinridge maintained services with the nurses and students she had until her British nurses were able to return, which many chose to do when the war ended. She was successful due solely to her political savvy and the social and political connections she enjoyed as a Breckinridge. Though the Service never claimed 'exemption' from the US government for anyone during wartime, the FNS was listed by the Emergency Management of the War Manpower Commission as 'essential.' The highest priority was for supplies but the FNS only became seriously short of two items: Horseshoes and Diapers. After exhausting all possible private suppliers, she used her 'high level contacts in Washington' for help, though none of them could see why horse shoes were essential for childbirth. One war production board official suggested that wear and tear on horseshoes might be minimized if the shoes were taken off the horse outside of working hours, recommending "unessential horse shoe styles should be eliminated." A Representative John Flannagan rescued the horses and their owners by asking on the house floor if they could be 'zipper' horseshoes. After the press joined in the laughter a factory was authorized to produce the shoes.[14] The fact that in wartime, a

---

[13] FNS Quarterly Bulletin 1946, 85M1: FNS, Box 29, Fol. 17. 'FNS Quarterly Bulletin, 1946.' This box also contained 'FNS Promotional & Fiscal Budget Material' for 1946, 1948 and 1951. University of Kentucky in Lexington, USA.

[14] FNS Spring Appeal 1942, 85M1: FNS, Box 29, Fol. 13. 'FNS Spring Appeal 1942', Breckinridge speaks of remembering women as well as men at war. She asks not to send extra money but rather use the attached letter, booklet and small leather saddlebag enclosed to win the interest of a friend in becoming a member for $2 annually. She asks forgiveness for not having the time or strength to make this a personal letter to each of her supporters but states she has affection for hundreds of them and a regard for each one. University of Kentucky in Lexington, USA.

factory was authorized to produce horseshoes for FNS horses, solely at the request of one middle-aged Nurse-Midwife living in Appalachia emphasized the kind of clout this woman wielded politically at a time when such power was a rarity and the respect that her organization garnered from those in power.

An appeal for diaper substitutes ran in the 1942 *FNS Quarterly Bulletin* but much that was received was old and fell apart after one wash. In 1943 a prominent friend of Breckinridge's, Representative Frances Bolton (who was active in public health, nursing education and other social service, education, and philanthropic work; vice regent for Ohio of the Mount Vernon Ladies' Association; member of the Republican State central committee, 1937–1940; delegate to Republican National Conventions and member of Resolutions Committee, 1956, 1960, 1964, and 1968; first woman appointed as congressional delegate to United Nations General Assembly, 1953; elected as a Republican by special election, 27 February 1940, to the 76th Congress to fill the vacancy caused by the death of her husband, Chester C. Bolton; re-elected to the fourteen succeeding Congresses and served from 27 February 1940, to 3 January 1969) presented the FNS's diaper problem on the house floor. Newspapers reported one congress member as saying in earlier times, 'millions of babies had been born without these conveniences,' Breckinridge wrote in her autobiography that she wondered how he happened not to have heard of "swaddling clothes, which took a great deal more yardage than diapers" [58].

Near the end of the war, personnel shortages became so acute that FNS Couriers took nurse aide courses and staffed the wards. Later, the first jeep acquired by the FNS was from the war department. One long time British FNS nurse who was unable to get back from Great Britain after the war because she wasn't 'priority' according to both the US and British governments wrote to Breckinridge in 1946 seeking her assistance in the matter. She stated, '… and my dear, I was back here in January and it was around October–November when I wrote her!' [59]. This same British nurse in an earlier interview also stated that when she left for England at the start of the war, Breckinridge purportedly reassured her that if she didn't like the British army all she needed to do was let her know and she'd get her back. The extent of her 'political pull' is evidenced by the fact that she made this same offer to an American FNS nurse who joined the Army in 1942.[15]

In the post-war years, the patriotic call to service was now gone and nationally women were either obliged (or forced) to leave the labour market in deference to home and family; resulting in even fewer women entering the nursing profession. A shortage of trained nurses at the conclusion of both World Wars and the labour turnover in the nursing profession after WWI became an increasing and perpetual problem for not only the profession but also the health care and government institutions that relied upon their industry.[16] It was also becoming apparent that it was

---

[15] Interview #82OH13FNS156 1982, Betty Lester, former long-time FNS Nurse (English): 3rd. Interview on 3 August 1978. Interviewer: Dale Deaton, FNS Oral History Project Interviews # 1978–1982.

[16] Alice Herman, American former FNS Nurse (1956–1978). Date interviewed: 23/05/2006. Interviewer: Edith A. West.

no longer possible to invoke monastic or militaristic ideals upon student nurses as social mores were changing with the arrival of emancipated women coming into the workforce who were now beginning to be offered more of a selection in their career choice. It was necessary instead to get the cooperation of the nurses rather than to enforce discipline [60]. Yet these realities did little to deter those within the rising institutional frameworks (hospital administrators, physicians or even the senior nursing staff) from continuing to impose them and instead of addressing these issues, institutions chose to entice new nurses and trainees with domicile incentives, which included large, pleasantly furnished dormitory rooms, the nicer of which had pools, recreation rooms and even tennis courts. They were also within easy access of the hospital and nurses and students alike had to maintain residences there.

These incentives illustrate the corporate culture that was rising to power as a direct result of industrialization on an international scale. This emerging culture required its members to put their 'heart and soul' into their work but unlike Appalachian culture, it offered no incentive to the 'heart and soul' of its workers nor did it provide a work environment in which such humanitarian endeavours would flourish and inspire [61]. For businesses, this was bad enough but for what came to be known as 'the health care *industry*' [italics added] within the United States this had a devastating effect due primarily to the fact that its service is humanitarian in both practice and principle.

By the 1950s, the discipline of medicine was a highly regarded profession and had established a value structure whereby intellectual achievement was highly prized both within its ranks and by the general public. One was not trained to be a physician; one went to medical school and was educated [62]. A doctor could choose from a range of burgeoning specialization areas in his discipline, professional medical associations existed in most industrialized countries and physicians had gained a powerful foothold of influence on all areas relating to health care policy making, care and distribution of services [63]. Medicine rapidly became the professional discipline, which was the 'gate keeper' to all of these burgeoning diagnostic and treatment resources, and the education of physicians began specializations in areas of study that did not exist a few short decades before. With the aid of substantial investments by governments and philanthropists, medical institutions for education, research and specialized patient care began to expand. This financial backing, coupled with overwhelming success in the treatment and cure of disease, brought physicians public recognition, confidence, authority and a very powerful political lobby [64]. Nursing at this time continued to be viewed as an occupation and the standard authoritarian approach to training coupled with low wages continued to reign supreme within the existing institutional setting. However, FNS nurses who were well outside of the institutional setting common in most hospitals outside of Appalachia, had done without a physician for so long and only called upon them when they came across situations they were not equipped within their scope of practice to handle, now found they had to go to or through doctors before being allowed to do virtually any treatment or educational counselling. These 'brought on' doctors also came with changes to the treatment regimes that were not always accepted by the nurses.

The FNS at this time also proved resistant to changing those cultural traits that were most valued by the people they served. Productivity at the FNS had more to do with people than numbers; hence FNS nurses were more productive, as well as more satisfied with their work environment, however 'harsh' such an environment became at times.[17] Indeed, perhaps the challenge associated with such an environment was the draw. All of the FNS nurses interviewed, both British and American, cited the 'adventure' aspect of their going to Appalachia as one of the top three reasons they went. They also valued the altruistic and travel aspects associated with the work but by far what made this practice culture viable were the benefits to the 'heart and soul' of the nurse and the professional value and autonomy placed upon her by both the organization and the community in which she served. These 'people orientation' aspects of the work were increasingly rare as the national health care environment began moving to centralized power structures, the business model, specialization and the institutionalization of technology. Most health care organizations in the nation at this time were centralized power structures and based upon the business model that had been so successful in the industrial revolution and it was a change that was occurring in every emerging industrialized country.

It took Breckinridge and her early nurses many years to earn 'rights' privileges in Appalachia, but they achieved it by subscribing to the following rule regarding the nurses' responsibility, 'If a father can make it to you to ask for help, then you can make it there to provide it.' There were to be no refusals to go when called upon by anyone in the community for help [65]. This created problems for the nurses and staff who did not come to Appalachia with a stronger sense of volunteer reciprocity (human service reward) than enterprise (socio-economic reward) frame-of-mind in its latter years. It also created friction between the nurses who were more 'human reward system'-oriented and those coming in to the area later who were, as it was claimed by 'earlier' FNS nurses, becoming less and less so. An early FNS nurse who was at the service on and off since the 1950s, till official retirement in 1978, ruminated on the changes at the FNS during her tenure and her observations of the region upon her return from a recent visit there. Though enjoying the trip back and seeing a lot of "her babies" (those grown whom she had delivered), she commented on the many changes, not all of them good that social security and governmental programs created. Of the huge unemployment problems existing upon her return visit she said:

> A lot of them are on unemployment [now] that's what I don't like about the modern day.... They [FNS] started to employ... people changed, and the higher uppers changed, and then they got... I don't know how they afforded to pay the doctors that they got afterwards. We had done with one doctor for so long, but then they gradually got a surgeon in, and a medical man, and then paediatrics. And you know when we started in the new hospital [Mary Breckinridge Hospital was built in 1975 to replace the old facility] you had to realize that we had to have these things, because they wouldn't have been accredited for one thing, and

---

[17] Elizabeth 'Hilly' Hillman, British former FNS Nurse-Midwife (1949–1954), Date interviewed: 04/05/2005. Interviewer: Edith A. West.

they were needed…But we had done our own necessitation on the babies…. until we had
the paediatrician.

Regarding the nursing staff, she lamented, '…But you see all these young ones
came and they wanted everything, the midwives themselves. I didn't like a lot of it
in the end'.[18] Many of these later nurses did not stay as long as the 'early nurses'
had, either leaving when their contract was up or before whereas most of the early
nurses stayed longer than they originally intended to and kept in contact with the
organization and people after they did leave. A few of the British 'early nurses' lived
their entire lives in the hills and are buried there.

The FNS and community it served often did not have clear boundaries, could not
identify shared solutions and did not reconcile contradictory beliefs and multiple
identities. Yet, these shared society members contend that they 'belonged' to a culture [66]. As one former FNS nurse put it:

> You were dependent upon other people to a certain extent (at FNS) and yet you were indepen-
> dent. But you saw other people they had a special value to them. They were important to you.
> It's a…. it's a feeling that I… I think it hard to describe. Well, now you know, you're kind of
> doing your own thing. It's… it's not in your job… job description [chuckle] (see Footnote 12).

The nurses and the community members for the most part shared a common
people orientation and overarching purpose, faced similar problems and had comparable experiences, more so in the organization's early years than in its later years.
They also shared differing orientations, purposes and accommodated different
beliefs, incommensurable technologies, implied different solutions that had multiple meanings for individual members. Though those working for the FNS certainly
never had the standard of living that others working for health care organizations in
the US had, they were also not living at the poverty level that the rest of the
Appalachian community did.

The nurses and staff who worked at the FNS came from different backgrounds
and all walks of life. They also came to the service for many different reasons,
among them humanitarian or Christian service, adventure, challenge and to 'experience some of life' or a 'different culture' before marriage. Those who claim to have
gleaned the most from their experience at the FNS also cite that their desire to work
for the Service was also motivated by a strong desire to 'live rough' or 'live out of
doors' and closer to nature and the rustic, rural isolation of the Appalachia's appealed
to them.[19] However, the overarching purpose which all of these early nurses had was
a desire to connect with the people they served in some way and on some level
despite any perceived cultural differences [67]. They also had a strong sense of
'spirituality,' that is of relatedness to the people that transcended the self in such a
way that empowered them while simultaneously valuing the individuals they cared

---

[18]Molly Lee, British former FNS Nurse-Midwife (1950–1970s), Date interviewed: 05/04/2005.
Interviewer: Edith A. West.

[19]Jean Corner-Rowan, British former FNS Nurse-Midwife (1964–1966), Date interviewed:
11/03/2005. Interviewer: Edith A. West.

for. Each expressed that their experiences at the FNS were ones that had deep meaning, had added purpose to their lives and had given them a sense of oneness with something greater than themselves, nature or the universe.

The 'factory-like' approach was described by Damman (1982) as coming into the hills of Kentucky and the FNS via the government and private agency projects of the 1960s when administrators became primarily interested in "numbers," telling FNS nurses to 'sign-up six patients per day (at the clinic, where they were now to be centrally located) leaving the nurses little time for home health care' [68]. A former American FNS nurse stated that she had a "great respect for all the administrators and people that were there (at the FNS)," as they believed in what was being done. She also stated that it was not a "*business*" [Italics added] then, which was what it had become "… or so it seemed to us when we were back (visiting) the last time".[20] The fact that a 14 year veteran and practicing nurse today made the following observation about her work environment when addressing what she disliked most about the work, "… the politics of management whose primary goal is to meet the bottom line… humanity suffers as a result," illustrates just how deeply embedded this culture has become in the provision of care in the US.[21]

The social and economic changes experienced in Appalachia since the 1900s have created deep seated problems within that culture, which persist today. Chief among them was the rise of the corporate culture prevalent outside of Appalachia and its subsequent infiltration into the region. The technological advancements and governmental control that altered the provision of health care in American society subsequently altered the provision of care in Appalachia as well. With the advent of money on a vast scale penetrating into Eastern Appalachia during and since the New Deal era, the people's culture has been weakened but not obliterated [69]. These two value systems mingled initially within the region and the people traversed both systems by continuing with subsistence farming while supplementing their incomes with 'outside' employment such as mining, factory work, and logging or even in some cases working for the FNS. However, eventually outside influences overtook and completely eradicated subsistence farming and created profound disruptions within the culture that persist today.

For both the Appalachian culture and the FNS, with the rise of a purely 'enterprise' form of economic system there also came a decline of traditional 'volunteer' reciprocity; more broadly defined as a 'human service reward' system. For rural Appalachia, this created a move from self-sufficiency to dependence that it is still struggling to free itself from today. For the FNS it created a shift from a community-based system (people focus) to a more institutionalised (object focused) provision of health care with an accompanying loss of independence in practice. This doing *for* instead of *with* people focus caused a break in the earned 'rights, place and

---

[20]Margaret (Maggie) Willson, British former FNS Nurse-Midwife (1955–1967).

[21]Shelley WC. Hospital telemetry nurse for 1 year; internal medicine & obstetrics-gynaecology office nurse for 5 years; labour & delivery room nurse for 9 years. Date surveyed 8/06/2007.

claims' status of the FNS and impeded the Service's ability to meet the health care needs of its community. It also lost the trust and loyalty of the community and created schisms within the organization which are further explored in the next chapter.

References

1. Obermiller J, Maloney M. The uses and misuses of Appalachian culture. J Appalach Stud. 2016;22(1):103–12.
2. Russ K. Working with clients of Appalachian culture. 2010. http://counselingoutfitters.com/vistas/vistas.
3. Puckett A. Seldom ask, never tell: labor & discourse in Appalachia. New York: Oxford University Press; 2002. p. 31.
4. Dammann N. A social history of the Frontier Nursing Service. Sun City: Social Change Press; 1982.
5. Breckinridge M. Wide neighborhoods: a story of the Frontier Nursing Service. Lexington: The University Press of Kentucky; 1952.
6. Abramson R, Haskell J. Encyclopedia of Appalachia. Knoxville: University of Tennessee Press; 2006. p. 1533.
7. Abramson R, Haskel J. Encyclopedia of Appalachia. Knoxville: University of Tennessee Press; 2006. p. 1533.
8. Encyclopedia of Appalachia. https://www.arc.gov/news/article.asp?ARTICLE_ID=287. Accessed 7 Jan 2019.
9. Yang Y, Kozhimannil K. Making a case to reduce legal impediments to midwifery practice in the United States. Womens Health Issues. 2015;25(4):314–7.
10. Obermiller J, Maloney M. The uses and misuses of Appalachian culture. J Appalach Stud. 2016;22(1):109.
11. West E. British and American Frontier Nursing Service (FNS) Nurses (1950–1960s): oral history narratives on nursing. J Oral Hist Soc. 2007;35(2):23–35.
12. Abramson R, Haskell J. Encyclopaedia of Appalachia. Knoxville: University of Tennessee Press; 2006. p. 149, 171.
13. Latimer M, Oberhauser A. Exploring gender and economic development in Appalachia. J Appalach Stud. 2004;10(3):269–91.
14. Farnham C. The education of the Southern Belle: higher education and student socialization in the Antebellum South, vol. 175. New York: New York University Press; 1994. p. 180.
15. Reynolds GP. Foxfire 10. New York: Doubleday; 1993. p. 224.
16. Abramson R, Haskell J. Encyclopaedia of Appalachia. Knoxville: University of Tennessee Press; 2006. p. 172.
17. Puckett A. Seldom ask, never tell: labour & discourse in Appalachia. New York: Oxford University Press; 2002. p. 210.
18. Salstrom P. Appalachia's path to dependency: rethinking a region's economic history, 1730–1940. Lexington: University Press of Kentucky; 2015. p. 1.
19. Reynolds GP. Foxfire 10. New York: Doubleday; 1993. p. 234.
20. Abramson R, Haskell J. Encyclopaedia of Appalachia. Knoxville: University of Tennessee Press; 2006. p. 444.
21. Abramson R, Haskell J. Encyclopaedia of Appalachia. Knoxville: University of Tennessee Press; 2006. p. 446, 151.
22. Bradshaw M. The Appalachian regional commission: twenty-five years of government policy, vol. 20. Lexington: The University Press of Kentucky; 1992.

23. Salstrom P. Appalachia's path to dependency: rethinking a region's economic history, 1730–1940. Lexington: University Press of Kentucky; 2015. p. 20.
24. Weller JE. Yesterday's people: life in contemporary Appalachia. Lexington: University Press of Kentucky; 1965.
25. Salstrom P. Appalachia's path to dependency: rethinking a region's economic history, 1730–1940. Lexington: University Press of Kentucky; 2015. p. 43.
26. Puckett A. Seldom ask, never tell: labour & discourse in Appalachia. New York: Oxford University Press; 2002. p. 95.
27. Kearny-Datesman M, Crandall J, Kearny EN. The American ways: an introduction to American culture. 4th ed. New York: Prentice Hall Regents; 2014. p. 106.
28. Schumann W, Fowler C. Globalization, identity, and activism in Appalachia and Wales: comparing the political economy of representation in two marginal "regions". J Appalach Stud. 2002;8(2):333–61.
29. Brogan H. Longman history of the United States of America. New York: Longman; 1985.
30. Appalchian Regional Commission. https://www.arc.gov/. Accessed 10 Jan.
31. Luu C. The legendary language of the Appalachian "Holler". JSTOR Daily. 2018. https://daily.jstor.org/the-legendary-language-of-the-appalachian-holler/. Accessed 11 Jan 2019.
32. US Census Burea. https://www.census.gov/quickfacts/lesliecountykentucky. Accessed 10 Jan 2019.
33. Center for Disease Control and Prevention. https://www.cdc.gov/niosh/mining/UserFiles/works/pdfs/shiim.pdf. Accessed 10 Jan 2019.
34. Crowe-Carraco C. Mary Breckinridge and the Frontier Nursing Service. Regist Ky Hist Soc. 1978;76(3):179–91. https://www.jstor.org/stable/23378979.
35. Schumann W, Fowler C. Globalization, identity, and activism in Appalachia and Wales: comparing the political economy of representation in two marginal "regions". J Appalach Stud. 2002;8(2):358.
36. Abramson R, Haskell J. Encyclopaedia of Appalachia. Knoxville: University of Tennessee Press; 2006. p. 1018.
37. Puckett A. Seldom ask, never tell: labour & discourse in Appalachia, vol. 209. New York: Oxford University Press; 2002. p. 210.
38. Knechtly L. Where else but here? Kentucky: Pippa Valley Printing; 1989. p. 2.
39. DeLong J. The economic history of the twentieth century. 1st ed. New York: Basic Books; 2018. p. 1–448.
40. Donelson-Moss G. America in the twentieth century. 5th ed. Upper Saddle River: Prentice Hall; 2010.
41. Davis J. A history of Britain 1885-1939. New York: St. Martin Press; 1999.
42. Goldfield D, Abbott C, Argersinger J, Argersinger P. Twentieth-century America. 2nd ed. New York: Pearson; 2013.
43. Lock S, Last J, Dunea G. The Oxford companion to medicine. 3rd ed. Oxford: Oxford University Press. https://doi.org/10.1093/acref/9780192629500.001.0001. Published online: 2006.
44. Rafferty AM, Robinson J, Elkan R. Nursing history and the politics of welfare. New York: Routledge; 1997.
45. Baly M. Nursing and social change. London: Routledge; 1995. p. 58.
46. Abel-Smith B. A history of the nursing profession. London: Heinemann; 1960. Published online: 2018.
47. Breckinridge M. Wide neighborhoods: a story of the Frontier Nursing Service. Lexington: The University Press of Kentucky; 1952. p. 32, 45, 59 and 11.
48. Dammann N. A social history of the Frontier Nursing Service. Sun City: Social Change Press; 1982. p. 28.
49. Wall R, Winter J. The upheaval of war: family, work and welfare in Europe, 1914–1918. New York: Cambridge University Press; 1988. p. 299.

50. Alitzer A. The establishment of the FNS: a resource mobilization approach. Unpublished Master's dissertation. Lexington: University of Kentucky; 1990. p. 8.
51. Criss B. Culture and the provision of care: FNS, 1925–1940. Unpublished PhD dissertation. Utah: University of Utah; 1988. p. 16.
52. Puckett A. Seldom ask, never tell: labour & discourse in Appalachia, vol. 19. New York: Oxford University Press; 2002. p. 31.
53. Heffner R. A documentary history of the United States: expanded and updated. 9th ed. New York: Penguin Group; 2013.
54. Braybon G, Summerfield P. Out of the cage: women's experiences in two World Wars. 5th ed. New York: Routledge; 2013. p. 260.
55. Braybon G, Summerfield P. Out of the cage: women's experiences in two World Wars. New York: Routledge; 2013. p. 123.
56. Abramson R, Haskell J. Encyclopaedia of Appalachia. Knoxville: University of Tennessee Press; 2006. p. 1019.
57. Corbin D. Life, work and rebellion in the coal fields: the Southern West Virginia miners 1880-1922. Morgantown: West Virginia University Press; 2015. p. 65.
58. Dammann N. A social history of the Frontier Nursing Service. Sun City: Social Change Press; 1982. p. 330.
59. Breckinridge M. Wide neighborhoods: a story of the Frontier Nursing Service. Lexington: The University Press of Kentucky; 1952. p. 62.
60. Hallum J. Nursing the image: media, culture and professional identity. New York: Routledge; 2013. p. 125.
61. Hudson-Jones A. Images of nurses: perspectives from history, art and literature. Philadelphia: University of Pennsylvania Press; 1988. p. 76.
62. Martin J. Cultures in organizations: three perspectives. Oxford: Oxford University Press; 1992. p. 102.
63. Dolan J, Fitzpatrick M, Herrmann E. Nursing in society: a historical perspective. 15th ed. Philadelphia: W.B. Saunders; 1983.
64. Cooter R, Pickstone J. Companion to medicine in the twentieth century. New York: Routledge; 2013.
65. Reid D. Saddlebags full of memories. Burt Lake Michigan, USA; 1992.
66. Meyerson D. "Normal" ambiguity?: a glimpse of an occupational culture. In: Frost P, Moore L, Louis M, Lundberg C, Martin J, editors. Reframing organizational culture. Newbury Park: Sage; 1991. p. 131–44.
67. Friedman L, McGarvie M. Charity, philanthropy, and civility in American history. New York: Cambridge University Press; 2003. p. 48.
68. Dammann N. A social history of the Frontier Nursing Service. Sun City: Social Change Press; 1982. p. 134.
69. Salstrom P. Appalachia's path to dependency: rethinking a region's economic history, 1730–1940. Lexington: University Press of Kentucky; 2015. p. 59.

Chapter 3
Place and Claims: Cultural and Communication in Appalachia

3.1 Cultural Diplomacy or Colonial Tendencies: Breckinridge in Appalachia

Breckinridge was a woman with a remarkable talent for being politic in all interests of concern to her organization. Her organization's interests were also intimately entwined with the interests of the local community. This was something that was not true of other organizational cultures entering the region. She used a unique form of cultural diplomacy to maximize the needed support for the service, which relied heavily on outside financial support and volunteer Couriers to work with her nurses. She also used it to garner the support of the local population. Therefore, to her aristocratic contributors she proffered the notion that it was not in-breeding but rather, un-mixed breeding of good English stock (of which she knew perfectly well most of them were) that contributed to research findings that indicated justification for her Service [1]. She made her argument to other health professionals using scientifically sound research generated from mental tests given to Appalachian children by a psychologist who was an expert in this field of study to argue against the eugenics crowd of her day [2]. To the local populous she was a distant relation. A former 20-year employee of the FNS and long-time resident said:

> There weren't no finer woman ever crossed the water than Mary Breckinridge was... she reported to us that she was across [her ancestors came from England].... across from the water. Well, my fore-parents was and so that... that just sat her up a little bit better and she began liking us all. She was more help to this country than any other person that ever been born in it. Now, I'll just be honest with you... see they was a helping us and we helped them. That's the way it went.[1]

---

[1]Kentucky Committee for Mothers & Babies Meeting Minutes. 85M1: FNS, Box 2, Fol. 2. Transcripts: Frankfort, Kentucky for Thursday 28 May 1925–2:30pm in Assembly Room of New Capital Hotel. Also in this folder are the 'FNS Resolutions. USA: forming the Service. University of Kentucky in Lexington; 1925.

© Springer Nature Switzerland AG 2019
E. West, *Frontier Nursing in Appalachia: History, Organization and the Changing Culture of Care*, https://doi.org/10.1007/978-3-030-20027-5_3

Yet though the use of her unique, many faceted brand of cultural diplomacy certainly troubled researchers studying both the Appalachia region and those who came into that region with the expressed purpose of helping the people, Breckinridge was never accused by anyone who actually knew her of being deliberately deceptive.[2] When asked if she was the same person at (local community) meetings as she was at Wendover, one former courier who originally went to the FNS for 6 weeks and ended up staying for 2 years stated emphatically, 'Yes, there wasn't a phoney bone in her body'.[3]

The many and varied narratives of her by employees, friends and the locals reveal a woman of wit and humour who knew her audience whether staff, nurses or community members and had a tremendous confidence in and respect for them all. She listened to what people had to say and never gave them the impression that she viewed them as 'beneath' her, whether that person was and adult or a child.[4] Still, she was known by her staff as well as the local population as 'Mrs. Breckinridge' and never 'Mary.' This fact appears to have troubled researchers (not the locals) in a number of interviews currently housed at the University of Kentucky in Lexington, USA for the FNS Oral History Project from 1978 to 1982 who implied that this was evidence that Breckinridge thought she was superior to the locals. This and the fact that she reportedly never had any local people to the 'Big House' for 'tea' as was her custom for her nurses and staff.

One former, long time FNS secretary summed it up best when she explained that the organization needed to maintain a professional distance and treat all of the local people alike as the work in the area 'depended on it.' No 'mixing' with the local men by the nurses was encouraged either.[5] Breckinridge was said to have frowned upon fraternization between the services mostly female employees and local men. Yet human nature being what it was, marriages did occur. A former FNS nurse who married a local man related her surprise and pleasure at receiving a hand-written note from Mrs. Breckinridge congratulating her on her recent marriage and wishing her a very happy future; when her first secretary married her brother she quipped, 'I wish I had brothers enough to marry all my secretaries'.[6] A few of the nurses who married while in the Service stayed on for a time or came back to help as their

[2]Interview #780H144FNS04 1978, Matt Gray, long-time resident of Appalachia, Interviewed 21 July, 1978, Interviewer: Dale Deaton.

[3]Elizabeth C. Walton, American FNS Midwifery School Graduate of 1945. Date surveyed: 22/07/2003.

[4]Interview #82OH39 FNS182. Beth B. Jones, former FNS Courier from Cincinnati, Ohio whose Aunt Margaret Rogan was a friend of Mary Breckinridge. She went for six weeks and stayed for two years. In: Interviewed: Unknown. Marion Barrett: Interviewer; 1982.

[5]Interview #78OH151FNS11. Georgia Ledford, former Secretary for FNS Community Committee & long-time resident of Appalachia, Interviewed 17 August. Carol Crow-Carraco: Interviewer; 1978. p. 1978.

[6]Interview #82OH03FNS146 1982, Agnes Lewis, former long-time FNS Secretary, Interviewed 5 January 1979. Interviewer: Dale Deaton.

schedules allowed. Those who did not were always welcome to come back to visit by their former employer and friends in the community and often did. It was also well documented that though the locals were never invited to tea they were certainly invited to the 'Big House' (Wendover) yearly for Christmas celebrations and the nurses as well as the organization's director had monthly 'meetings' at the clinic cites where food and socializing also occurred.[7] Overall, Breckinridge's shortcomings were attributed by those that knew her best and longest to her forceful personality and the pressures of running the Service.[8] Even when leading language was used to frame many of the questions for the Oral History database at the University of Kentucky in the late 1970s and early 1980s such as, 'Would you describe her (Breckinridge) as moody?' responses tended to mirror this one made by a former courier, 'Moody? No. Angry when mothers and children were suffering? Yes' [3]. Another long-time secretary wrote that Breckinridge, "like a chameleon" could change her personality to match the culture she was in; gentle, humble and cheerful with the locals, sophisticated when in cities or speaking with old friends from the 'outside.'

Varying accounts of her by former staff, nurses, midwifery students, friends, supporters and local residents suggest a formidable, commanding and decidedly controlling woman whose administrative style could be viewed by some as micro-managerial. The FNS was, after all, Breckinridge's Service and it most definitely had her image imprinted upon it. However, the truth was that though she certainly maintained firm control regarding the oversight of the organization, by all accounts the day-to-day provision of health care at the FNS was placed squarely into the hands of its nurses while the financial and administrative duties were those of its director. It was well documented in a variety of sources and restated by former FNS nurses as well as others connected with the organization that Mrs. Breckinridge had only three rules for her nurses regarding the community, 'You don't talk politics, religion or moonshine'.[9]

She also had complete confidence in her staff and nurses, even when they did not share her faith in them. A former long-time personal secretary to Breckinridge said that she had placed quite a bit of confidence in her and allowed her 'great freedom in her work.' She attributed this to the mutual confidence and compatibility that the two of them shared, though she felt she had 'nothing like her (Breckinridge's) background' but rather a very 'mediocre' background because she 'had not been to college'.[10] Breckinridge garnered, not demanded, respect from those that knew her well. A close friend of Breckinridge said of her, "she had the mind of a man and a heart of

---

[7] Roberta Stidham, American former FNS Nurse (1960–1961), Date surveyed: 13/03/2003. Date interviewed: 17/05/2006. Interviewer: Edith A. West.

[8] Interview #78OH151FNS11 1978, Georgia Ledford.

[9] Interview#82OH34FNS177, 1982, Mary Stewart.

[10] Anne Lorentzen, American former FNS Nurse (1963–1965), Date surveyed: 29/12/2003. Date interviewed: 11/03/2005. Interviewer: Edith A. West.

a mother, no patience for a laggard and no time for an idealist. She would say, 'Ideas not ideals are what matter in the world. Don't give me theories, give me facts'".[11]

Yet Breckinridge has been accused of treating the locals, 'like children' by researchers outside of Appalachia after her demise [4]. Perhaps a more accurate statement about the woman would be that she treated everyone like her child; bullying or nurturing depending on what was needed for their own personal growth or that of her beloved Service. New employees were acclimated via mentorship with more senior, seasoned and experienced employees who had already established a relationship with the local people. The system worked satisfactorily with all parties knowing and doing their respective roles within the organization with a minimum of interference but quite a bit of mingling between its branches (administration, staff, students and community residents). One resident's description of a local committee meeting intimated that though business matters were discussed, there were also story telling, refreshments and a lot of socializing that took place between the FNS's staff and the local people. All of these narratives taken in sum represent the various character facets of the FNS, the organization's founder and her dealings with the local population. Just as a portrait painted from the side or from the front though different are still faithful representations of the woman; who for all intents and purposes was as multi-faceted and seemingly paradoxical as the rest of us despite the need of some after her death to paint her as a caricature [5].

In many ways Breckinridge was a conglomeration of what could be considered both the 'old' and 'new' American woman and her organization's culture reflected this diversity. As a consequence, her service was often labelled as one or the other by opposing factions both inside and outside of the organization from its inception, though it was in the late 1950s and beyond that this dichotomy became most pronounced. She has been criticized for harbouring latent elitist, 'racist' and 'colonial' tendencies and fostering them in Eastern Appalachia. She was chastised in an interview with one of the many prominent FNS visitors who observed the woman and the work first-hand for not allowing a black man, the chauffer of one of the other visitors who also supported the work, to stay in the main house. Instead, the driver slept in the adjacent barn [6]. It is interesting to note that later in the interview this same visitor made a rather prejudicial comment of her own regarding the locals when she labelled them 'rabbits' in reference to the average number of children each family contained. Still, the observation certainly had merit though Breckinridge's personal correspondence suggested that there may also have been other motives for her actions.

In a letter from Kate Hyder, Director of Nurse-Midwifery at Flint-Goodridge Hospital of Dillard University in New Orleans dated March 4, 1943, Hyder requested that a 'Negro Obstetrician, a Dr. Segre,' be allowed to accompany her on a visit to observe the FNS Midwifery School, outposts and hospital; and work with Breckinridge's resident physician, Dr. Kooser. Breckinridge's response was that she

[11] Interview#82OH11FNS154, 1982. Wilma Duvall Whittlesey, FNS Secretary from 1929–1936, Interviewed 30 November 1979, Interviewer: Dale Deaton.

could not ask Dr. Segre,' 'though personally she would be very glad to invite him.' She explained her dilemma thus, '… there is literally no place up in here where he could be a guest. In central Kentucky where several leading coloured citizens, among them an Episcopal Minister, a man like Dr. Segre' could be properly entertained in between his visits to a hospital, there are literally no such homes here and I am truly sorry that I cannot ask him'.[12] Though it could certainly be argued that Breckinridge was hiding behind the perceived disapproval of her other guests, the local population or both, one has to remember that this was, after all, the South in 1943; not only the American South but the more isolated, rural Appalachian South.

In this carefully worded letter, Breckinridge may have been using the 'diplomacy' she has become legendary for to hide her prejudice but her statements here taken in conjunction with the housing of the black chauffeur suggest that perhaps the issue was less about race and rather more concerned with the existing class issues within the culture. Breckinridge intimates a man of Dr. Segre's position should be properly entertained by a county's leading citizens and laments that this would not be possible in the poor rural area where her home and hospital are located. One could argue, as many have done after her death, that this reflected as badly on Breckinridge's view of the local people as it did on her view of the people of Dr. Segre's race. Yet she defied this label as well by choosing to live in the impoverished area her organization serviced for the last 40 years of her life where she purportedly fed chickens, pigs and horses, kept dogs, visited these poor homes on a regular basis and lived as simply as the people to whom she provided health care.

Breckinridge gave assistance whenever needed from whom ever requested it. She also gave direction as to where to get support if the FNS was not able, for whatever reason, to directly provide it. She received requests from many medical as well as nursing organizations throughout the years and responded to them all. One such correspondence was a letter to a Miss Findley at the Tuskeegee School of Nurse Midwifery in Alabama, which agreed to their request to be placed on the Service's mailing list.[13] The Tuskeegee School of Nurse Midwifery was one of the first such programs at a historically black college or University in the nation and remains one of the oldest predominantly black schools of nursing in continuous operation in the US. In addition, the bulk of Breckinridge's nurse midwives who graduated in the 1940s and 1950s went on to serve in many non-Western countries, chief among them, Africa, India, Indonesia, Nepal and Honduras where they not only worked along side but also trained the local people. Some of the FNS's 1960s graduates are still doing this work today.[14]

---

[12]Letter to Kate Hyder from Mary Breckinridge, 10 March 1943, 85M1: FNS, Box 198, Fol. 3. 'Letter from Kate Hyder, Director of Nurse-Midwifery, Flint-Goodridge Hospital of Dillard University, New Orleans, Dated: 4 March 1943 to Mrs. Mary Breckinridge', University of Kentucky in Lexington, USA.

[13]Correspondence between Miss Findley and Dorothy Buck 1945, 85M1: FNS, Box 199, Fol. 1. 'Correspondence between Miss Findley and FNS Nurse Dorothy Buck 1945', University of Kentucky in Lexington, USA.

[14]Madonna Buret-Spratt, American FNS Midwifery School Graduate of 1960. Date surveyed: 14/06/2003.

Breckinridge's upbringing in the segregated South, the daughter of what could be considered 'Southern Royalty' may have had considerable bearing on her decision to house a black driver in her barn instead of the main house. This choice can hardly be viewed as out of character for any Southerner to do at this time in the nation's history. What her organization contributed over the years to the Tuskeegee School of Nurse Midwifery in Alabama, numerous other organizations and countless rural areas within the non-Western countries that her nurse graduates serviced was equally within character for her organization and was something remarkable for its time. Breckinridge shared a cultural trait with the local populous that was an anomaly elsewhere in the nation in regard to the treatment of unwed mothers. One former FNS nurse said of the Appalachian culture that the attitude toward these mothers, the support of family and community, was singular when compared not only to US cultural norms but also with what was going on in England at the time as girls in this condition 'would have been sent away'.[15] One of the first two students admitted into her midwifery school was Native American [Cherokee] (see Footnote 11). Even so, Breckinridge has been categorized since her death by some researchers as one of the many single, white, childless, 'elite,' 'progressive-types' who belonged to a generation educated to believe that marriage and career were incompatible and who in their efforts to help the poor and needy have done irreparable damage to the 'objects' of their benevolence [7].

One such view suggested that solely due to her pre-existing social position upon arrival in Appalachia, Breckinridge sought to 'deliberately construct the mountain people and culture for purposes of strengthening her ability to raise funds for her Service.' Further, she is accused of believing that though she thought the local people could be educated she also felt they could never reach the same 'level of development enjoyed by those who came from the outside' [8]. Essentially, the charge is that Breckinridge adhered to the controversial 'eugenics' movement that was being supported throughout the US from the 1880s to 1940s that was replete with references to and studies of 'poor white mountain folk' [9]. Most often associated with the racism and Nazi medicine of the 1930s and 1940s, eugenics programs focused on the belief that selective breeding practices amongst whites could ensure the mental, physical and moral health and fitness of their children and future generations. Breckinridge believed, as did most people by the start of the First World War, that evidence strongly indicated most infant and childhood deaths were not the inevitable result of inherent defects but were a consequence of prenatal and postnatal environmental conditions that could be improved. It was one of the principal reasons for organizing her Service in the region.

Though it was certainly true that Breckinridge was prolifically diplomatic in her desire to keep the service operating in the midst of opposing cultures and the myriad of friction created between these forces it is also well documented that she had a deep affection, respect and high regard for the people she was serving. In fact, in

---

[15]Margaret (Maggie) Willson, British former FNS Nurse-Midwife (1955–1967).

direct contradiction to the suggestion that Breckinridge saw the locals as 'inferior' intellectually to those outside Appalachia, she did research to prove the exact opposite to be true. When others were saying that these people had lower intelligence than the rest of the nation due to their poverty, isolation and 'in-breeding' she conducted a research study that proved otherwise and published the information entitled, 'Midwifery In The Kentucky Mountains: An Investigation' in 1923. Her investigation into childbearing practices and survey of the 'granny midwives' in the Eastern Appalachian region was extensive and innovative for its time. The report said of the people that they were the direct descendents of British immigrants who came 200 years before, have lived a more remote existence than the general populace due to geography and contrary to popular opinion had been found to have 'I.Q. averages slightly above that of the rest of the nation, even where illiteracy flourished' [10].

It has been suggested, again citing latent 'colonial' tendencies as the cause, that Breckinridge used the local people in a 'menial labour' capacity, yet made no effort to train the locals or provide the same sort of scholarship monies to them to get training that she offered outsiders coming into her organization. It has also been argued that had she done so, it would have allowed the people to stay instead of having to leave the region due to the economic hardships [11]. Though it is true that Breckinridge rarely offered scholarship monies to locals, it is equally true that at the height of the depression when her nurses were receiving no salary to stay (most did anyway and she was eventually forced to discharge seven nurses and leave the work for those remaining) she became the sole employer for roughly 30% of the local population with those 'menial labour jobs' at a time when the choices were to leave or starve (see Footnote 1) Though in both in never forgot how that incident upset The only other time the FNS was 'sued' was when a FNS has been cited as a cause for many.

The organization was always plagued with economic crises and sending a girl for nurses training and then, graduate nurses training was not cost effective. Breckinridge's early employment requirements were that a nurse had to have completed training (not be a student) and come to the organization with some public health, district nursing and midwifery experience; preferably with equestrian experience as well. If they lacked some of these qualifications yet were well suited to the work, she provided scholarship monies toward their education to get qualified even though it often meant that nurses had to go to England to do so.[16] Later, her midwifery school was a graduate program that necessitated not only nurses, but diploma and later only bachelor degree nurses. This precluded the local girls as there was no nurse training school and the hospital Breckinridge sponsored was never designed to be anything but a place for the very ill; those in need of special nursing or medical attention and emergency cases.

---

[16] FNS Quarterly Bulletin; 1928.

Virtually all nurse training schools at the time were hospital-based and those coming to the FNS had received training outside of the region. In addition, schools, especially schools outside of the region, were believed by a fair number of Appalachian people to teach children to 'get above their raisin' making some communities sceptical of education beyond the eighth grade, even into the middle of the twentieth century [12]. This contrasted the existing education system outside of the region, which reflected the nation's value regarding the ideal of equality of opportunity. The American idea of individual success based on equality of opportunity or 'working your way to the top' was not shared by most Appalachians. These communities valued more practical, vocational types of training which would offer the skills necessary to provide for a family close to home [13].

Though nursing was something that could be done close to home at the FNS, it was also viewed at this time both in and out of the region as temporary work for girls that would out of necessity be abandoned once a woman married and had a family. Even so, in the Service's latter years as views about education began to change in Appalachia, many former 'FNS babies' did choose to go outside of the region to receive nurses training and came back to the area to live and work. Many of them credited the fine work done by the FNS and the role models that these nurses were in their formative years as the reason why they chose to become nurses. Breckinridge did not hire married women or women with children throughout her tenure as director. She urged the nurse-midwives she hired not to 'fraternize' with the local men and after her own divorce never sought remarriage, considering her work her life and in so doing implied that her nurses follow her example.

Breckinridge employed and educated single, childless, mostly white females, as was the norm at the time both inside and outside of the region [14].

3.2 FNS 'Place' Communicative Repertoire in Appalachia: The Early Years

In the case of Appalachia, even when consensus confirms that individuals are within their 'rights,' they must also conform to their 'place' within family or community social organizational structure. 'Place' is an extremely complex construct in Appalachian discourse. 'Place' assigns an individual to a geographical locale. However, a more dominant meaning of 'place' that restricts and redefines this primary geographical one refers to an individual's position within a complex set of relationships with others in a 'belonging' network. In this sense, 'place' is negotiated, asserted and developed over a lifetime of community life with others rather than assigned statically on the basis of discursive practices involving a specific space. Often a negotiated 'place' is linked to a physical place (for example, a woman's place with respect to her husband is to be home while he is out providing for her and his children, and an elderly woman's place at a family picnic is at the head of the table while a newly married younger daughter sits to the side). Though one may have the right to show someone how to do a task, it must be his or her 'place' in relation to the other to perform that demonstration in Appalachia [15].

Breckinridge's organization had earned its 'place' within the Eastern Appalachian community by virtue of its permanence physically, culturally and socio-economically there but this 'place' had limitations, hence Breckinridge's rules regarding the taboo subjects of politics, religion and moonshine. One overstepped ones 'place' at one's own peril. The nurses had also negotiated both 'rights' and 'place' outside of the usual ones appointed to women, but these too had their limitations. FNS early nurse, Helen Browne, who later became the director of the FNS, related a story of a home visit she did where she found it necessary to slap a hysterical patient to get her to listen only to have the woman's husband pull a gun on her and order her out of the house. Terrified, she calmly informed him she had to deliver the placenta before leaving. He stood over her with the gun while she finished the job but she had the fortitude to return the very next day to care for the patient. Thankfully, by then the man had calmed down.[17] Another early nurse penned that a local man said that she had 'talked his eye out' in reference to her persistent urgings that he have his unattended eye infection looked at that he would not allow her to treat before he lost the eye entirely [16]. The fact that this local man eventually heeded her advise was testament to the unique 'place' that these women earned in what was decidedly a patriarchal society; one in which women did not advise men.

When Appalachian residents made requests or demands on others within these networks, they were essentially constructing the local socio-economy. These 'rights,' 'place' and 'claims' practices were the tools necessary to construct communication networks for the purchase of commodities or to maintain commodity market activities within the culture. They also usually interfaced directly with county and regional political power networks. These goods and services, which were circulated and obtained in capitalistic markets as commodities or as payment for wage-labour, increasingly depended upon other patterns and organizations of request practices within the socioeconomic communicative repertoire in Appalachia, first with the arrival of the FNS and later in a much more accelerated fashion with the advent of government initiatives that came into the region [17]. The FNS in its early years was much closer to the existing socioeconomic communicative repertoire than the incoming government initiatives that came into the region in its latter years. Later, the Service was forced to adopt many of the corporate culture characteristics that were imbedded within these incoming initiatives and subsequently were in direct opposition to those which the Appalachian people were struggling to maintain at the time and much like the Native American, the people of Appalachia eventually found themselves studied by scholars, local, state and federally funded governmental and private sector researchers all wanting to help alleviate their economic woes while simultaneously, either purposely or unintentionally engineering cultural assimilation [18]. The FNS unwittingly played a role in this first by encouraging the people to accept government assistance in the depression via New Deal

---

[17]Madonna Buret-Spratt, American FNS Midwifery School Graduate of 1960.

projects and later by moving away from its philanthropic roots and into the emerging health care system. It should also be noted that neither move was completely unavoidable for the service if it wanted to keep its doors open as well as meet the community's needs.

FNS nurses recognized the need for the technological, social and economic advancements that entered their practice environment for the good of the quality of life and health of the community. The Appalachian people were also not opposed to the changes coming into the hills initially. After all, their culture had already managed to successfully find a way to 'make a deal' for services provided by the FNS. Services were obtained through the exchange of cash and the prevailing 'barter' system by which 'haggling' or 'makin' a deal' was the established modus operandi for doing things. It was not unusual in the FNS's early years for staff to be given a pig, eggs, food or service in kind in exchange for health care provided by the nurses as cash was not readily available in the hills.[18] Service in kind might involve handy-man services, such as the father of the child delivered by the nurse fixing the nurse's roof or doing some work in her barn or on the health clinic she resided in. The people were not opposed to using this new 'cash only' system but what it was not prepared for or willing to embrace was the *impersonal* [italics added] treatment that such a system fostered [19].

In the Service's latter years, when radios and other technological advances began to come into the hills, there are two stories told by a former personal secretary of Mary Breckinridge, Ms. Agnes Lewis that adequately summed-up the effect that this new culture was having on the local population. In the first, a man had fallen, having toppled over a pig, on Wendover property. He was refunded the $1.86 he'd come to pay for FNS services as compensation. He wrote Breckinridge that he was going to 'law' (sue) her. Breckinridge wrote him that 'there was nothing that couldn't be settled between neighbours' and to come see her. He eventually came but insisted he was going ahead with the lawsuit. Breckinridge informed him that she refunded the money he'd owed her even though he hadn't been hurt in any way from the fall and that she didn't know what else she could be expected to do. "She also told him that her lawyer would charge her no fees but that he would be expected to pay the court fees for the lawsuit. She told him she didn't want a lawsuit but if he felt he must 'law' then 'law' he must." Lewis challenged this man asking him how he could do this to Breckinridge. He said he didn't want to 'law' her (personally), but wanted to 'law' the FNS (business). Lewis explained to him that Breckinridge had put everything into the FNS and that there was simply no money to pay lawsuits, whereby he dropped the suit. "Lewis attributed both this man's attitude and actions to the fact that the people now had 'radios' and she was sure that someone had found out how much money you could get by 'lawing' and put the man up to it'.[19]

---

[18] Molly Lee, British former FNS Nurse-Midwife (1950–1970s).

[19] Interview #82OH03FNS146 1982, Agnes Lewis, former long-time FNS Secretary.

The only other time the FNS was 'sued' was when a man falsely accused Breckinridge of sending a horse back unshod. Breckinridge had sent an 'unsuitable' horse back to a man who stated that he'd sent the horse to her shod and it was returned to him un-shoed. When all attempts to reason with the man had failed and she was forced to go to the county courthouse, it was purported that she very cleverly and subtly used her age and back injury to garner sympathy from the court. A lawyer in Hazard who handled the case said of Breckinridge, 'She's the best lawyer we have in Kentucky.' Though she won the case, Lewis reported that she 'never forgot how that incident upset her (Breckinridge)' (see Footnote 19). Though in both instances Breckinridge did not hesitate to use (successfully) her diplomatic prowess or powers of persuasion to move her audience she lamented the need to do so and later to have to do so through a third-party mediator (both 'impersonal' and 'governmental') to effectively, fairly and equitably communicate with a local person on a matter of business.

The FNS has been cited as a cause for many of these negative changes in Eastern Appalachia by researchers since the 1970s. Breckinridge's character, in much the same way as the Appalachian people's, was also cited as a cause for the region's social, cultural and economic descent. She was accused of being a 'colonizer' who brought capitalistic ideology and corporate oppression into the area and of creating a negative image of the people to those outside the region. However, the case could certainly be made that Breckinridge did not inflict these tendencies upon the people or her nurses but rather that her organization was eventually forced into the unenviable position of being the agent through whom they came into the region.[20] She acquired this dubious distinction by virtue of being one of the very few organizational entities who refused to abandon the community in the wake of the misery inflicted upon it by most of the businesses that came into the region, stripped the land, made the people dependent upon them and promptly left when more money could be made elsewhere with little regard to the cultural and economic dearth they left in their wake.

3.3 FNS 'Place' Communicative Repertoire in Appalachia: The Latter Years

The community members, who saw the changes occurring at the Service in its latter years, retained a sense of loyalty to Breckinridge and continued to identify themselves with the woman and her service even after she died. One woman had the following to say when an interviewer suggested that she didn't want to admit to their being any 'bad' FNS nurses, 'Breckinridge probably got out gals who could

---

[20]Interview #82OH09FNS 152, 1982, Sherman Wooten, long-time resident of Appalachia, Interviewed 7 November 1979. Interviewer: Dale Deaton.

do the work… some now complain that they don't come, but they are only human'.[21] She also cited the 'turn-over' of new nurses as part of the problem with the communities acceptance of the nurses stating you'd need to 'get used to different nurses… learning to trust all over again.' She as well as other community members interviewed who had utilized the service or been FNS babies themselves also cited the 'hospital's coming in' and the people's 'getting used to going to the doctor' as the reason for the move away from the FNS after Breckinridge's death. The coming of usable roads that made access to health care facilities and physicians outside of the county and the doctors now at the FNS referring patients to 'specialists' outside of the county also contributed to the 'patient load just falling off to nothing'.[22]

One community member said the nurses had so much more paperwork to do and more people to handle all of that. The move from barter to cash and the steady increase in the amount of cash required for the services was also mentioned as a change not perceived by the community as for the better. Yet most community members interviewed were still reluctant to find fault with the FNS when asked about the changes, even when they chose to use health care services outside of the county in the Service's latter years. When the increase in costs was mentioned, it was also stated, 'Well, everything is going up and they have to go up to meet the bills' or 'the way times is, you know, you can't do things free no more'.[23]

In much the same way that the early nurses cited the negative changes in the people within the community due to 'welfare' and not the people themselves, so the people blamed the changes at the FNS in its latter years on outside forces and not the character of its founder or her nurses. There was discomposure on the part of both the nurses and their female patients when asked directly about the changes experienced by them in the FNS's latter years and a good deal of ambivalence about them. One book on feminism and autobiography that looks at the texts, theories and methods associated with oral histories explains this phenomenon thus, 'that the narrator of discursive repertoire selects a set of concepts and definitions which allow them psychic comfort when telling their pasts' [20]. So, ultimately though the economic indebtedness of continued business on the part of the recipient (community) did begin to crumble as the role of the FNS (benefactor) changed the bonds of loyalty and gratitude were much harder to sever than the political fidelity of the community. In the end, one female community member explained the cold, hard facts best when she quipped:

> "They (FNS) are getting more commercialized like other hospitals, you know, and their fees are getting to be enormous (chuckle).. it's just 'cause they have to do that, I guess, to keep up with the trend or the other hospitals that are doing this.

> But it seems to me that it takes a person with a really good income or else they're on welfare to afford any of the hospital services, even the FNS."[24]

---

[21] Roberta Stidham, American former FNS Nurse (1960–1961).

[22] Alice Herman, American former FNS Nurse (1956–1978).

[23] Phyllis Long, American former FNS Nurse (1964–1967; 1973–1976; 1993–1996). Date surveyed: 11/07/2005.

[24] Interview#78OH150FNS10, 1982. Mary & Clyde Brewer, long-time residents of Appalachia who wrote a book on it called "Of Bolder Me "and later called "Rugged Trails of Appalachia", Interviewed 10 August 1978. Interviewer: Dale Deaton.

After Breckinridge's death in 1965 many of the local residents commented on the fact that they didn't think anybody could have taken her place.[25] Others attributed the early success of the FNS to the fact that Breckinridge kept a tight rein on the workings of the organization, people and its employees.[26] For the most part, the local people were loyal to the service and cited the woman who founded it as the underlying reason for the overall success of the organization and blamed any negative changes that occurred later on 'inflation,' 'changing times' and 'money problems' within the community.[27]

The FNS has been accused by researchers since the 1970s of being a contributor to Appalachia's dependency, economic and cultural decline. Its founder, Mary Breckinridge has also been charged with harbouring elitist and racist tendencies and 'colonizing' Eastern Appalachia by non-Appalachian scholars studying the region. What is perhaps overlooked by these scholars is that the FNS experienced the same type of changes as the people via governmental interference and adoption of the corporate model. The Service was also displaced socially, politically, culturally and economically from the community, its symbiotic relationship with the people forever disrupted and its unique, innovative, superior brand of care completely obliterated in the Service's latter years.

The fact that the people who knew Breckinridge and benefited from her organization were reluctant to blame the Service for the negative changes to their culture demonstrated the Services' 'place' status within the community. Breckinridge's decentralized; people-focus approach was demonstrated in her dealings with staff as well as the local community and was one that the community valued as well. Thus, the FNS's 'place' had been negotiated, asserted and developed over a lifetime of community life as well as service in Eastern Appalachia. This 'place' status was reciprocated by the nurses' unwillingness to blame the people for their dependence in the Service's latter years. This type of loyalty is also a trait associated with strong cultures [21].

An examination of the lack of clarity and disruptions that developed within the FNS's strong cultural place within the community when it was forced to move from a decentralized to centralized power structure in its latter years is more fully explored in the ensuing chapter. Further, how this move from community based to institutionalized care, and the adoption of a corporate approach to health care practices impacted the FNS and continues to impact the profession as a whole with regard to nurse-physician relationships, nurse education and work environments, professional recruitment and retention practices, and public image are addressed in subsequent chapters.

---

[25] Interview #78OH147FNS07, 1978. Frank Bowling, long-time resident of Appalachia/Community Committee Member, Interviewed 1 July 1978, Interviewer: Dale Deaton.

[26] Interview #78OH144FNS04, 1978. Matt Gray, long-time resident of Appalachia.

[27] Interview#78OH150FNS10, 1982. Mary & Clyde Brewer, long-time residents of Appalachia.

References

1. Goodnow N. Outlines of nursing history. New York: Saunders; 1921. p. 275.
2. Breckinridge M. Wide neighborhoods: a story of the Frontier Nursing Service. Lexington: The University Press of Kentucky; 1952.
3. Knechtly L. Where else but here? Kentucky: Pippa Valley Printing; 1989. p. 73.
4. Dammann N. A social history of the Frontier Nursing Service. Sun City: Social Change Press; 1982. p. 108.
5. Harris H. Constructing colonialism: medicine, technology and the FNS. Unpublished Master's thesis. Virginia: Virginia Polytechnic Institute and State University; 1995. p. 8.
6. Thompson B, Bornat J. The voice of the past: oral history. 4th ed. Oxford: Oxford University Press; 2017.
7. Alitzer A. The establishment of the FNS: a resource mobilization approach; 1990. vol. 8. p. 39.
8. Harris H. Constructing colonialism: medicine, technology and the FNS; 1995. p. 8.
9. Abramson R, Haskell J. Encyclopaedia of Appalachia. Knoxville: University of Tennessee Press; 2006. p. 169.
10. Wall R, Winter J. The upheaval of war: family, work and welfare in Europe, 1914–1918. New York: Cambridge University Press; 1988. p. 370.
11. Breckinridge M. Wide neighborhoods: a story of the Frontier Nursing Service. Lexington: The University Press of Kentucky; 1952. p. 120.
12. Abramson R, Haskell J. Encyclopaedia of Appalachia. Knoxville: University of Tennessee Press; 2006. p. 1519.
13. Datesman M, Crandall J, Kearny EN. The American ways: an introduction to American culture. 3rd ed. Upper Saddle River: Prentice Hall Regents; 2005. p. 172.
14. Breckinridge M. Wide neighborhoods: a story of the Frontier Nursing Service. Lexington: The University Press of Kentucky; 1952. p. 32.
15. Puckett A. Seldom ask, never tell: labour & discourse in Appalachia. New York: Oxford University Press; 2002. p. 32.
16. Reid D. Saddlebags full of memories; 1992. p. 95.
17. Puckett A. Seldom ask, never tell: labour & discourse in Appalachia. New York: Oxford University Press; 2002. p. 209.
18. Ford T. The southern Appalachian region: a survey. Lexington: University of Kentucky Press; 1962. p. 10.
19. Weller JE. Yesterday's people: life in contemporary Appalachia. Lexington: University of Kentucky Press; 1965.
20. Cosslett T, Lury C, Summerfield P. Feminism & autobiography: texts, theories and methods. London: Routledge; 2000. p. 105.
21. Kotter J, Heskett J. Corporate culture and performance. New York: Simon & Schuster; 2011.

Chapter 4
Centralized Versus Decentralized Structures in Appalachia

4.1 Centralized Versus Decentralized Structures

The term 'knowledge is power' came to prominence as formal knowledge began to be linked with political clout and the people who created, transmitted and applied this knowledge became the formal agents of it. With growth in the magnitude and complexity of formal knowledge came the development of professional disciplines. These disciplines became institutions with political, socio-economic and cultural identities of their own as well as the driving forces, which provided education to its members within other, larger institutional settings. Institutions began to address the increasing number of areas of human life to which their particular brand of knowledge could be applied and with this shift in a tendency toward rule by public debate and participation in decision making toward a rule by the new 'knowledge brokers' (intellectuals) came the inevitable move away from egalitarianism toward a more intellectual monocracy [1].

A profession is also an occupation that has special forms of protection from competition in capitalist labour markets and is one that benefits from a 'social closure' [2]. This is where nursing has fallen short of its goal. Nursing has been able to regulate the profession from within to some degree. For example, certified midwives have gradually replaced 'granny' midwives and nurses have needed to be licensed as early as the 1920s. Yet nursing has not been able to assert itself as a profession fully in the marketplace as institutions with greater political clout have marginalized its distinction and position within society. Throughout the years, nursing like many other struggling professions, has tried to emulate those characteristics thought to be indicative of occupations deemed professions of longer standing by society, such as medicine and law [3]. This effort to emulate other professions has been viewed by some nursing scholars as taking on the persona of the oppressor but could also be interpreted as a strategic move of cultural survival through acquisition of a fictive kin categorization, which would allow for status within the community (in this case the professional community) from which to relate, and otherwise communicate and

© Springer Nature Switzerland AG 2019
E. West, *Frontier Nursing in Appalachia: History, Organization and the Changing Culture of Care*, https://doi.org/10.1007/978-3-030-20027-5_4

interact or, in other words, belong [4]. The discipline of nursing has been hampered by the schisms that persist within its own discipline. The debate continues to rage between rank and file nurses and nursing leaders surrounding issues of professionalism versus unionism but the truth is that despite its goals and tactics unions and professional associations alike respond to market changes in much the same way [5]. A dichotomy also exists regarding what value (if any) should be placed on the concepts of compassion and care (people focus often attributed to females) when the virtues of intellect and technological skill mastery (object focus often attributed to males) are so obviously more highly valued by society.

Manifestation of the existing ambivalence within the profession on the complex issues surrounding what nursing requires, who nurses are and even what the definition of nursing really is has been most noticeable in the recent surge in literature aimed at 'debunking' the supposed 'Nightingalism,' which purportedly not only exists but is 'holding professional advancement back.' Some opinions of the influence of Nightingale are so strong as to suggest that due to the 'crisis' in nursing it is time to 'retire Nightingale as a symbol' [6]. One historical analysis seeking to determine the power utilized by Nightingale concluded that though she did demonstrate the leadership required to achieve major reforms she was 'not able to empower other nurses and this continues to have a lasting impact on nursing's development' [7]. Other nurses doubt how a woman who was decidedly nursing's first theorist, researcher, statistician, administrator, educator, visionary and nursing's first public image as well as patient care reformer could possibly be considered to have 'not been able to empower other nurses' [8].

Breckinridge was a staunch admirer of Nightingale and embraced many of her philosophies. She emulated Nightingale's commitment to research and kept excellent records that later proved invaluable for many and varied research and scholarly works pertaining to epidemiology, sociology, nursing, public health, midwifery, obstetrics, paediatrics, gerontology and statistics. Breckinridge sponsored a research project to send two nurses out to the Ozark Mountains to see if her organizational model could be duplicated in this area, which was one that most closely resembled that of Appalachia. Unfortunately, the Depression struck, and as there were no funds, the project was abandoned in its infancy and was never resumed.[1] The FNS also did its share of research in the local community. Of the largest, lengthiest and most well-known was the ENOVID birth control study from 1959 to 1967 whereby the efficacy and possible side effects of ENOVID (oral contraceptives) were first done in the US. Breast cancer research was also done from 1961 to 1965.

Former FNS physicians ruminating on Breckinridge's motives seemed mystified by her decision to allow the first birth control trials to be done in her districts as they essentially obliterated the amount of 'business' being done by the midwives by severely curtailing the number of births being attended by FNS Nurse-

---

[1] FNS Summary of Executive Committee Minutes 1925–1935. 85M1: FNS, Box 2, Fol. 1. Includes resolution made on 10 March 1928 to invite the Dr. and Mrs. MacKenzie to the FNS and Breckinridge's request for time off due to 'exhaustion', 14 November 1930. University of Kentucky in Lexington, USA.

Midwives.[2] This decision also had an adverse effect on the education of FNS student nurse-midwives as the number of deliveries dropped dramatically. One researcher suggested that the reason Breckinridge permitted the ENOVID birth control study, which spanned the years 1959–1967, was due to the longstanding friendship that Breckinridge had with Doctor Roc; that she was 'captivated by his charm' and not a crusader of family planning at all [9]. The idea that Breckinridge was a woman who could be swayed to make such a monumental decision concerning not only her organization but the community based upon something as superficial as 'charm,' and a physician's charm at that, makes no sense whatever based on what we know of her character. Breckinridge may not have been an 'activist' in any modern sense of the word, her upbringing, social class and absolute dedication to the FNS precluded it; she certainly saw the condition of these women as evidenced by her dealings with them and writings about them and her Service. She realized the value that birth control could provide to their quality of life as well as the quality of life of their families and community as a whole in the face of such grinding poverty. After the trials were completed, one of the first family planning programs began in Eastern Kentucky via the FNS in 1964. Yet, by 1966, Breckinridge's successor noted at a staff meeting that though people 'on the outside' were very interested in their Family Planning Program, she felt it had been going on long enough now and that the district nurses should sit down and talk with the families about having another child. She didn't want them (the people) to forget that they could stop the pill or have the IUD removed if they would like to have another baby. She also stipulated that this education should be done by the district nurse and not left to the family planning clinic.[3] Perhaps by this time, Breckinridge's statement at the organization's inception that the ultimate goal was to 'surpass itself' proved to be more prophetic than she had originally intended.

Breckinridge and Nightingale were both a product of their appointed times in history. Breckinridge appreciated Nightingale's zeal to change and improve health care and nursing by using the means that were at her disposal and did the same. Breckinridge, like Nightingale, often found herself at odds with those in power within the existing establishments that were often part of the problem as a result of her efforts. A former FNS physician said of Breckinridge, 'she was really not behind in her theory, just in some of the other things going on (culturally) but she was so far ahead in her conception'.[4] One nurse put it most succinctly when she wrote, 'the legend of the lady with the lamp may have been debunked, but Florence Nightingale's zeal is needed to pull the National Health Service (NHS) out of a crisis' [10]. Much the same can also be said of the current

---

[2] Interview #82OH05FNS148, 1982, Dr. Mary Weiss (former FNS Medical Director) & Dr. Pauline Fox (former County Health Officer/Appalachia Regional Health Officer), Interviewed 14 February 1979. Interviewer: Dale Deaton.

[3] 85M1: FNS, Box 70, Fol. 9. 'FNS Staff Meeting Minutes, 30 September 1965', University of Kentucky in Lexington, USA.

[4] Interview #82OH05FNS148, 1982, Dr. Mary Weiss (former FNS Medical Director) & Dr. Pauline Fox (former County Health Officer/Appalachia Regional Health Officer).

American Health Care System. Visionaries like Nightingale and Breckinridge saw reciprocal benefits for all as a result of their efforts and endeavored to change the organizational and wider-environment's culture when they failed to meet this expectation.

4.2   Managers, Leaders and Visionaries: Strong Versus Weak Cultures

Florence Nightingale, whom Breckinridge greatly admired, was, like Breckinridge, a founder and leader. Both of these women made remarkable achievements in the advancement of nursing as a profession against very powerful forces within the established medical, hospital, military and governmental institutions of their day. Nightingale brought nursing out of the dark ages, garnered for it the respect it deserved as a profession and greatly improved patient care practices in the process. Breckinridge brought the concept of Nurse-Midwifery to the US, established its first professional body and also brought a unique blend of district, public health and midwifery nursing to rural Eastern Appalachia and many third world countries as well. Both Nightingale and Breckinridge were revered by nurses and the general public throughout history as a result of their individual leadership capabilities and styles in much the same way as leaders have in other disciplines. Perhaps it was inevitable then, that they would also eventually have their reputations challenged and in many cases unfairly besmirched by those outside of nursing who have neglected to consider their epoch in history when examining them and their achievements and who had neither the talent nor the tenacity to accomplish nearly as much. What astounds was that these women should also be accused by those within the discipline of nursing, by nurse scholars and leaders as having in some way harmed the discipline. Perhaps this phenomenon should not be surprising considering that the majority of nursing's leaders are within institutional settings of one sort or another, where they are very rarely founders or leaders but rather managers of the institutional establishment or status quo. This condition can create a phenomenon called 'groupthink,' which was a term coined by social psychologist Irving Janis and was said to occur when a group made faulty decisions because group pressures lead to a deterioration of "mental efficiency, reality testing, and moral judgment." Groups affected by groupthink tend to ignore alternatives and take irrational actions that *dehumanize* [italics added] other groups [11]. This phenomenon described not only what occurred within health care institutions but also what transpired within the FNS in its latter years, as it struggled to maintain its early years' values, beliefs and cultural identity within a decidedly 'corporate' culture shift from its 'philanthropic' roots. Managers are concerned with the problem at hand; they focus on what has to be done. Leaders on the other hand, notice what has to be done, but spend their time figuring out how to get it done. Breckinridge illustrated this point of leadership when she encountered governmental bureaucracy in getting her Nurse-Midwives into the US. Two former

British FNS Nurse-Midwives stated that they had more difficulty with 'immigration' than they had with the FNS when they came. Both of them recalled having to send references. One of them recalled filling out an application form and certainly having a 'medical, rudimentary though it was' prior to joining the FNS. She had received literature on the FNS from a Matron at the British Hospital for Mothers and Babies when she expressed to her the desire to 'travel before she reached the age of 30'.[5] She was sent $200 from the FNS for her fare by sea and rail from New York to Lexington, Kentucky, changing trains in Washington DC. She was met in New York by an organization called 'Travellers Aid' who then got her to the railroad station. Before leaving Britain, she had to visit the US Embassy in London, where she was finger printed and interviewed, before being granted a visa to enter the US. She also remembered having to have a Small Pox vaccination. She recollected that at the time she came, 1955, Kentucky did not recognise UK qualifications (i.e., SRB and SCM) but the state of Arkansas did. She explained:

> So we Brits were registered to practice in the latter, but "got in" to the Kentucky registration system via Arkansas. I did have to take a midwifery exam, the same one that the students I had been teaching (prior to coming to the US) were taking!! Thankfully I did pass!!! (see footnote 5)

Breckinridge, a divorced, widowed socialite and bereaved mother of her only two children was not the typical student nurse, nurse practitioner or philanthropist of her day. Breckinridge's philanthropic contemporaries as well as benevolent humanitarians today rarely, if ever, lived in the same manner as their employees or the local community they sought to assist. The most they were expected to contribute was a sizable personal check or perhaps a substantial amount of money they were able to raise for their cause [12]. Breckinridge's Service was at its prime when its volunteer director was in her mid-fifties and sixties, an age when most are looking to retire. She brought a wealth of more than just currency into the hills. She brought a culture that viewed both personal and professional experience as a precious asset rather than a liability. She also understood exactly what was needed for both her midwifery school and practice environment because she had been a student nurse, she researched the needs of the community and she had actually done the work that she was asking her nurses to do.

Breckinridge grasped the essential facts and underlying forces that determined the needs of the community and her nurses. Unfortunately, she did not anticipate trends in the *business* of medicine and the magnitude of the government's future involvement. She also did not foresee the coming health care *industry*, added costs therein created by the companies that would rise and become a part of the existing establishment; nor the multitude of technological, pharmacological and biological breakthroughs sufficiently enough to generate a vision and strategy that would bring her organization into the future with its people-focus intact. Indeed, based upon the circumstances surrounding and engulfing the FNS in its latter years it is reasonable to assume that no one could have done so. The regional control (generalized power structure) the Service had had since the organization's inception was handed over

---

[5] Margaret (Maggie) Willson, British former FNS Nurse-Midwife (1955–1967).

to the federal government (centralized power structure). Centralized power structures tend to foster coping, planning, budgeting, organizing and controlling effective action while discouraging the promotion of sustained, positive change through realistic and exhaustive analysis of surroundings coupled with appropriate direction setting. Institutional power structures also tend to discourage the alignment, motivation and inspiration of people toward meaningful action choosing instead to adopt a truth from others and then implement it without probing for the facts that reveal underlying realities [13]. Perhaps long time Breckinridge secretary, Agnes Lewis summed up the difference between managers and leaders best when she said the following in answer to the question, 'what kept people in (FNS) service?'

> Dedication to the work in the beginning. Dedication to both the work and the woman in later years.[6]

Leaders, not managers earn this type of dedication. Breckinridge inspired this dedication in her staff by giving her best and by 'somehow having a command over everybody in the room and the place, even when she was not in the room!' These statements were made about her when she was 90 years of age by a graduate of the school of midwifery.[7]

A former long-time FNS secretary called her employer a 'Renaissance woman, able in so many directions' and in whose company one could not be long before *'developing a social conscience'* [Italics added].[8] Long time FNS nurses also said that all 'respected' her even if some 'liked' her better than others.[9] An FNS nurse who had been with the Service for many years said, 'I didn't have the devotion to her that some people had for her, *she didn't want it really* [Italics added] but you never gave her second best because she always gave it her best (see footnote 8). It was also said of Breckinridge that her 'main interest was not in "training" but rather "guiding and stimulating" people who could follow her and in whose judgement she would have confidence'.[10] These are all hallmark traits of a leader and these traits not only garnered the respect and loyalty of her staff but also the community her organization served for so many years. Locals, even when prodded by over-zealous researchers to say the contrary, ultimately said of FNS's founder that though she may not agree with you, she was always interested in what everybody's ideas were, which she would then 'take back and get off to herself and think over' prior to making any decisions.[11]

---

[6] Interview #82OH03FNS146, 1982, Agnes Lewis, former long-time FNS Secretary.

[7] Interview #78OH148FNS08 1978, Martha Lady, FNS Midwifery School Graduate of 1960.

[8] Interview#82OH11FNS154, 1982. Wilma Duvall Whittlesey, FNS Secretary from 1929–1936.

[9] Interview #82OH12FNS155, 1982, Betty Lester, former long-time FNS Nurse.

[10] Interview #78OH147FNS07, 1978. Frank Bowling, long-time resident of Appalachia/Community Committee Member.

[11] Reprint from Midwives Chronicle 1965 (p. 471). 200547M: FNS, Box 203, Fol. 1. 'Are We Needed? by Helen E. Browne', from Midwives Chronicle, the Official Journal of the Royal College of Midwives, Autumn.

Breckinridge's successor due to the series of social, political and economic circumstances that converged upon Eastern Appalachia in the Service's latter years
was reduced to the role of 'manager' to the federal government's presumed role
of 'leader' and this role was by proxy. Where Breckinridge's leadership was about
innovating an initiating in its early years, her successor finished her tenure at the
FNS by managing the institutional government's status quo. Indeed, in the late 1960s
when Breckinridge's successor asked the people if they wanted the Service to continue and was given an affirmative answer, she was hoping to help the people adjust
to the 'new' while maintaining what was best about the 'old,' namely the people's
'family solidarity.' She also hoped to maintain high standards and broaden education programs to be of help to people of the area, nation and the world. After all,
foreign countries were still coming into the area to observe the FNS [8]. She could
not have anticipated the speed at which these changes would occur, the degree of
change that would be required of the Service as a direct result of them nor the overall
affect these changes would have on the Service and the community. She had not been
Breckinridge's first nor second choice as her successor. Breckinridge had outlived
them both and Browne, though certainly as good an administrator as was possible
amidst such crushing change did not possess the vision or the relational standing
within the local and non-local committees to lead effectively (see footnote 7).

Sanborn [14] suggested leadership was all about taking an organization to a
place it would not have otherwise gone without you, in a value-adding, measur-
able way [14]. When you 'vision,' you think your way into a situation and it is the
approach in visioning that separates managers from leaders. Breckinridge's style of
administration was singular in that it was based on a human process at a time when
the national move was toward the business model. The business model focused on
management, which in essence was a process of resource allocation. Indeed, every
business model cites the necessity of a 'results-oriented culture' in building a 'spirit
of high performance into an organization' [15]. The different strategies used by
managers and leaders in terms of their use of human resources can also differentiate
for us the major factors that influence each position. Managers are required to monitor, supervise, and get tasks done in a certain amount of time. Managers must be
efficient, and thus time is the most important human resource for them. By improving their efficiency, managers can improve their managerial success. Leaders, on
the other hand, must strategically use not only their time, but energy as well. Thus,
leaders should use their energy efficiently because there is only a certain number of
tasks that can be done in 1 day. By using these resources strategically, leaders can
also efficiently use the time and energy of others. Sanborn stated, "Managers try to
put more time into life, whereas leaders try to put more life into their time" [16].
Breckinridge lived by the latter of these two values and her 'early nurses' held them
as well. A British former FNS nurse said, "…and that's the thing I value, is the work
people have put into life".[12]

Leaders must carefully plan out strategies they will use to accomplish given tasks
because strategy is not the consequence of planning, but the opposite—its starting

---

[12] Molly Lee, British former FNS Nurse-Midwife (1950–1970s).

point. Managers and leaders have different strategic approaches in utilizing their human resources. It is the approach that separates the one from the other. It is evident that by 'visioning' the appropriate outcome and by using human resources purposefully, goals can be met efficiently as well. As mentioned earlier, time is the most valuable resource for managers because they must be efficient, therefore it is can be said that the managers are focused on time. The prime focus in a managerial position is the speed at which tasks are completed. Leaders conversely are and should be more focused on being effective, that is their intentions are on doing the right thing. Managerial power is positional power; it is power *over* people whereas leadership is supportive power, and it is power *with* people.

Breckinridge, though obviously a manager was also able to distinguish herself and her organization by being more than that. Breckinridge was something that was not common within organizations either then or now. The distinction within organizations between leaders and managers are key to understanding 'weak' and 'strong' organizational cultures. The managerial approach attempts to impose upon its organization's members the philosophy, values, beliefs and norms of the institutional culture whereas leaders elicit these essentials from their members voluntarily. The former method relies upon systems, controls, procedures, policies, and structure, whereas the latter relies upon trust and people [17]. Both Breckinridge and Nightingale possessed and demonstrated evidence of leadership, understanding and wisdom. What is more, they were both visionaries as well. These are traits necessary for strong organizational cultures. They are also traits that are lacking in centralized, institutionalized power structures.

Organizational culture is a system of shared meaning and beliefs held by members that determine, in large degree, how they act. They represent a common perception held by the organization's members. The more employees accept the organization's key values and the greater their commitment to those values, the stronger the culture tends to be [18].

Strong cultures in which the key values are deeply held and widely shared have a greater influence on employees than do weak cultures. Further, there are some basic traits within a culture that can be learned: stories/history; rituals; material symbols and language [19]. For the FNS, these core values and cultural traits within the organization were also intricately entwined with that of its founder. Breckinridge formulated only two goals for the organization: improving the health of children and pioneering a system of rural healthcare that could serve as a model for healthcare systems serving the most remote regions of the world. Both of these goals were highly successful as long as she was director of the Service, which essentially was as long as she lived. The unique community she served, the staff, students and nurses she recruited the people who supported her financially outside of Appalachia also held the same values as the organization's founder. Thus, there was an alignment to the organizational values of the Service. This was demonstrated in the language used by the local people, former FNS staff, nurses and students embedded within their oral history narratives to describe the organization and its work. Language which, for the nurses included descriptors such as, 'freedom, camaraderie, and 'thrilling', 'stimulating,' 'adventurous' and 'the people,' to illustrate what was best about working at the Service. A British former FNS nurse interviewed went as far as to say, "… a lot of freedom, we had. I'm so glad I lived when I did and not when you live. I wouldn't be you for two big apples" (see footnote 12).

Strong cultures are said to exist where staff respond to stimuli because of their alignment to organizational values. Where cultures are strong, people do things because they believe it is the right thing to do [20]. This was certainly true of FNS nurses in the organization's early years, who often went without sleep, worked with far less equipment and supplies; and never achieved the salaries that nurses garnered outside of Appalachia. It was remarkable that all of these nurses also either inferred or stated outright that they received far greater non-tangible rewards while working at the FNS than they ever did when they were working set hours, had proper equipment, supplies and support personnel; and good salaries within institutional settings elsewhere. Feeling that they made a huge, positive impact on the health of the community and had the respect of those they worked with and served. These features together with their professional autonomy were consistently rated higher than having sufficient institutional equipment, supplies or support personnel, salary or even personal comfort. It is perhaps more remarkable that all of these values, both tangible and intangible, persist in the discourse of nurses in practice settings today. "Salary, staffing, autonomy and respect remain key issues with the understanding that nursing has achieved much by way of the more tangible rewards, while either not having or in some cases losing those less tangible rewards, such as autonomy, respect and professional 'stimulation,' stating instead that they feel like 'factory' workers or little girls in pyjama-like scrubs and pony tails."[13] The descriptions expressed by nurses to explain the change at the FNS in its latter years mirror those made by nurses in practice today.[14] They too equate the change at the FNS as being similar to the environments they worked in outside of Appalachia as early as the 1940s and refer to the 'priority' given to 'paper work.' Words used to illustrate the change included, 'business,' or 'corporate' culture; over-regulation; a focus on 'the bottom line' and the prioritization of the paperwork it generated, which created a "factory-like experience" that proved detrimental to quality patient care [21].

The characteristics of a weak culture are many subcultures, few strong traditions, few values and beliefs widely shared by all employees and no strong sense of company identity [22]. The death of Mary Breckinridge in the early 1960s and influx of governmental programs such as Medicare and Medicaid are cited by both the local and FNS staff as the 'breaking point of the old and the new' in Appalachia as well as at the Service. Loss of autonomy occurred for the local people when they became dependent on the welfare system. It occurred for the nurses with the

---

[13] Richard, Hospital emergency room staff nurse for 5 years; home health nurse for 4 years. Date surveyed: 31/12/2004; Loan, MS, Hospital operating room staff nurse for 2.5 years, research 5 years. Date surveyed: 21/01/2005; Morrison, S., Hospital staff nurse for 1 year, critical care for 10 years, pain management for 13 years. Date surveyed: 17/06/2005; Slamp, L., Hospital staff nurse for 2.75 years. Date surveyed: 08/10/2005; Ann, J., Hospital oncology nurse <1 year. Date surveyed: 05/09/2006; Scarfe, B., Hospital staff nurse for 6 years, critical care 2 years. Date surveyed: 9/10/2006.

[14] Jean Corner-Rowan, British former FNS Nurse-Midwife (1964–1966).

advent of government monies coming in that were also tied with the hierarchical institutional set-up that was the norm outside of Appalachia. This social hierarchy had vastly differing values to that of the FNS and a much more bureaucratic system of health care delivery.

A former British FNS nurse stated, "I found it a little strange at first expecting to collect money for fees, you know, annual fee, which was little enough, and to know that they have to pay. I remember feeling awkward about charging for things, because… people did have to pay".[15] The 'bottom line,' which for so many years at the FNS, a philanthropy, focused solely on community care 'from cradle to grave' for the *people*, now had to centre on functioning within the business model, where the focus was on *things;* such as technology, tasks and efficiency as measured by time and cost management. As a direct result of these changes, the FNS had to meet more stringent criteria regarding its personnel as well as its provision of health care. A long time British former FNS nurse mused, "… later on, they (the FNS) had all these people with expensive degrees and that's your problem, you see… learn too much." An American former FNS nurse who was at the Service in its latter years admitted to "rivalry" between the British and American nurses developing that mainly focused on level of education. This was something that was not evident in the Service's early years between the American and British nurses. With the advent of these more highly educated nurses came the expectation of a higher salary, more structured working hours and better working conditions. This created a gulf between the 'older' and 'younger' staff that had little to do with 'age' and much more to do with a fundamental value shift in American society and the value orientation of these nurses within the culture (see footnote 12). It also created schisms within the Service between departments that had never existed before. The people bond upon which fidelity and loyalty was anchored had been replaced with something far less personal and much more commercial. One nurse recounted that, "We got called for (the midwives)… midwives were the only solid basic people, because some of us stayed a long time." However, later in her discourse, she bitterly recounted that in the Service's latter years, the local people no longer wanted home deliveries but wanted deliveries back in the hospital. "Can you believe that, after all Mrs. Breckinridge's efforts on (behalf) of mothers and babies they wiped out the midwives".[16]

4.3   The Institutionalization of Childbirth

By 1950 heart disease, cancer and stroke became much more prominent causes of death as most Western nations experienced a substantial decrease in acute infectious diseases and life expectancy increased.[17] In Western Europe, the United States and other developed countries political pressure increased to ensure that individuals

---

[15] Elizabeth 'Hilly' Hillman, British former FNS Nurse-Midwife (1949–1954).

[16] Anne Lorentzen, American former FNS Nurse (1963–1965).

[17] Guthrie D. A history of medicine (Bibliolife DBA of Bibilio Bazaar II LLC, Aug 8, 2015).

had access to medical treatment and care. Hospitals became the points of care and research [23]. Maternal mortality was in the region of 5% per one thousand total births and women began to feel that they might have a better chance of survival in the hospital. It should also be noted that from 1951 to 1965, FNS Nurse-Midwives attended 6325 maternal cases without losing a single mother. In addition, since 1934 there have been one third less stillbirths and one third less infant deaths within 1 month of birth than was occurring in the general population of Kentucky through the work of the Service.[18] Cultural attitudes however, were changing at this time and it was only later that the psychological drawback of separation from family supports, which occurs with institutionalised births, was fully realized [24].

The political gains made by nursing in both America and Great Britain were intricately linked with those empowered from without the discipline and were more often than not contingent upon their endorsement to succeed. This was due primarily to the similar political, socio-cultural and economic hardships that existed for women prior to and well after they secured the right to vote, the ever-widening schisms within nursing ranks regarding ideas on hospital versus community-based education practices and issues relating to elitist ideology versus the rank and file nurse on what type of woman should even be a nurse [25]. It is worth noting that the position of the British Nurse-Midwife was the one exception in that it built a profession with potential and status long before nursing was able to do so because it had established itself long before the golden age of medicine helped to establish physicians. The inherent independence associated with midwifery in its public health role within the community was also an asset as was the fact that the first Midwives Act in 1902 secured a statute that ensured that eventually the original aim of the midwives' institute would be fulfilled, that is, that all women in Britain were entitled to the service of a well-trained corps of midwives. In the US, where there was often no opportunity to bend the ear of men in power, or to fight the rising tide of power and influence on the part of doctors, the role of the midwife was relegated to that of handmaiden status, where it still struggles to free itself even today. Though rivalry existed for centuries between physicians and midwives in Great Britain due to the parallels between the subordinate role of an all-female profession and the position of women in society, a power-base already existed prior to medicine's rise [26].

British Nurse-Midwives had an independent practice, which initially included acceptance of fee for service from their clients. A strong precedent already existed in Britain whereby midwives were recognized as practitioners of normal childbirth and doctors were only called to labours with complications. However, in the US, gaining the trust of the more rural public proved difficult for midwives and 'Handywomen' who tended to be older and known to all in the community were often more highly regarded than the certified midwife, who was likely to be young, middle-class and wearing a uniform. Prevailing folk remedies included the use of cow dung to treat a breast abscess and the overall feeling within the rural com-

---

[18] 'FNS, The First Forty Years', 1925–1965. 85M1: FNS, Box 29, Fol. 29. Mary Breckinridge, University of Kentucky in Lexington, USA.

munities was that experience meant more than training. This cultural aspect also existed in the Appalachia's where 'granny women' utilized the local remedy for haemorrhage, which was placement of an axe, blade side up, beneath the bed of the afflicted woman [27]. Unfortunately, it was not long before the shift from home births to antenatal clinics and hospitals created a turning point for Nurse-Midwives in the US as doctors took over much of their practice. One nurse lamented that the biggest problem facing midwifery was in convincing modern doctors that they were not 'rivals' and wanted to work with them, and by that she meant:

> Give them their time and skills and training to take care of the high-risk patients and let us do the normal ones. I think we could do an awful lot in helping doctors in the teaching of patients too.[19]

When asked the biggest opposition that midwives had in America this midwife answered, 'doctors.' The changing cultural climate in which it was thought a mother had a better chance of survival in hospital also created changes in the existing nursing regulatory boards and the British Nurse Midwife, once quite independent in her practice, now also began finding herself hampered by the institutionalization of childbirth.

The national standards had increased by 1938 and required 1 full year of supervision for trained nurses and 2 years for the untrained. The number of Central Midwives Board training failures was also high this year.[20] The midwifery revisions of the Central Midwives Board in 1947 presented the following conclusions to all training authorities after reviewing the available syllabi for midwifery training, 'subjects which include the symptoms and signs of cancer of the breast and womb and the part a midwife can play in persuading women to seek advice early when suspicion is aroused cannot be properly regarded as an integral part of a course of training in midwifery and should be deleted'.[21] The Board also advised that to attend clinical demonstration on venereal diseases and to receive instruction in the prevention and treatment of opthalmia neonatorum frequently involved pupil-midwives in long absences from the wards, with results that time available for practical instruction, witnessing and delivery of cases being further reduced. Attendance at demonstrations was therefore to be deleted. They also suggested the second exam be mainly oral, clinical and practical. Also set forth by the new rules was that if a hospital was approved as a midwifery training school, then the assistant nurses would be replaced by pupil-midwives.[22] Though this would certainly be an incentive to hospitals, as it would benefit them financially, it could hardly be thought to improve the midwife's educational environment. Most of the increases in tutorial classes

---

[19] Interview #78OH148FNS08 1978. Martha Lady.

[20] QNI Report 1938. Nursing Student Records 1920–1950. Queen's Nursing Institute, Surviving Student Records Spanning the Years 1920–1950. Royal College of Nursing Archives in Edinburgh, UK.

[21] QNI Report 1938, (Nursing Student Records 1920–1950), p. 9.

[22] Written Correspondence from the Central Midwifery Board to Queen Charlotte's Maternity Hospital 1938. QNI Reports for the Years 1920–1946. Queen's Nursing Institute Annual Reports to the Executive Committee. Royal College of Nursing Archives in Edinburgh, UK.

were scheduled to fit in with the pupil-midwife's off duty hours as the ward work 'fully occupied their working hours.' Comments by physicians who were sent to facilities to evaluate the 'new' midwifery scheme pointed out that the 'question of continuity of care was raised with the frequent absences of midwives from the ward, from the medical standpoint, as they are essential for Obstetric doctors to rely on in noting changes in the patient's condition or progress of labour' when students were off the floor for classes. One physician wrote:

> "It is apparent at this hospital that training of pupil-midwives suffers from the fact that it occupies a less important place in the day's routine than hours off duty and on no account must it be allowed to interfere with the latter." He goes on to note that the hospital in question is "understaffed and only has two sisters on day duty."[23]

FNS Nurse-Midwives attempting to go back to train for new certifications or advanced degrees that were coming into vogue in the Service's latter years often found themselves hampered by too much experience or just not being particularly 'academically minded' enough to do well on the certification exams. One nurse stated that she had gone back to England via a scholarship from the FNS to study for the midwife teaching diploma, which at the time was a 6-month residential course. She passed all of the course work and came back to be the Dean of the Midwifery Graduate School at the FNS though she never did 'qualify' via licensure because, 'I get into a twit over taking examinations' (see Footnote 5).

Another FNS nurse who also was sent to Great Britain for a teaching certification experienced a similar problem and though she did finally pass the certification exam, had to take it more than once. This particular nurse suffered the humiliation of being demoted to that of 'assistant' to a nurse whom she taught in the midwifery school toward the end of her tenure at the FNS. She stated, 'my pupil, or student that I'd helped get her midwifery, she was accepted as a midwife. Did she deliver babies? I don't think she did. She was an Obstetrical Nurse and I was only a... I've forgotten what I was, but it was quite a joke really' (see footnote 12). The student apparently held the degree requirement that was deemed necessary to teach and be an administrator of a school of nursing in the US. This nurse explained her reasons for finally leaving the FNS:

> My time was up because things had changed and I didn't have the freedom. But you know there were two young doctors there and one of them didn't know very much midwifery and we actually taught medical students. Nurses always do, don't they?... Wherever they are.

In the mid-1960s the costs of delivery for patients in labour were only reimbursed if they saw a physician, not a nurse-midwife. Deliveries outside of a hospital setting were excluded from coverage thus ensuring that most women would have to give birth at hospitals rather than at home [28]. Both lay midwives as well as certified nurse-midwives have experienced pressure from legislative bodies seeking to limit or control midwifery. In addition, powerful lobbies such as the American Medical Association have attempted to influence legislatures to bar the practice. Certified nurse-midwives have been denied privileges at hospitals and obstetricians who

---

[23]Written Correspondence to the Central Midwifery Board 1942, QNI Reports for the Years 1920–1946.

wanted to partner with them have found that to do so would put them at risk of having their malpractice insurance cancelled. In one high profile case, where a group of certified nurse midwives sued an insurance company in Tennessee, it was found that the company which controlled more than 80% of the State's malpractice insurance market was owned and operated by physicians [29]. In contrast, Kentucky remains one of the few states in which nurse-midwifery has been recognized as a valuable part of the health-care delivery system. This reality was due in large part to the political, economic and social network that was forged by Mary Breckinridge long before the institutionalization of health care penetrated and transformed care delivery there.

Hospitals, and physicians in particular, have always had a keen interest in how nurses practice and have introduced statutes and provisions that prohibit medical diagnosis and treatment by nurses, including prescription and dispensing of medications, which hinder nursing's efforts to be recognized for services independent of medicine and to implement the full scope of nursing practice. Though these regulations certainly existed for FNS nurses, one of the functions of the FNS's 'medical advisory council' was to create a 'medical directives' book for the nurses to use with standing orders, which included treatments and medications that the nurses consulted so that physicians were not called upon unless there was a complication, emergency or consultation needed by the nurse, which warranted it. The directives were updated continually and nurses were given in-service training on any new treatment regimes. When the incoming system challenged this system, FNS physicians and nurses responded by partnering to create one of the first certificate programs to prepare family nurse practitioners (FNP), which for all intents and purposes was a nurse specifically trained and certified to do the work that had always been done at the FNS, namely: district nursing, home health nursing and midwifery (In 1970, the name of the School was changed to the Frontier School of Midwifery and Family Nursing (FSMFN) to reflect this addition of the FNP program). This collaboration was done at a time when physicians outside of the FNS vehemently opposed the nurses' role being 'expanded' in this way, opting to support the formation of Physician Assistants instead.[24]

4.4   The 1960s: 'War on Poverty' or Corporate Colonization?

In the 30, September 1965 FNS Staff Meeting Minutes the language used to describe the incoming Peace Corps Volunteers and US Public Health Service team was 'invasion.' The FNS was told the Volunteers in Service to America (VISTA) workers would 'help at the district' (outposts). The US Public Health Service was to send a

---

[24] W.B. Beasley Letter to K.L. White at Johns Hopkins University, 14 April 1966. 2005M547: FNS, Box 227, Fol. 9. 'W.B. Beasley Letter to K.L. White at Johns Hopkins University, 14 April 1966.' This folder also contained a letter from Dr. Robert R. Huntley at the University of North Carolina dated, 26 April 1966 and a letter from Dr. Kurt W. Deuschle at the University of Kentucky dated, 16, May 1966 also vehemently opposing support of developing a Nurse Practitioner Program. University of Kentucky in Lexington, USA.

team of two full time doctors, five nurses, assorted health educators, sanitation and social workers and a psychosocial worker. Specialists were to hold clinics at the closest city, Hyden. The FNS recorded at the meeting that they were told, "until the team got started it would not know how the FNS was to fit into this program."[25] It quickly became apparent that the intention was never for the incoming volunteers and government workers to 'fit into' the existing decentralized power structure but rather for the FNS to 'fit into' the centralized power structure that was the norm outside of the region. Outsiders used the well-established 'place' status of the FNS within the Appalachian culture while disenfranchising the Service at the same time.

The FNS staff meeting minutes for August of 1965 was cautiously optimistic regarding the arrival of the federal government into the area stating, 'We must help the people of our area adjust to these programs in such a way that they may have a better way of life, and yet still keep the good things which are here, the greatest of which is their family solidarity.' The meeting minutes go on to say, almost as an afterthought, that any referrals made by the government workers would be made to the FNS and the local doctor first. At another staff meeting the minutes reflect the Service's belief that hosting these programs will put the FNS in the 'eyes of this country more than it has been ever before' and seemed enthusiastic that 'the Peace Corps, the US Public Health team and the Surgeon General are interested in the kind of nurse we provide here'.[26] However, the change coming was not to bring the FNS model of decentralized, generalized and personalized community based health care to the nation and the world but rather to bring the monolithic, ever-expanding, fragmented, institutionalised system of health care into Appalachia.

Perhaps what affected the Service in its latter years most, aside from the federal government driven changes was the erosion of the socio-political network that had worked so well for the FNS in the past. Prominent women of social standing on urban committees who had the social conscience of their mothers and grandmothers were much harder to find. One young woman from a wealthy family who worked for the FNS briefly said of Breckinridge:

> I hadn't any idea of doing anything more for the FNS and I didn't know much about it, but I immediately was put in touch with all these important people on the Pittsburgh Committee, which was wonderful for me socially.[27]

Social 'connections' with 'important people' were viewed as desirable but the work of the committee was admittedly viewed as secondary or perhaps only as the means necessary to achieving it. This woman stated that the committee consisted of 'younger' people and that the work it did was really 'not needed anymore.'

---

[25] FNS Staff Meeting Minutes, 30 September 1965, 85M1: FNS, Box 220, Fol. 9. 'FNS Staff Meeting Minutes (1965–1966)', Including 18 March 1965, 30 September 1965, 1 September 1966, 20 January 1966. University of Kentucky in Lexington, USA.

[26] FNS Staff Meeting Minutes, 30 January 1966, 85M1: FNS, Box 220, Fol. 9. 'FNS Staff Meeting Minutes (1965–1966)'.

[27] Interview #79OH229FNS121, 1982, Mary Martin & Phoebe Hawkins, former FNS Committee Members outside of Appalachia in the Service's 'latter years', Interviewed 23 May 1979. Interviewer: Anne Campbell Ritchie.

The political landscape had changed due in large part to the cultural shift from decentralized to more centralized power structures. Many of the FNS's improvements in its latter years were achieved via government, university and or business grants, all of which had 'strings' attached in some fashion in order to either procure or maintain them [30]. In the same way that the relationship between the organization and its wealthy patrons changed in the Service's latter years so did its relationship with the people. The local people used to donate time and volunteer labour to keep the nursing centres up and running in their areas but by the 1970s this was not being done anymore. When asked why, one resident stated that there was 'too much prosperity' and that all the government programs made the people 'sorry.' He also cited the fact that a lot of the land was now owned by the government.[28]

Daiski [31] in a Canadian study which examined the views of hospital staff nurses about their relationships with nursing colleagues and other health care professionals and their ideas for change concluded that change for the better needed to come from within the nursing profession [31]. Yet is this really possible if nurses become embedded within the establishment and embrace the values that are keeping sustained positive change from occurring? Within any organizational culture there are deeper elements that are unseen and not consciously identified in everyday interactions between its members. Additionally, these are the elements of culture which are often taboo to discuss inside the organization. Many of these 'unspoken rules' exist without the conscious knowledge of the membership. Those with sufficient experience to understand this level of organizational culture usually become acclimatized to its attributes over time, thus reinforcing the invisibility of their existence. Schein [32] called this paradoxical organizational behaviour. It explains why an organization can profess highly aesthetic and moral standards in its slogans, mission statement and other operational creeds while simultaneously displaying curiously opposing behaviour at the deepest level of the culture. Indeed, merely understanding culture at the deepest level may be insufficient to institute cultural change because the dynamics of interpersonal relationships (often under threatening conditions) are added to the dynamics of organizational culture while attempts are made to institute desired change [32].

A self proclaimed 'debutant' who hailed from Breckinridge's Cincinnati Committee and came out to the FNS in the 1951 as a courier, later becoming 'head' of this division in 1961, said of the organization "We hadn't played our game well enough," referring to the political savvy necessary to function within the incoming centralized power structure. She also attributed the FNS's decline to not having enough senior staff and 'too few chiefs to run the organization in the health care field of today'.[29] This statement stands in stark contrast to most of the rank-and-file nurses interviewed who were senior staff that left the Service who tended to see the problem as being too many chiefs with too many rules and regulations impinging on their practice autonomy.

---

[28] Interview #78OH147FNS07, 1978. Frank Bowling.

[29] Interview #82OH08FNS151, 1982, Kate Ireland, former FNS Courier (1951), Interviewed 1 November 1979. Interviewer: Dale Deaton.

A former US Senator, whose grandmother was Mrs. Thurston Ballard, a socially 'connected' and very active committee worker for the FNS outside of Appalachia, accused Breckinridge of 'wanting things as they were, resisting the move to jeeps, accepting Medicare/Medicaid and the building of a dam in the area,' all of which purportedly was viewed by the Senator as 'progress' despite the fact that the Buckhorn Dam, though providing some small measure of economic assistance by providing guides, fisherman and boat dock worker jobs for the locals, also obliterated an entire local community and cultural life, one in which the FNS had an outpost [33]. Yet it should also be noted that this was the same woman who was the first to bring electricity, indoor pluming and the telephone into the area. She had no objection to these for either her staff or the local people. She also brought the idea of wellness-focused community based care into Appalachia when the rest of the country was focusing on institutionalized, sick patient care and she brought it into an area that had no care at all. This was innovative. Indeed, the trend today has been to move back towards not only wellness care as a means to keeping the populace healthier longer but also back toward community-based health care delivery systems in order bring down the high cost of health care.

When examined from both an historical and cultural perspective one can see that the model Breckinridge brought into Appalachia was neither wholly 'Appalachian' nor 'national' and as such the organization was never fully able to satisfy the demands continually being made upon it to conform to either culture. From the organization's start, Breckinridge encountered resistance from the existing power structures when attempting to procure public funding for the development of her project. This was the reason it began as philanthropy. In a letter denying her state public funding (the tenor of which was both condescending and paternalistic) Breckinridge was told her project would be considered only when all other project applications had been evaluated with preference to be given to those applications viewed 'in the eyes of the committee' as being from a 'county.' This stipulation obviously excluded FNS since its plan was designed for geographic reasons, to span three counties.[30]

In the organization's latter years, when financial assistance was sought from the Federal Government the FNS was once again excluded because many of the programs that were being funded as 'new and innovative' by the government had been being done by the FNS for years, and as such could not be funded as new projects. An example of this was family planning which had been done through the FNS as a pilot project for the rest of the country in the late 1950s, long before it became an 'in' program elsewhere in the US. It didn't seem to matter that the reason it became an 'in' program was because of the trials done at FNS, no government money was forthcoming. Another example cited by Dr. Mary Weiss, former FNS Medical Director and Dr. Pauline Fox, a former Regional County Health Officer was when the University of Kentucky announced their conception of the parent being allowed to stay and help take care of the child on the hospital unit. They

---

[30] Letter to Mary Breckinridge from Courtnay Dinwiddle, 24 February 1923, Denial of public funds for FNS, Frontier Nursing Service 1789–1985, 'Mary Breckinridge Series: Correspondence 1925–1970', University of Kentucky in Lexington, USA.

stated, 'This made all kinds of national news and the FNS had been doing this since 1929'.[31] One physician blamed Breckinridge's successor, Helen E. Browne for "holding back progress" and "getting grief for trying to improve hospital care and upgrade equipment." This physician also blamed other medical people who came into the area and "should have pushed for change but did not" (see footnote 31). FNS physicians coming to the Service in its latter years also felt that Obstetrics and Nurse Midwifery were "favoured" over all else and blamed the "British nurses" for wanting to do things "the British way."

The idea of the spouse and children being allowed to stay and help during the birthing process that was being embraced by the rest of the nation in the 1980s had been done at the FNS since 1929. Still, in the end fathers were coming for the nurses in cars while the nurses still had horses as their primary means of transportation.[32] Perhaps the reluctance to move from horses to jeeps was due to the fact that many of the FNS's potential employees came into Eastern Appalachia looking for adventure and driving a jeep didn't have the same mystique as riding horseback in the Kentucky Mountains.[33] Breckinridge had traded on the unique environment for free medical care and personnel for many years.[34] She resisted those changes that would either adversely affect the recruitment and retention of staff or had the potential to harmfully affect the local people, believing that 'once the people are out of it you are lost.' When the question of what the people's needs are was no longer asked but rather what should be done for them it created dependency and Breckinridge felt strongly that people should be self-sufficient.[35]

Breckinridge was an equal opportunity diplomat. Though a staunch Democrat, many of her friends and political allies were Republicans as well as Democrats. She contacted Thurston Morton, a former Republican US Senator whose grandmother was a close friend of Breckinridge's and very active in FNS committee work outside of Appalachia, to secure at the US governments' expense, the moving of one of her existing clinic/outposts to higher ground when the state opted to construct the Buckhorn Damn. Though Breckinridge was asked to run for office by the Democratic Party, she declined citing the need to maintain political neutrality as being in the best interests of her organization. Morton said of Breckinridge that he envied her ability to move an audience and described her as 'poetic,' 'emotional' and as having the ability to bring an audience 'to tears'.[36]

A former FNS courier said that the FNS had continual financial problems partly because "… it could not explain its program to the government and foundations as they spoke a different 'language' than most health agencies," and as a result seldom

---

[31] Interview #82OH05FNS148, 1982, Dr. Mary Weiss & Dr. Pauline Fox.

[32] Interview #82OH08FNS151, 1982, Kate Ireland.

[33] Interview#82OH11FNS154, 1982. Wilma Duvall Whittlesey.

[34] FNS Spring Appeal 1942, 85M1: FNS, Box 29, Fol. 13.

[35] Interview#82OH37FNS180. Thurston Morton, former Senator & Grandson of Mrs. Thurston Ballard who was very active in FNS committee work outside of Appalachia, Interviewed 24 October 1978. Interviewer: Carol Crowe-Carraco.

[36] Interview#82OH37FNS180. Thurston Morton.

fitted into their funding requirements.[37] It was often the case that the service relied on philanthropy to offset the lack of financial support of the state or federal government in order to continue to provide service to the community as the people were not in a position to meet the financial demands created by technological advances, new treatment modalities and the ever-increasing government rules and regulations associated with their arrival. This eventually placed the FNS in the unenviable position of trying to meet the health care needs of the people through more and more outside financial help and manpower over which they had less and less control, while simultaneously trying to keep the care as culturally congruent as possible for the local people. Breckinridge's reluctance to accept government funding when it was offered in the 1960s was alleged as substantiation by one researcher of her development of a 'colonial' system 'from whence she wielded complete control' [34]. This proved to be a paradoxical interpretation of Breckinridge's motives when one considers that her encouragement of the Appalachian people to accept federal government help in the 1930s via Roosevelt's New Deal works projects had also been cited by researchers as a major cause for Appalachia's complete dependency on the US government and ensuing cultural ruination.

Breckinridge has been either credited or accused, depending on which side of the argument one is on, for having persuaded the locals to change their point of view regarding government assistance during the depression and to accept the help (see footnote 33). This helped to improve roads into the area and brought much needed jobs to the men who had lost them to industry and could no longer subsidise their family's subsistence-based farming lifestyle, which alone could not support them all adequately. The New Deal programs of the depression era were later thought to have hurt more than they helped Appalachia by starting the cycle of dependency by the local population upon the US government, which later ushered in the 'war on poverty' initiatives of the 1960s that completed the socio-economic destruction of the region. Questions began to arise regarding whether Breckinridge's organization was part of the problem instead of the solution it was thought to have been after her death.

Many scholars in recent years have attacked missionaries, mission schools and various organizations that have been accused of shoving their own values and tastes upon Appalachia and manoeuvring these people into accepting mainstream cultural values. These perspectives view cultural politics as a manifestation of basic American imperialism [35]. It could be argued that Breckinridge did not attempt to manoeuvre people into accepting all of the outside values coming into Appalachia but rather only those health or social services she felt could help meet the needs of the community. She had always expected some form of payment for services provided to the people, albeit cash or bartered goods or services though she realized the necessity for the New Deal programs in the short term in order to ensure the people's survival as did most people struggling through the great depression. Mining collapsed in the 1930s and the crisis of the depression shattered factory employment and mercantile trade so subsistence farming made a come-back at this time

---

[37] Interview#82OH34FNS177, 1982, Mary Stewart.

but because of the great economic maladjustments in Appalachia's major industries, particularly coal mining and agriculture, large numbers of people were able to qualify for welfare benefits and circumstances drew many Appalachian people into the welfare system [36]. This system undermined the Mountaineer's traditional independence and had corrupted Mountain politics. The New Deal policies of the 1930s ultimately did not improve rural persons' conditions unless they owned a lot of land. The plan was market-oriented and domestic allotment focused, which proved to be a very impersonal solution for the small family farm problem. This left rural Americans dependent on outside forces (such as the Farm Bloc, National Farm Bureau Federation and various state Agricultural Colleges) and governmental policies [37]. The result was that powerful new county political machines were built throughout the region that based much of their power upon the control of welfare.

Political success in Appalachia depended upon how well a candidate manipulated the language and images of family, God, country and community that are important to the culture, regardless of the incumbent's personal ideology or particular party affiliation. In the four decades surrounding the turn of the twentieth century, control of mountain resources has been transferred to the industrial elite and the legal and political authority shifted from traditional leadership to a corporate representative who significantly altered the methods of political communication but only subtly changed the message [38]. Exploitation of coal and timber required mines, mills and company towns to be located near water sources and the resources themselves but often the towns were further planned for corporate goals, which sometimes included dividing racial and ethnic groups or creating a paternalistic atmosphere. Corporate manipulation of the imagery and language of kinship instructed Appalachian employees to promote and protect the financial health of the corporate 'family' and in so doing ensure the security of their own families as well. This was a successful strategy as it resonated within the core belief system of the Appalachian peoples.

By the 1960s, President Kennedy's Economic Opportunity Act established a plethora of human programs that included job training, head start (children program), domestic Peace Corps and VISTA, job corps and upward bound (high school dropout program). These government initiatives were designed to break the cycle of poverty but were limited by the fact that they were conceived by and administered from the nations capital via developmental economists and managers who were also largely from outside of the region. This flaw proved to be fatal as a number of these programs seriously collided with the projects that were already in power within the region [39]. Also, the federally designated 'Appalachia Region' proved to be far too complex socio-economically for such a broad definition and a one-size-fits-all approach. Here we see the folly of powerful, albeit well-intentioned, institutions who engage in absentee problem-solving using an 'objectification of people' approach. Indeed, it was arrogant to think that the economic problems of the region alone could be adequately addressed while simultaneously excluding the cultural values that this society held dear and their intertwinement within the local economy. Another example of this type of omission is evident in a letter sent by Mary Breckinridge in response to a booklet sent to her for use by the FNS entitled,

'Our Daily Food' by a Mrs. Thomas who offered to send more. Breckinridge graciously explained in the letter that it had been the Service's experience that as the charts within these booklets are all designed for 'people who live in cities' who obtain 'milk in bottles instead of right from the cow… and have things like grapefruits featured in them,' which were unheard of in Appalachia and that as a result, her nurses did not find them of much use. She was, however, profuse in her thanks to Mrs. Thomas for sending them though they could not be of use to her there.[38]

This one-size-fits-all way of doing businesses was regarded by the local population as impersonal and thus hostile. It eventually served to make Appalachian people suspicious of government, state and federal agencies, and social workers [40]. FNS nurses who saw these changes come into the hills said that welfare 'ruined' the people. Those there long enough to see what negative effects this had on the society attributed the rise in drinking, domestic violence and 'laziness' on the part of the Appalachian men to these changes and not the men. One nurse who came in the early 1960s and left before her contracted tenure at the FNS used the term 'hillbillies' to describe the people. She also described their squalid living conditions and ignorance in humorous vignettes, which accompanied a slide presentation that she had shown back in England when asked of her experiences at the FNS. She intimated that the people in Kentucky preferred this way of life.[39] This nurse, however, was only at the FNS just under a year in 1960 when she opted not to fulfil the 2-year commitment that she signed on for because she 'had her eye on a farmer back home.' Her interpretation of the people was a singular one among those former FNS nurses (American and British) that were either surveyed or interviewed. This nurse also left nursing to become a farmer's wife directly after leaving the Service. Her tenure there fell within the time frame in which many of the older nurses interviewed felt that 'newer' staff could not really call themselves FNS nurses, as the practice conditions as well as the calibre of the nurse coming into the region had changed so significantly (see footnote 12). Indeed, one nurse refused to be taped for an interview citing that she had been misquoted by an interviewer in the past who had written negative things about the people she loved and cared for during her tenure at the FNS. She explained her reason as a desire not to 'exploit' them any more than they had already been in the past.[40]

In the early 1960s, with 55% of Leslie County's 2713 families living below the poverty threshold, Breckinridge adamantly refused to honor government program vouchers (welfare) from the locals preferring to continue the barter for services form of payment if the patient could not pay the greatly reduced fees her organization continued to offer. It was commonly referred to as the 'Happy Pappy Program' by Service members. This program put fathers to work at $1.25 per hour to clean out

---

[38] Breckinridge letter to Mrs. Thomas, 29 May 1952. 85M1: FNS, Box 119, Fol. 2. University of Kentucky in Lexington, USA.

[39] Judie Pridie-Halse, British former FNS Nurse-Midwife (1960–1961), Date interviewed: 09/04/2005. Interviewer: Edith A. West.

[40] Alice Herman, American former FNS Nurse (1956–1978).

creek beds, cut roadside weeds and perform miscellaneous chores assigned to them by the school board, county or city supervisors.[41] The hospital provided free care for any child under the age of 16 years and a greatly reduced fee for adult's due to subsidization of the services by patrons outside of the region. However, the people, who appreciated having the hospital so much, usually made a donation when they took their children home.[42] Later, due mostly to federal government grants, local efforts and various 'war on poverty' state initiatives many hospitals and clinics were established and enlarged in the region. Simultaneously, Appalachia's major industries forced large numbers of people to be eligible for welfare benefits and these circumstances drew many Appalachian people into the system [36]. This coupled by the fact that the people now had greatly improved access to these other health care providers, also began to draw the local people away from the FNS to places where they could use welfare benefits to pay.

Breckinridge based her organization on the principle that nothing of value is free and you have to pay for anything you get. Her philosophy was everybody "pays something and in so doing they also 'buy into' something (see footnote 16)." The payment needn't have been currency and it usually wasn't in Appalachia but the value of the doing was intimately connected with the human dignity of both the doer and recipient. Further, it was a reciprocal and ongoing relational process between both the giver and recipient. Some local people viewed it differently in the Service's latter years. As one local explained it:

> Sometimes you go to a hospital and sometimes you're welcomed in and sometimes you ain't, so there you go…. See they was a helping us (FNS) and we helped them. That's the way it went…. We stood by them, they shoulda' stood by us (see footnote 40).

In the FNS's latter years the people felt that the organization had forfeited its 'place' as sole beneficiary when they were turned away and that if the Service expected the locals to remain loyal to them, then they needed to remain loyal to the community. Other Appalachian residents echoed this feeling of abandonment in the Services' later years, only from a different perspective. One resident recounted that they had been taught that the nurses took care of a lot but when the hospitals came in, people 'got to going to the doctors and somewhere along the way we got to thinking that maybe the doctor is the one to day when in reality the nurse could still do so much for you' (see footnote 32). Therefore, it could be argued that the people's abandonment of the FNS also played a role in this shift in the economic and social realities experienced by both the peoples of Eastern Kentucky and the Service in its later years. The cultural shift regarding the provision of health care by physicians as the point of access, which was well established outside of Appalachia, began to infiltrate the hills and continues nationally today. Another resident of the county described this advance thus:

---

[41] Anne Lorentzen , American former FNS Nurse (1963 1965), Date surveyed: 29/12/2003. Date interviewed: 11/03/2005. Interviewer: Edith A. West.

[42] 85M1: FNS, Box 25, Fol. 6. 'Letters from a Frontier Hospital by Charlotte Duggar, RN', Reprint from 'FNS Quarterly Bulletin, Spring 1940 (Vol. XV).

The doctor I saw decided I needed a specialist... I kept going to Lexington because they referred me, you know? And I didn't know the patient load had just fell off to nothing (at the FNS). We just... we had a change of nurses too often. I think that hurt.[43]

It is clear that the changes in the economic structure, FNS personnel, and cultural attitudes regarding health care within society created a tenuous relationship between the people and the FNS, a relationship that heretofore had been crucial for the survival of both. The continuing growth in technology and medical advances also furthered the fragmentation of care, which warranted consultations with any of a host of specialists. All of these factors further forced the service from its generalized care roots into the wider world of modern specialization that the rest of the country had already embraced. It was also true that this unique environment lent itself to 'trade offs' that were necessary to keep the organization running that included hosting visiting specialists, researchers and writers in the hopes of garnering free medical care, positive press and financial assistance. This did garner the assistance needed but it also did not always work for the region or the Service's ultimate benefit in regard to the 'relational' ties that both cultures were struggling to maintain in the midst of such rapid and enormous economic and social change. An Appalachian community member who served on an FNS committee for 20 years and witnessed these changes first hand perhaps illustrated it best by relating the following story told him by an old Appalachian man when he was a young man.

When these old, poor people comes around you, you see, you have to help 'em but make 'em do a little something. Make them think they earned it 'cause you can't keep it up and when you cut it off they be your worst enemies you got (see footnote 28).

This former FNS committee member imagined that this old man had the right idea. Breckinridge resisted government assistance for as long as she could, realizing that acceptance also meant unprecedented change to both the local as well as her organization's cultural climate but her successor, Helen E. Browne, was ultimately forced to honor welfare benefits after her death or the organization would have ceased to exist (see footnote 40). As Breckinridge's Service exists today as a 'federally operated' health care service, it would appear her reticence was justified. An examination of the Service's 'early years' organizational chart (Appendix B) to what currently exists today illustrates the power shift from a nursing focused, nurse operated entity to a corporation, complete with more than one Board of Directors and the creation of a 'President and CEO' designation. The hierarchy is one in which nurses and nursing are considered one of the many 'human resources' necessary to the 'industry' of care provision within the organization (Appendix C). Breckinridge's 'early years' chart has national medical and nursing councils with equal input to the Director (Breckinridge), Board of Governors over the Director and Medical Directors beneath the Director. The lower portions of the chart have nurses supervising nurses, though reporting indirectly to the medical directors via the Hyden Hospital Supervisor (a nurse). Within the organizational chart today, all boards of directors, as well as all departments below, report to a President and

---

[43] Interview #82OH09FNS 152, 1982, Sherman Wooten.

CEO. The sole exception is the nurse education piece of the equation, which is bypassed entirely within the organization's power and control structures.

Health is a political issue because health care must be a part of socioeconomic plans developed at the national level and nurses are directly influenced by these matters [41].

After Breckinridge's death in 1963 her chosen successor, Director Helen E. Browne, found the Service at a crossroads. Foreseeing the inevitable, she asked all of the FNS's district committees (community representatives in each of the district outposts) if they wanted the FNS to stay [42]. This question was shocking to the locals who stated emphatically that 'of course we want you to stay.' It was then that the FNS began to accept more of the state and federal government programs. The new government health regional regulations prohibited the construction of a hospital for small populations of approximately 18,000, which the FNS served [43]. The Service managed to get around this stipulation by documenting the need for training primary health care personnel in their underserved area. Of all the incoming government programs, the Federal Government Medicare and Medicaid Programs of the 1960s had the largest and most destructive impact on the Service [44].

The advent of Medicare and Medicaid inundated the nurses with a mass of paperwork and incomplete charting resulted in rejected claims for payment. As a result, clerical personnel were added. The government also determined where patients could now be treated, as Medicare and Medicaid would not reimburse for deliveries done outside of the hospital (see Footnote 16). When the State Health Commissioner recommended closure of the existing hospital due to 'fire code violations' in the late 1960s and a lack of water made it impossible to install the sprinkler system necessary to keep it open, it was determined that a new hospital was to be built but not before Medicare/Medicaid payments were halted for all except outpatients being seen at the existing hospital [45]. While the new hospital was under construction, the FNS was faced with the prospect of closing the existing hospital down and terminating its employees but realized that doing so would wreak havoc on an already depressed region as few of the locals could have been absorbed into the local economy. At the time, FNS employed [46] persons of whom approximately 75% were local citizens. In addition, most of the outsiders (physicians and nurses) would have accepted jobs elsewhere, thus making it difficult to staff the new hospital once it opened. So, FNS chose to keep the hospital open which meant accepting and treating Medicare and Medicaid patients at no charge since most could not afford to pay even minimal fees. To do so the FNS borrowed from the endowment fund and increased its fund-raising efforts. Donors responded generously [45]. In 1975 the new hospital opened, but it was designed for something the FNS never really wanted, sick people. Wellness, preventative medicine, delivery of mothers safely in their homes with well supervised prenatal care before and after delivery had become a thing of the past. The FNS now delivered medical care in much the same way the rest of the nation did [45].

It is of interest to note that it was not till after the FNS began receiving government funds that there was an increase in the number of premature births and deaths in the first week of life. This change in health of infants was attributed to the fact that patients now had to be ill before Medicaid would pay for treatment. The FNS's financial problems were compounded by the fact that over 55% of the Leslie County families had incomes below the poverty level. Since the FNS never refused patients regardless of their ability to pay, it became impossible for the Service to support itself through medical fees. Medicaid and Medicare did not solve this predicament as they did not cover 'preventive care' and would no longer cover many of the types of district and home care services that the FNS provided within the community (see footnote 14). This forced the nurses to resort to creative charting and transporting mothers in labour via jeep to the facility to deliver babies in order to secure payment for services.[44]

This way of doing business adversely affected the FNS as evidenced by excerpts from an FNS Staff Meeting for 1 September1966, lamenting the fact that most of the staff meetings had become 'un-educational, gripe-sessions.' It goes on to state that *the Service had broken down into 'little departments and not enough thought had been given to the problems of the others.'* [Italics added][45] This shift of focus was also evident in these minutes as the remaining half of the first page was devoted to procurement of ancillary staff, such as X-ray technicians and equipment and the final two pages to Medicare payment protocols, paperwork and billing. This was a distinct change from previous meeting minutes that dealt with the people issues of employment of physicians, nurse recruitment, increasing nurse salaries and discussions regarding the midwifery school, scholarships or fund-raising efforts (see Footnote 45).

The whole work load of the Service had changed in a few short years. No longer were the district nurses the most hard-working branch of the staff. The hospital became the central repository for pre, intra and postnatal care in addition to all medical and surgical patient care. District nurses were told they now had to plan their own work and their own off-duty time. It would no longer be done for them elsewhere and only one nurse at a centre could relieve the other for week ends. The hospital staff could not plan their own off-duty time many of them now working overtime and those on duty were working 'very hard.' The load of patients at Hyden Clinic had increased vastly in the last few years. The economy of the area had improved greatly, but it had come too quickly. In 1966, Director Helen E. Browne, called for the staff to 'help the people whenever we can and urge them to pay their bills in full while accepting gratefully less if that was all the Service could get.' This particular meeting had three pages of minutes, most of which dealt with efforts to figure out the new government (Medicare and Medicaid) paperwork and how much to charge patients for services. The 'gripe sessions' and 'break down' of FNS departments allude to the internal organizational culture shift that was occurring due to the changing socioeconomy in the region and the simultaneous shift from community to hospital based, institutionalized care [47]. One of the things research has found that nurses are most dissatisfied with when salary is good are 'co-workers who don't provide good care, feeling overloaded and factors that interfere with job and patient care' [48]. For the

---

[44] FNS Staff Meeting, 1 September 1966. 85M1: FNS, Box 220, Fol. 9. University of Kentucky in Lexington, USA.

[45] FNS Summary of Executive Committee Minutes 1925–1935. 85M1: FNS, Box 2, Fol. 1.

FNS nurse, when the care benefits associated with 'relationship' to both the people and the organization began to wane, so did satisfaction with the work environment. This is when the organization's senior nurses began to leave. For them, the organization no longer met the cultural expectations that they saw as 'what they stood for' and 'who they were' as nurses and specifically FNS nurses. This was ironic as nearly all cultural identities within organizations are focused on business relevance and economic agreements. Its members have distinct and recognized corporate identifications [49]. For the FNS, when it began to take on the corporate persona as an organization it adversely affected both recruitment and retention of its nurses who came on board when it was a philanthropy with a heart and soul. They were unable or unwilling to make the transition in the organization's latter years.

Some characteristics of low performance cultures are a politicized internal environment, hostility to change, promotion of managers who understand structures, systems and controls better than vision, strategies and culture-building and have an aversion to looking outside the organization for superior practices. Conversely, high performance cultures emphasize achievement and excellence, produce extraordinary results with ordinary people and emphasize an intense people orientation. The FNS under Breckinridge's tutelage was clearly a high-performance culture. It purveyed policies and practices that inspired ordinary *people* to do their best and was certainly results oriented. By 1958, FNS nurse-midwives had attended over 10,000 births. All maternal and infant outcome statistics for FNS's first 30 years of operation (1925–1954) were better than for the country as a whole. The biggest differences were in the maternal mortality rate (9.1 per 10,000 births for FNS, compared with 34 per 10,000 births for the US as a whole) and low birth weight (3.8% for FNS, compared with 7.6% for the country). The people orientation was certainly evident to both the FNS nurses as well as the general populace. Moreover, the FNS was a strong culture in that the philosophy, values and beliefs of the organization were not only clear and explicit but also widely shared and deeply rooted in not only the organization and its nurses, but also the community that it served with the 'rewards' to all parties abundantly apparent in their oral history narratives. Further, it could also be argued that the FNS's organizational culture was more closely aligned to the discipline's philosophy, values, beliefs than other health care organizations as evidenced by comparison of the FNS's philosophy and objectives (Appendix D) and the American Nurses Association (ANA) Code of Ethics (Appendix E). As long as Breckinridge lived, the organization had a sincere commitment to operating according to tradition and perpetuating the organization's values and legendary stories. Indeed, the community created a 'Mary Breckinridge Day' in the late 1960s that continues today as the 'Mary Breckinridge Festival' in Eastern Kentucky [50].

A low-performance culture may be strong or weak and a strong low-performance culture may actively inhibit necessary competitive re-alignment. Hospitals are certainly described by nurses today as strong, low-performance cultures where managers as well as nurses are actively discouraged from exercising initiative to alter status quo and where avoiding risks and not screwing-up are deemed more important than innovativeness. They are also entrenched, multi-layered bureaucracies where people are promoted who understand structures, systems and controls better than vision, strategies and culture building. In the FNS's latter years, it too clearly exhibited the characteristics of a weak culture, with many subcultures (departments) developing within the organization which resulted from the move from decentralization to a centralized power structure and fewer strong traditions such as afternoon teas or even the wearing of the FNS uniform within the organization. Also, with the unique, symbiotic relationship it had with the local community weakened as a direct result of the culture shift, there was no strong sense of identity and few values and beliefs widely shared by all of its employees after Breckinridge's death. It was at this time that many of the long-time staff nurses chose to leave the FNS. Yet though there was certainly a lowered performance culture after Breckinridge's death, it cannot be said that the FNS was ever a 'low performance culture.' The innovation that created and sustained the organization prevailed in its greatest crisis with the advent of the Nurse Practitioner Program and its tenacity to not quite fully surrender its uniqueness to the establishment. The FNS continues to combine education and service through a hospital, home health agency, rural healthcare clinics and a school of nurse midwifery and family nursing. This continues to be a collaborative effort of nursing and medicine supported by thousands of friends across the country that provides financial assistance to fulfil their mission through a foundation. A hospital that now exists there bares Breckinridge's name and is a private, not for profit, sole-community hospital that continues to meet the challenges facing small rural hospitals. It should also be noted that its staff were not among the nearly 700 nurses who went on strike recently at nine Appalachian Regional Healthcare (ARH) hospitals in Kentucky and West Virginia [51].

The history of the formation of professional disciplines goes part and parcel with the rise of institutional hierarchies, where power and political clout is wielded within the market place. These institutions have a culture as well as reflect elements of the societal culture from whence they sprang. The use of formal knowledge to order human affairs is, of course, an exercise of power, an act of domination over those who are the object [52]. For the discipline of nursing this has proven to be problematic as its cultural identity is rooted in humanitarianism and service, values that are people as opposed to object focused and are not as highly regarded by society.

The regional control (generalized power structure) the FNS had had since the organization's inception was handed over to the federal government (centralized power structure) in the late 1960s. Centralized power structures tend to foster coping, planning, budgeting, organizing and controlling effective action (managers) while discouraging the promotion of sustained, positive change through realistic and exhaustive analysis of surroundings coupled with appropriate direction setting (leaders). Institutional power structures also tend to discourage the alignment, motivation and inspiration of *people* (visionaries) toward meaningful action choosing instead to adopt a truth from others and then implement it without probing for the facts that reveal reality. The degree to which the people focus is shifted toward the objectification of the work determines how strong or weak and how high or low a particular organizational culture performs.

Nurses within centralized power settings are forced to take on the persona of the culture in which they practice. It has been said that the management and organization that was useful on a day to day basis when in crisis has the negative effect of siphoning responsibility away from individual human beings who find themselves trapped by structural and bureaucratic rigidity within the organization [53].

The strong organizational culture that existed at the FNS was based on a philanthropic, not a corporate value structure. When this value structure shifted from its original goal of individualized care and working *with* its community to doing the work and meeting the requirements *of* the institution *for* the community, it was no longer fully congruent with its nurses or the local community's needs. In a larger sense, the FNS's forced move from its philanthropic and 'nursing model' roots to the more established corporate approach (business and medical model) being used outside of Appalachia, which resulted in a lack of community, professional and institutional congruency could also be proffered as a source of the cyclic crisis problems so often cited as causes for nursing shortages. This was strongly evidenced by the remarkably similar language used by both the former FNS nurses to describe how their practice environment *changed* as well as nurses in practice today to describe their *present* work environment. The moral inhabitability of this environment and its relationship to the cultural identity of its nurses is explored in depth in the subsequent chapter.

References

1. Lipset S. Political man: the social bases of politics, expanded edition. Worthing: World Books Ltd.; 1981. p. 12.
2. Cunningham S. Review essay, Schumpeter's capitalism, socialism and democracy. Int J Cult Policy. 2010;16(1):20–2.
3. Andrist C, Nicholas P, Wolf K. A history of nursing ideas. Burlington: Jones and Bartlett Publishers; 2006. p. 23.
4. Puckett A. Seldom ask, never tell: labour & discourse in Appalachia. New York: Oxford University Press; 2002. p. 31.
5. Olsen T. Historical case study of apprenticeship of nurses at Saint Luke's Training School for Nurses (1892–1937). Unpublished PhD dissertation. Minneapolis: University of Minnesota; 1991.
6. Nelson R. Good Night, Florence: with nursing in crisis, some say it's time to retire Nightingale as a symbol. Can J Nurs Leadersh. 2003;16(2):46–50.
7. Selanders LC. Florence Nightingale: the evolution and social impact of feminist values in nursing. J Holist Nurs. 2010;16(2):227–43. https://doi.org/10.1177/0898010109360256.
8. Easson-Bruno S. Don't blame Florence. Can J Nurs Leadersh. 2003;16(4):8–9.
9. Harris H. Constructing colonialism: medicine, technology and the FNS. p. 73.
10. Salvage J. The legend of the lady with the lamp has been debunked but Florence Nightingale's zeal is needed. Nurs Times. 2001;97(30):18.
11. Rahim M. Managing conflict in organizations. New York: Routledge; 2017. p. 132.
12. Nasaw D. The Gospel of wealth essays and other writings (Penguin Classics). New York: Penguin Books; 2006.
13. Schein EH. Organizational culture and leadership. 5th ed. San Francisco: Jossey-Bass; 2016.
14. Sanborn M. You don't need a title to be a leader: how anyone, anywhere, can make a positive difference. New York: Vintage Books; 2006. p. 86.

15. Thompson A, Strickland A. Strategic management: concepts and cases. Boston: Irwin/McGraw-Hill; 2001. p. 503.
16. Sanborn M. You don't need a title to be a leader: how anyone, anywhere, can make a positive difference. New York: Doubleday Broadway Publishing; 2006. p. 11.
17. Thompson A, Strickland A. Strategic management: concepts and cases. Boston: McGraw-Hill Irwin; 2001. p. 56.
18. Robbins S, Coulter M. Management. 9th ed. New Jersey: Prentice-Hall; 2009.
19. McKiernan P. Historical evolution of strategic management volume I. New York: Routledge; 2017. p. 18, Chapter 13.
20. Rahim M. Managing conflict in organizations. New York: Praeger; 1992. p. 133.
21. Cohen J. Minority report: working party on the recruitment and training of nurses. His Majesty's Stationery Office: London. Royal College of London (Metropolitan Library Archives, London, UK, 1948).
22. Thompson A, Strickland A. Strategic management: concepts and cases. Boston: Irwin/McGraw-Hill; 2001. p. 572.
23. Leathard A. Health care provision: past, present and into the twenty-first century. 2nd ed. Cheltenham: Stanley Thornes Ltd; 2000.
24. Borsay A, Hunger B. Nursing and midwifery in Britain since 1700. London: McMillan Education; 2012.
25. Davies C. Rewriting nursing history—again? Nurs Hist Rev. 2007;15:11–28.
26. Leap N, Hunter B. The midwife's tale: an oral history from handywoman to professional midwife. Pen and Sword: Barnsley; 2013.
27. Reid D. Saddlebags full of memories (Burt Lake Michigan: USA; 1992). p. 41.
28. Abramson R, Haskell J. Encyclopaedia of Appalachia. Knoxville: University of Tennessee Press; 2006. p. 1650.
29. Abramson R, Haskell J. Encyclopaedia of Appalachia. Knoxville: University of Tennessee Press; 2006. p. 1652.
30. Dammann N. A social history of the Frontier Nursing Service. Sun City: Social Change Press; 1982. p. 134.
31. Daiski I. Changing nurses' dis-empowering relationship patterns. J Adv Nurs. 2004;48(1):43–50.
32. Schein EH. Organizational culture and leadership. 5th ed. San Francisco: Jossey-Bass; 2016. p. 87.
33. Baird K. Raising the bar on service excellence. Fort Atkinson: Golden Lamp Press; 2011.
34. Harris H. Constructing colonialism: medicine, technology and the FNS. p. 74.
35. Whisnant D. All that is native and fine. 2nd ed. Chapel Hill: UNC Press Books; 2018. p. 231.
36. Drake R. History of Appalachia. Lexington: University Press of Kentucky; 2003. p. 169.
37. Drake R. History of Appalachia. Lexington: University Press of Kentucky; 2003. p. 170.
38. Abramson R, Haskell J. Encyclopaedia of Appalachia. Knoxville: University of Tennessee Press; 2006. p. 209.
39. Drake R. History of Appalachia. Lexington: University Press of Kentucky; 2003. p. 177.
40. Weller JE. Yesterday's people: life in contemporary Appalachia. University of Kentucky Press: Lexington; 1965.
41. Roux G, Halstead J. Issues and trends in nursing: practice, policy and leadership. Burlington: Jones and Bartlett Learning, LLC; 2018. p. 17–26.
42. Dammann N. A social history of the Frontier Nursing Service. Sun City: Social Change Press; 1982. p. 123.
43. Dammann N. A social history of the Frontier Nursing Service. Sun City: Social Change Press; 1982. p. 122.
44. Dammann N. A social history of the Frontier Nursing Service. Sun City: Social Change Press; 1982. p. 133.
45. Dammann N. A social history of the Frontier Nursing Service. Sun City: Social Change Press; 1982. p. 137.
46. Dammann N. A social history of the Frontier Nursing Service. Sun City: Social Change Press; 1982. p. 58.

47. Carayon P. Handbook of human factors and ergonomics in health care and patient safety. 2nd ed. New York: CRC Press; 2012. p. 122.
48. Schultz M, Hatch MJ, Larson MH. The expressive organization: linking identity, reputation and the corporate brand. Oxford: Oxford University Press. p. 14.
49. Campbell A. Mary Breckinridge and the American Committee for Devastated France: the Foundations of the Frontier Nursing Service. The Register of the Kentucky Historical Society. 1984;82(3):257–76. https://www.jstor.org/stable/23380341.
50. Mary Breckinridge Festival. https://leslie.ca.uky.edu/files/calendar_oct_2018_0.pdf. Accessed 14 Jan 2019.
51. Pridemore A. Appalachia Regional Healthcare Hospital Strike. 2007. https://www.register-herald.com/news/local_news/nurses-ok-contract-arh-strike-set-to-end/article_b8b5f2d8-cafb-532f-bb71-506dd574f005.html. Accessed 14 Jan 2019.
52. Freidson E. Professional powers: a study of the institutionalization of formal knowledge. Chicago: University of Chicago Press; 1986.
53. Thierry P, Mitroff I. Transforming the crisis-prone organization: preventing individual, organizational and environmental tragedies. San Francisco: Jossey-Bass Inc.; 1992. p. 6.

Chapter 5
Moral Inhabitability and Work Environments

5.1 Moral Inhabitability and Work Environments

In Great Britain, a 1948 Report issued by the Ministry of Health, the Department of Health for Scotland, the Ministry of Labour and National Service, on the recruitment and training of nurses to address yet another post-war nursing shortage, indicated that not much had changed for nurses except the steady increase in clinical skill and responsibility [1]. The report called for, amongst other things, the 'humanizing' of hospital discipline for nurses. It also included several comments from nurses who were interviewed by the committee at the time about their reasons for leaving the nursing profession before completing training. This statement made by one of them illustrates the type of work environment which still existed at the end of the 1940s.

> Bewildered by the thousand and one duties, many futile, finding no sympathy in those above the probationer stage and not given credit for a grain of intelligence…. Any attempt to justify oneself was insubordination [2].

This probationer's remarks underscore the uncaring atmosphere that existed within an institutional culture that purportedly provided care. Other descriptors used by these former probationers, which emphasized how little the institutional culture had changed are the 'boarding school mentality', 'tyrannical' matrons and the 'do as you are told' mindset of the institution's physicians, administrators and nursing supervisors while being treated like 'little girls' [3]. These probationers described the work environment as 'unfair, unduly harsh' with 'long hours and little leisure time, unnecessarily strict' with 'patient-focused care deferred in preference of the all encompassing institutional routines and record keeping.' Cohen went on to suggest in this report that any reform which may seem to imply criticism of the senior nursing staff or may require a curtailment of their power over the student nurse will likely meet a wall of resistance. This is insightful and forward thinking for the time as systems founded on 'business values' certainly do not change due

© Springer Nature Switzerland AG 2019
E. West, *Frontier Nursing in Appalachia: History, Organization and the Changing Culture of Care*, https://doi.org/10.1007/978-3-030-20027-5_5

primarily to the fact that they protect and benefit the very people who hold the power to fix the problem and very often simply refuse to do so if they are a part of the problem [4]. Cohen added that the institution itself also had a policy or established interest to defend and that only those who could view the situation dispassionately, even when their own interests seemed affected were likely to welcome change. Cohen identified the barriers to change that these bastions of power created and suggested a 'scientific approach' to hours of work, conditions, energy or output of the nurses required and staff ratio of nurse to patient and compared this new health care system to an 'industry.'

Cohen noted, using business terminology generally used to describe objects or machines, that 'productivity' (in this case total man or woman power) and the national economy, not just health or nursing service alone, should be evaluated [5]. He also suggested a discipline for students befitting a professional life, salaries based on consideration of 'productivity' and working arrangements, which would not be subordinate to the existing ties and routine of medical ward visits that constituted one of the chief obstacles to introducing a workable three-shift working day for nurses. Cohen's assessment subscribes to the prevailing twentieth century business model that was and still is being used to deliver health care on both sides of the Atlantic. It subscribes to a reward system for employees based on organizational performance which links skills-based pay to performance and increased productivity [6]. It is disheartening to note that many of these calls for reform, particularly those made about appropriate length of professional education, public acknowledgement and recognition, adequate working conditions with appropriate nurse to patient ratios and salary, made over half a century ago in both America and Great Britain are still being called for today [7].

This continues to be the case even after much has been done since that time by way of 'scientific approaches' to study nursing's recruitment, retention and work environment problems since the Rockefeller Foundation Nurse Labour Market reports (spanning the years 1923–1963) in the US and the Cohen Report in the UK in 1948. Time has proven that though pay incentives and benefit packages with paid vacation leave will certainly draw nurses into the profession, it will do little to keep them there if their work environment can be described as, "harsh, humiliating and futile" [1].

The combination of hard work and poor educational conditions made nursing a particularly unattractive field for young women and received the blame for creating a shortage of qualified applicants to schools of nursing in America, which prompted the Rockefeller Foundation (RF) to conduct the first significant national study of the nurse labour market in the early twentieth century known as the Goldmark Report [8]. The 500-page report outlined the dismal working conditions, uncertain or inadequate periods of employment, little opportunity for advancement and low income as the primary sources of the problem. Few tangible outcomes resulted from this report, and the two that followed it over a 30-year period, even though the 'more cautious approach' suggested by a Dr. David Edsall, Dean of Harvard Medical School, 'for further analysis of the situation before advocating changes in the educational system' demonstrated repeatedly the obvious need for reform to not just nursing education, but nurses' practice environments as well [9]. What was also needed was a 'considerable commitment of funds' similar to what was given to medicine, which the Foundation was not willing to extend nursing. Alan Gregg of the RF's International Health Division provided significant moral support for the findings and recommendations of the second report done by the RF called the Brown Report and inferred that little would be accomplished unless nursing received adequate funds. However, he also formally denied any such funding to the National League for Nursing (NLN) when they solicited assistance. Gregg expressed doubts that the League could complete the proposed work satisfactorily and explained that it was 'not in the interests of medical science to take up the subject of nursing education' [10]. The Rockefeller Foundation went on to provide well researched and documented consistency for the suggested improvements over a 30-year period by three separate studies, which not only indicated an irrefutable validity to each study's findings but also aptly illustrated the causes for hesitancy to help on the part of the RF. Fear of implementing reforms or imposing measures unwelcome to other health care groups, namely the American Medical Association, the American College of Surgeons, the American Hospital Association and the American Public Health Association was to be avoided at all costs.

Substantial investments were being made by governments and philanthropies to help create the expansion of medical institutions for education, research and patient care and to improve public access to these institutions. Yet even though as early as the turn of the century, the battle for control of nurse education, better standards, practice environments and recognition also raged on both sides of the Atlantic by nurse leaders and professional nursing organizations, and with it a debate concerning the resulting nurse shortages that perpetually existed in hospitals; governments and philanthropies were not as forthcoming with funding for nurses unless their interests coincided with the best interests of medical, hospital or governmental institutions [11].

Hospitals in both Britain and America at this time consisted of nursing education and practice environments that were defined, structured, reformed and re-structured in large part by non-nurses who saw nursing as a means to an end in the provision of health care [12]. In both countries the primary problem surrounding recruitment and retention issues in nursing education and practice was a continual lack of adequate financial and public support, a shift to the institutionalisation of health care with accompanying paternal or maternal hierarchy (often both), a military style of training, and an overemphasis on recruitment and under-emphasis on retention reforms necessary to maintain an adequate supply of nurses in practice. Breckinridge saw her work as her life, a clearly monastic outlook and also had a history of service in the Red Cross, a disciplined organization. These clearly influenced her. Yet she was able to bring to her organization the discipline associated with a military style without the oppressive regulatory component that could chafe and the rewards of a monastic way of life that was not devoid of human interaction, connectedness and a sense of belonging and purpose that gave meaning to life.[1]

---

[1] Interview #82OH03FNS146, 1982, Agnes Lewis.

Job dissatisfaction continues to be a key issue contributing to the crisis related to recruiting and retaining nurses and it is not merely a national occurrence. Nurses in Germany and Hong Kong also cite 'organizational climate' as a key cause for their dissatisfaction [13]. Dissatisfaction occurred not with salary issues, but rather in relation to feelings of being 'overloaded' or due to factors that 'interfered' with job and patient care such as a lack of resources or a lack of a feeling of 'achievement, recognition and respect' [14]. Though historically salary, hours of work and tangible benefits have always been considered important issues for nurses, it is interesting to note that they have never been the sole indicators of satisfaction. In fact, they are more often than not deemed secondary to issues of professional autonomy, good working relationships and nurse-patient interactions. Yet these secondary considerations have been and continue to be the driving forces for change within the existing organizational culture. This reality is illustrated best when the order of importance within the work culture is reversed. For example, in the UK where good relations existed between physicians and nurses and a team approach to care was valued within the institutional culture, nurses were found to be most dissatisfied with their salaries [15]. Also, for Chinese nurses, though the 'organizational climate' was found to contribute to an increase in absenteeism because nursing is a valued career with high pay and job security within their society and national economy, nurses there, though dissatisfied with the organizational climate would not even consider leaving the profession [16].

These recent studies when taken in totem with those done in both the US and UK some 80 years prior suggest that a purely 'scientific' or 'corporate' approach to these issues alone are not sufficient as they do not address the humanity nor the empowerment pieces of the equation fully enough to make sustainable positive change possible. One former FNS nurse recalled that after lunch, as was her custom, Breckinridge asked the 'new nurse' to accompany her to the stable to feed the kitchen scraps to the barn cats and to talk. This nurse, a city girl, stated that she thought barn cats caught mice, to which Breckinridge responded: 'If you expected someone to do their job, you fed them well.' Breckinridge clearly had the same philosophy concerning her employees as she has been quoted as saying that her nurses needed more than a 'fair salary or decent living accommodations and extra days of holiday for the long hours spent in working overtime,' all of which she provided. She also stated: 'People have to grow. If they stand still their work is static too and the FNS would be missing its mark altogether if its work stood still.' Breckinridge led by example and gave the impression that she would never ask her staff or her nurses to do something that she was not willing to do herself.[2]

Institutional work outside of Appalachia at the time was described by nurse recruits as 'routine,' 'domestic' and a drudge. By contrast, FNS nurse recruits described their work both within the hospital setting and out in the district as, 'the first time we used an education', 'more independence (in Kentucky) than anywhere

---

[2]Roberta Stidham, American former FNS Nurse (1960–1961).

else that I've ever worked', 'hard, to be sure, but it was freedom that I had not experienced before or since', 'enjoyable' and 'unique.' As opposed to the descriptors such as 'rude, harsh, petty and tyrannical', which were being used to describe the matrons at a London Hospital, the following words were used to describe FNS administrators, 'kind and an excellent teacher with a good sense of humour and was just enjoyable to be around', 'having high expectations and yet facilitated students'' 'development of skills in a gentle manner', 'warm hearted', 'fair and just', 'having a positive attitude', 'a gracious and effective *leader.*' [Italics added] [17].

Hospitals in both Britain and America at this time consisted of nursing education and practice environments that were defined, structured, reformed and re-structured in large part by non-nurses who saw nursing as a means to an end in the provision of health care [18]. In both countries the primary problem surrounding recruitment and retention issues in nursing education and practice was a continual lack of adequate financial and public support, a shift to the institutionalisation of health care with accompanying paternal or maternal hierarchy (often both), a military style of training, and an overemphasis on recruitment and under-emphasis on retention reforms necessary to maintain an adequate supply of nurses in practice. Breckinridge saw her work as her life, a clearly monastic outlook and also had a history of service in the Red Cross, a disciplined organization. These clearly influenced her. Yet she was able to bring to her organization the discipline associated with a military style without the oppressive regulatory component that could chafe and the rewards of a monastic way of life that was not devoid of human interaction, connectedness and a sense of belonging and purpose that gave meaning to life.

5.2   The FNS and 'Morally Inhabitable' Work Environments

Breckinridge was a Christian woman and took her religion seriously enough to put it into practice. The motto for the FNS since its inception has been, 'He shall gather the lambs with his arm and carry them in His bosom and shall gently lead those that are with young,' a direct quote from the Bible's book of Isaiah.[3] Her organization was only philanthropic from an economic perspective. From a social perspective, the organization was a charity in the broadest sense of the word. Indeed, it was the organization's desire to connect, 'love thy neighbour as thyself' so-to-speak, that distinguished if from being a purely philanthropic endeavour. It was also what made it successful. In many ways, this organizational duality mirrored that of the Appalachian culture's 'people orientation' associated with mutual work, reward and relational reciprocity. It was what made the early years of the service go beyond successful to become so deeply meaningful for both its nurses and the community. Many of Breckinridge's nurses shared her Christian beliefs, as did many of the

---

[3]FNS Quarterly Bulletin. 85M1: FNS, Box 36, Fol. 15. 'Motto and purposed of the FNS', May 1927, vol. III. Lexington: University of Kentucky in Lexington; 1927. p. 32.

graduates from her midwifery school. Most of those seeking to come for the distinctly rural training afforded them via the School went on to foreign mission fields after their training was completed. However, a particular religious affiliation was not a pre-requisite for working for the FNS either and 'not talking religion' with the locals was one of the few rules that Breckinridge instituted. There were over 200 different Christian denominations in Appalachia at the time that she founded her Service [19]. Appalachian values are intricately tied to roots in the Protistant faith and are steeped in traditional adherence to God, family, and community. These roots are linked to religions sects that have historically experienced persecution, such as Calvanism, Quakerism, the Mennonite faith, and the Moravian Brethren. Many early Appalachia settelers were in rural areas that had no formal church or pastor so they oranized themselves and welcomed uneducated traveling ministers who shaped the spiritual beliefs of those in this isolated area. Hence, the mountain church's rural heritage is one less concerned with actual church attendance and more concerned with how faith permiates the lives of the individuals within the community. Values that are similar across the various religious sects which permiate the area include a religious world view, moral codes, Biblical interpretations, egalitarianism, independence, individualism, familism, neighborliness, love of the land and conflict avoidance [20]. Fatalism, which is the belief that what happens to one that is outside of the individuals control may be from God's hand, is also prominent in Appalachia. It is not uncommon to hear, "It must be God's will" when untoward circumstances occur.

For Breckinridge, religion was viewed much like every other facet of her organizational culture, as an extension of the person in the doing with and for another person. Christ was to be shown through the doing of the work and was not dogma to be foisted upon the person as a work in and of itself. This was a remarkably similar credo to that of the Appalachian people with regard to the official structuring or institutionalisation of any form of industry albeit mental or physical. The Appalachian phrase, 'around here honey, we work with our hands, not with our heads' aptly described the way both the nurses and their patients were likely to interpret and assign value to their labor [21]. Perhaps a fuller interpretation of this concept would be to say: the work that moves our hearts are the actions done for one another, not our intentions, however good they may be. This singular and ingrained relationship to nature, God and other people was as strong in the Mountains as it was in those early FNS nurses. One resident explained it thus:

> Even though they [Appalachian people] don't have an official structure [Religion] … there is more God consciousness in this society than almost any society in America. Almost everyone believes in God. The reason for this is you're close to nature, alone with the stars, the mountains, and with the streams. Young people here feel a stronger sense than the more sophisticated urban young person who is almost totally diverted from reality in the sense that he is an urbanic. When you have concrete buildings and concrete streets and all your food is out of cans, how can you have a strong sense of your identity with nature? If you can't identify yourself with creation you can't possibly identify yourself with the creator. Here we do [22].

This desire for relationship whether it is towards nature, man or God could well be defined as spirituality. Nursing scholars continue to debate the definition of spirituality because it is such a broad, encompassing and abstract term. Reed defines spirituality as 'the propensity to make meaning through a sense of relatedness to dimensions that transcend the self in such a way that empowers and does not devalue the individual' [23].

It is also that which gives meaning and purpose to an individual's life. Finally, it is both the means for escaping the constrictions of life into a broader spectrum or experience and the reason for living. It is more than simply what makes life worthwhile; spirituality leads to a sense of oneness or connectedness with something greater than self, nature or universe [24]. All of these facets of spirituality deal with the inherent value of *relationship*. One resident in describing the problems associated with Appalachia said it most succinctly when he supposed that the Appalachian problem doesn't seem to be political, economical or social but rather a "spiritual problem and its name is greed" in reference to the motivation behind many of the supposedly 'charitable' acts being done by outsiders *for* the community [25].

A form of organized or institutionalised philanthropy had already replaced charity by this time in most of the nation but had not totally eliminated the urge for personal service or the spirit of volunteerism. The Peace Corps and VISTA in the 1960s are examples of the 'spirit' that still inspired to help people in distress. The trouble was that the hunger for personal connection to others had been left out of most academic accounts of these charitable acts [26]. And to perpetuate this omission is to undermine the very enterprise of helping others. In Appalachia, to have reciprocal relations, individuals must have 'claims' to each other, meaning they must be in an active ongoing, face-to-face and personal relationship with someone who meets 'rights' and 'place' criteria and who can be expected to fulfil each other's 'needs' to some degree. For example, family members could 'claim' time, labour, goods and information from each other. In addition, these relationships must be nurtured and reaffirmed on a regular, often time-consuming basis. Many Appalachian residents felt that 'loving one's neighbour' also meant being responsible *to him* as well as *for him*, and being willing to be affected by him as opposed to just being willing to affect him. Because of this, locals objected to a great many of the church and federal programs that came into the hills. The work was seen as a, 'I'm here to help though I don't know what all you other slobs are here for, but I'm here to help,' mentality on the part of the so-called 'professional do-gooders' [22]. The basic problem with the philanthropic endeavours perpetrated by those outside of the culture was that they were outside of the culture and as such, lacked the 'people' connection necessary to have the 'right' and 'place' to make any 'claims' for fulfilment of time, labour, goods or informational 'needs' within the community. This difficulty was mirrored in the following correspondence from Dr. Karl E. Yaple, M.D., Paediatrician to long time FNS Physician, Roger Beasley, M.D., which addressed the host of 'volunteer' workers coming into the Appalachia's in the 1960s to help provide health care there. In the letter, he cites the common problem that urban trained professionals (outsiders) had when going into rural Appalachia to 'help out':

> When the VISTA workers come in here; when Berea College volunteers come in, when volunteers from the council of the Southern Mountains come in; and, well, the list is very long, but they all wind up falling flat on their faces because they don't know anything about

the area. They refuse to accept the status quo here, and because of this they obviously do not do any good here and get frustrated and leave, actually very quickly.[4]

When scholarship began to be focused mainly on the institutions of philanthropy, the ideas of leaders and issues of public policy it distorted the benevolent enterprise. Without direct mutual bonds between givers and recipients, philanthropy sacrifices practical effectiveness and moral purpose [27]. In stark contrast, an example of how these bonds were reciprocal between the FNS and the local community can be found in the story of how the 'Grassy Clinic' was built. The FNS nurse discussed building a clinic for the use of 50 families in that district and found they were 'keen to have it.' The nurse wrote, 'We have no money. I have none and you have none but you have the logs and you have the chinking…you the roof board and the saw mill can donate the floor boards'.[5] The clinic was literally built from the ground up by 'volunteer' labour and goods; some from the FNS and some from the community; some donated currency coming in from outside the region helped to purchase those commodities that were not available in the hills but most of the donated goods and services were done by the locals. The nurses even helped to build the structure they would live in and serve from alongside the people. The people, in turn, became a structure for the nurses before there were roads or ambulances by becoming 'Mountain Ambulances.' If a patient needed to go to the hospital, people would make stretchers with their coats and two tree branches and carry their neighbours down the mountain with the nurse walking along beside.[6] The community was expected to form a local committee that would look after the interests of the clinic once it was built. This committee would meet with the nurses regularly and the volunteer director monthly. If a community had no vested interest in supporting a clinic then a clinic was not built in that community for them. This sentiment is mirrored in the following excerpt from a 1935 FNS *Quarterly Bulletin*, 'We work through rather than for the people.' In fact, if local participation ceased, so did the clinic as evidenced by the closing of the 'Wolf Creek Centre' owing to the lack of promised local support.[7] Indeed, all of the FNS nurses expressed a strong sense of

---

[4]Dr. Karl Yaple Letter to Dr. Roger Beasley, 10, February 1966, 2005M547: FNS, Box 227, Fol. 9.
[5]Reprint from FNS Quarterly Bulletin 1932, 2005M547: FNS, Box 40, Fol. 2. 'Building of Grassy Clinic by Edith Marsh. Marsh came to the FNS in 1930, then went to Scotland for midwifery training. She then returned to Kentucky and was posted at the Flat Creek Clinic, Hyden. She was transferred to the Frances Payne Bolton Centre at Confluence in December of 1932. University of Kentucky in Lexington, USA.
[6]FNS Film, Forgotten Frontier 1927, FNS Audio Visual Series, This is a silent, black and white film, the first made of the FNS. It was filmed by Breckinridge's cousin, Marvin Breckinridge. Factual stories were re-enacted by the FNS nurses and the families they served in the actual homes of the local people, depicting the work of the Service. University of Kentucky in Lexington, USA.
[7]FNS Lexington Kentucky Committee Report 1925, 85M1: FNS, Box 11, Fol. 22. Comparative reports on all outposts citing number of sick visits, duty hours, inoculations given, etc., This box also contained 'FNS Comparative Reports from 1950–1959.' University of Kentucky in Lexington, USA.

spirituality as a motivating factor to their joining the Service. Though all of them held deeply Christian values, there was no one denominational affiliation and a few did not identify themselves to any particular denomination. However, a long-time FNS nurse made the following comment regarding the impact of faith and how these values not only transformed the work environment but also the worker within such an environment:

> I got into the midwifery training school on a bit of a fib... really because in those days, midwifery training to be fully qualified, you did it in two parts of six months, and the first part was always in hospital and the second six months was either by all district or part district. And I had no intention of doing more than the first six months. I was surprised how much I enjoyed it and how kind all the top knob staff were to us pupil midwives as we were called in those days. Because, I don't know whether it happens in the States or not, but you hear stories of how awful such and such a place is and how dreadful they treat you as a trained nurse but as a pupil midwife at this particular hospital where I went, the British hospital for mothers and babies, they just didn't expect you to know anything and they taught you gentle and lovingly and really got through to you and it was built around Christian principles which I hadn't a clue about in those days and I became a Christian while I was there.[8]

The focus on external motivators such as salary and other more tangible benefits to recruit nurses to the exclusion of other, less tangible benefits has harmed and not helped the profession by causing some nurses to leave and those who remain to do so with feelings of disillusionment, dissatisfaction, frustration and entrapment.

A ground-breaking Canadian study by Peter et al. [28] identified the by-product of the discipline's crisis cycle as *'moral inhabitability'* that existed in nurses' institutional work environments [28]. This study focused on the difficult work environments of nurses and concluded that these environments had significant *ethical* [italics added] implications for nurses, chief among them, feelings of oppression, powerlessness, exploitation, marginalization, and interpersonal hostility. Work environments were perceived as dominated by medical or business values where nursing perspectives were marginalized and the study concluded that the work environment was 'morally uninhabitable' for nurses. Yet even in these conditions nurses had still managed to find meaningful ways to resist this culture and influence the moral environment positively [29]. Perhaps what is most telling about this particular study is the patronizing, vitriolic commentary it generated from a male, medical assistant who saw the issues raised in it as merely something 'endemic to modern organizational life.' He argued that nursing's account of 'familiar, everyday experiences as evidence for an erosion of something specific to nursing' in the study as not being 'authoritative' as it was based on 'self-report and the nurses' self-justifying of (these) accounts' [30]. Without being conscious of it, he reinforced the marginalization complaint raised by the nurse authors. He also held the view that the 'moral inhabitability' being generated in the work place was 'endemic to modern organizational life.' It is certainly true that nurses have been forced to try and provide humane

---

[8]Margaret (Maggie) Willson, British former FNS Nurse-Midwife (1955–1967).

care within an ever-expanding and increasingly inhumane institutional environment, like others do in major corporations in the US.

Unfortunately, Paley implies that this state of affairs is not unusual or 'surprising' and therefore, should not be questioned or challenged. The business model used by institutions has an inexorable, symbiotic economic relationship with the medical establishment. Therefore, one must wonder if perhaps this is the reason that Paley so readily accepts the status quo as merely being 'endemic to modern organizational life.' After all, his is a career that was created by physicians specifically for use within such a framework. Perhaps the success of the FNS as a work environment stems from the fact that a uniquely developed 'nursing model' and not the medical or business models was at its core and a nurse was at its helm in the organization's early years. Nursing there was inherently viewed as both a vocation and a profession not a vocation *or* a profession. Its nurses were valued by both the organization and the community as health professionals and were completely autonomous in their practice and thus knew exactly who they were within both cultures. Therefore, what was 'endemic' to its organizational life was a culture that proved to be the direct opposite of what existed elsewhere, regardless of the demands of the Appalachian practice environment and perhaps as a direct result of it as well as its relative isolation from the rest of the nation. The FNS provided a 'morally habitable' environment for its members as well as the local community it served and in this way, it adequately compensated for any tangible benefits lacking as a direct result of its practice environment being harsh, rural and isolated. The reverse of this condition is much more difficult to achieve and in fact, in the Service's later years, as the cultural complexion of the region as well as the organization began to become more and more indistinguishable from the rest of the nation, professional autonomy waned and dissatisfaction escalated not only within the organizational structure, but also between nurses and the community.

5.3 'Morally Uninhabitable' or Just 'Modern Organizational Life?'

Moral values, along with traditions, laws, behaviour patterns and beliefs are the defining features of a culture. Moral values are things held to be right or wrong or desirable or undesirable. Though Breckinridge was quoted as saying she valued 'ideas' (facts) not 'ideals' (morals)' she was able to provide an ideal, that is to say morally inhabitable, health care environment for both her nurses and the local community due solely to the fact that she made a point of acquiring and considering all of the available facts (ideas) prior to making any decision, choosing a deliberate course of action or offering her opinion [31]. As a result, there was a profound difference between the organizational culture and ultimately the work environment, which existed outside of Appalachia andthe one that existed in her Service's early years. The approach Breckinridge had taken was also crucial in the identity formation of those early FNS nurses. For FNS nurses it was the difference between being controlled by the institution or inspired by a trusted leader; coping with a difficult and complex work environment or promoting change within it; providing effective nursing actions or experiencing meaningful nursing practice.

An organization's culture can contribute to or hinder successful strategy execution. In the case of the FNS, the culture initially contributed significant and successful district, public health and midwifery services to the people of Eastern Appalachia as evidenced by the nurses as well as community members' many positive comments concerning its provision of care in the organization's early years. The negative comments made by both the nurses and community members about the Service after Breckinridge's death also illustrated how the organizational culture changed and hindered the provision of care by creating a morally uninhabitable environment for its nurses and ultimately served to alienate its patrons as well. The FNS's ability to successfully implement health care to the peoples of Eastern Appalachia in the organization's latter years was certainly curtailed by government interference but its demise was not blamed entirely on the move from community to institutional provision of care that this change dictated as the sole cause of this failure by either the nurses or the community. They also saw the change in the organization's culture as a contributing factor as well. The organization's beliefs and strategies were no longer compatible with the community's and furthermore, with its community service and humanitarian focus gone it was no longer compatible with that of its 'feeder' culture (wider society) for either its physicians or its nurses.

Historically, the true nature and complexity of the recruitment and retention issues in nursing practice lies embedded within the complexity of these changes within its practice and education cultures. Have nurse leaders within institutionalized care environments defined themselves by the same attributes that they believe defines the institution in order to create a meaningful 'relationship' with it and thus identify with and belong to it? Has this 'corporate' identity impeded nursing leadership's ability to impact the culture from within by improving the work environment of nurses as well as the care delivery environments of patients? [32] If this is indeed the case, the tragedy has become that the defence mechanism being used to protect this identity, which has been namely to blame others for it, has lead to further crisis with tragic effects on the discipline of nursing, nurses, patients and the health care delivery environment [33]. The 'crisis prone' manage in the belief that they can handle a crisis by increasing their power or technology, denying the possibility of a crisis or involving fate as an excuse to do nothing about it [34]. Nurse leaders who find themselves working within such situations may well feel trapped by the same structural and bureaucratic rigidity as their employees and end up merely trying to survive within it in much the same way that their employees that stay do [35].

The idea that there even is a crisis in the health care industry and that it is escalating exponentially in relation to both the dominant culture and technological advances is just beginning to enter the collective psyche of the general population as evidenced by an article that ran in the Pittsburgh, PA *Tribune Review*. The article, entitled 'Stress puts health-care industry in crisis,' begins with the statement that most people are aware that there is a national shortage of nurses and that doctors often experience serious depression that put them at a higher suicide rate than males in other professions. It then goes on to lament the fact that "talented and skilled workers are entering and leaving the health-care professions in a revolving-door-fashion." The authors credit 'stress' as the symptom and cite the cause as "problems from every facet of society falling on health care workers" [36]. This article was different than most in that it does not cite stress as a cause, but rather a symptom of a much larger issue. FNS nurses described very similar stresses at the Service in its latter years citing that though the FNS always had some difficulty recruiting nurses and physicians, after the advent of the massive changes associated with government interference, the problem escalated. A former FNS nurse who was at the Service from 1964 to 1967 as a public health nurse, 1973–1976 as faculty in the Graduate School of Midwifery and from 1993 to 1996 as part-time faculty in the Community-Based Nurse-Midwife Education Program stated that one of the worst things about working at the FNS was "interpersonal conflicts," She stated that "cliques" developed, "feelings were hurt," every "relationship magnified" and the teaching staff had to sort out all of the problems.[9]

A newer twenty-first century phenomenon cited in the *Tribune Review* article not experienced at the FNS was the rise of inter-workplace violence and verbal and in some cases physical abuse, which are attributed to the increased pressure that is being placed upon those health care workers who choose to remain in the 'health care industry.' Nursing research has also identified this phenomenon and attribute it to numerous causes, among them oppressed group behaviour [37]. This situation was credited for having created the cyclical crisis of nurses leaving the profession, thereby generating an environment that was even more difficult for the nurses remaining. In a recent study completed by the Federation of Nurses and Health Professionals (FNHP) it was reported that as many as 50% of currently employed registered nurses have considered leaving client care within the past 2-year period. Another study completed by the American Nurses Association (ANA) found as many as 54% of nurses reported they would not recommend nursing as a profession. The reasons for this were inadequate staffing, heavy workloads and increased use of mandatory overtime [38]. In addition, educators, administrators and staff were also cited as sources for the departure of nurses from the discipline and for not working together to create a "culture of caring" that would serve to keep nurses from leaving [39].

It has also been pointed-out that though many of these studies done by nurses underscore the problem, identify some causes for the problem and even makes recommendations that provide direction in what needs to be done, however, *how* these recommendations are to be met was lacking. Turkel [40] stated a *culture* [italics added] of caring within the work place must be created if the art and science of nursing was to survive [40].

---

[9]Phyllis Long, American former FNS Nurse (1964–1967; 1973–1976; 1993–1996).

The proliferation of studies that exist which cite the causes for nursing shortages illustrates the difficulties inherent in creating sustained positive institutional change and also explains why fidelity to institutions as well as other nurses within them has not been forthcoming.

It can also be said with confidence that most nurses have always hoped to receive more from their labour with human beings than a wage or they would not have chosen nursing as a career, regardless of where they stand on the 'vocation' versus 'profession' debate. A former FNS Midwifery-Nursing Student had this to say about her time working at one of the district outposts (Brutus Centre): "Everyone that was there wanted to be there. It was like an extended family… There was little clock watching, except for timing contractions. Excellent *care* [italics added] was the reward".[10] This 'reward' is something that nurses today are finding harder and harder to achieve. A nurse with seven years of experience expressed her disappointment with not being able to meet the many expectations of the institution (i.e. administration, managers, physicians, families, patients, ancillary departments and other health care areas such as physical therapy, etc.) even though she fully realized that they were totally unrealistic expectations, even in the most optimal circumstances. Still she admitted, "This is my chief complaint and source of discontent".[11] Another former FNS nurse who presently still practices as a Nurse Practitioner, a degree she earned at the FNS, explained why she would not consider working for the FNS today:

> The memories of how *enriching* [italics added] it was when I was there,… it's not that place anymore, you know? The delivery system, the health care delivery system is totally changed and it still has a few district clinics but it's not the same. It's like working in a primary care clinic somewhere that you could plunk down anywhere and those *connections* [italics added] to the community are not the same anymore because of that, because it's just a place to go do a days work.[12]

It is difficult to know how to approach fixing what was once described as an enriching environment that has become 'a work place.' It is even more difficult when the environment has come to be described by nurses today as 'a shock,' 'anticlimactic,' 'disillusioning,' 'factory-like;' the negativity therein 'a daily struggle to rise above' and generally lacking in 'enthusiasm, motivation and professional growth'.[13] Science and technology are embodied within corporate culture making methodical, systematic and controlled environments the norm and observable, objective, experimental and empirical evidence highly prized within the institution.

---

[10] Jean Corner-Rowan, British former FNS Nurse-Midwife (1964–1966).

[11] Topcat TC. Primarily hospital staff nurse for 5 years; brief stints in newborn nursery, occupational nursing, physicians' office (family practice) and as a campus nurse. Date surveyed 24/11/2007.

[12] Judy Haralson-Rafson, American former FNS Nurse (1971–1976; 1971 Graduate of FNS Family Nurse Practitioner Program).

[13] Sloan MS. Hospital operating room staff nurse for 2.5 years; research .5 years, Sable, J., Hospital staff nurse for 2 years, Slamp, L., Hospital staff nurse for 2.75 years, Ann, J., Hospital oncology nurse <1 year, and Smar, R., Hospital obstetrics nurse for 5 years.

Those things deemed unscientific such as intuition or instinct, and unempirical, that is individual, personal and subjective are not. Nurses have attempted to quantify those aspects of their work that are an 'art' and not a science for decades with minimal success. An article in the 1935 FNS *Quarterly Bulletin* attempted to show statistically how the nurse spent her day. However, Statistician Marion S. Ross admitted that there was no such thing as a "typical" day as "no 2 days were the same" for FNS nurses, making quantification extremely difficult.[14] In much the same way quantification of non-task oriented technical skills such as advocacy, education, care management, comfort, counselling or just listening to a patient still remains elusive to quantify and thought of as merely 'hand holding' by some nurses and non-nurses alike. Staffing tools developed for hospitals claiming to calculate accurately the "full time equivalent nursing establishment required for a ward or unit" often reward the higher tech areas that require more skill tasks on the part of the nurse working with equipment, while the medical and elder care units continue to have deficits [41]. This demonstrates both the worth placed upon these values by society as well as the business sector to which the modern health care industry definitely belongs.

The Second World War served to advance many surgical techniques and medical treatments particularly in emergency care, trauma, intensive care, wound care, burn treatment, mental health and rehabilitative care. As medical technology, steadily advanced hospitals became the central repository for costly equipment and people began to expect a level of quality in the care these facilities provided. This shift in focus caused many that previously viewed public health or community based services as the way to best meet the health care needs of the population as somehow second rate to the larger, technologically sophisticated institutions that had sprung up in their place [42]. Those in America and Britain unfortunate enough to warrant medical care in isolated rural areas often had to find either the money, transportation or both necessary to get to a doctor or hospital. They more often than not either did without or relied on the existing herbal or 'folk' remedies [43].

By the 1950s, the quest for health services was steeped in the belief in the powers of medical science, the availability of private insurance and the needs of the 'baby boom' generation in the US. Meanwhile, declining enrolments in nursing schools and the loss of graduates through marriage at a time when hospitals were admitting millions of patients every day led to yet another critical nursing shortage but despite this fact, hospital administrators continued to pay nurses inadequate salaries [44]. Nursing leaders on both side of the Atlantic, albeit reluctantly at first began to discuss the use of collective bargaining techniques to obtain the salaries and working conditions that nurses needed in order to adequately care for patients, consolidate power and achieve their goals outside of a system in which existed numerous centralized power structures, each with its own agenda and the political clout to impose them [45]. Eventually, researchers and the general public began to question whether biomedical advances alone created the phenomenal decrease in morbidity and mortality that had occurred over the last century as it was already becoming clear that

---

[14]FNS Quarterly Bulletin 1935, 85M1: FNS, Box 25, Fol. 2., 50.

some antibiotics often encouraged the development of additional resistant strains in bacteria. Research began to suggest that perhaps environmental changes, higher standards of living, better housing, nutrition and the emergence of family limitation had also impacted the decline in morbidity and mortality in the first half of the century. An approach to care which began to address these 'non-biomedical' issues began to emerge in the modern provision of health care from which a host of health care providers evolved. Yet the physician remains the central figure through which all of this care is disseminated. The relationship between nurses and physicians and their roles, hierarchy and value assignation within the institutional setting is more fully explored in the following chapter.

5.4 Institutional Environments: Why Nurses 'Eat Their Young'

Three nurses presently in practice used the same terminology in reference to how nurses related to one another declaring that we '…eat our young.' This is remarkable as both the perspective and the language used by all three nurses were unsolicited and in answer to questions regarding what they 'didn't like about nursing' and was nursing 'all they thought it would be.' Two of these nurses were US nurses, one with 2 years and the other with 5 years of experience. Neither of these nurses liked the attitude of the 'older' nurses that they practice with nor felt particularly supported by the profession. The third, a Master's prepared Canadian nurse had 23 years of experience and began her practice as a graduate of a hospital school of nursing. Her description of training echoes those made by US and UK nurses alike in similar educational environments. She attributed the 'eat our young' nursing phenomenon to a 'sense of inferiority that makes us (nurses) uncomfortable and threatened by anyone or anything new'.[15] She goes on to state that nursing likes too much the 'old' ways and has 'difficulty with change' that 'contradicts the way we've always done it.' This comment ostensibly made about nurses and the profession of nursing more adequately reflects the entrapment by structural bureaucracy and rigidity within the institutional culture that continues to dominate where nurses practice [35].

A long time FNS nurse was quoted as saying the following regarding crisis management at the Service:

> We (FNS) have always had crises, the depression, the war, Mary Breckinridge's death… Sometimes we didn't know if we could make it, but we always pulled through. The FNS will always make it [46].

---

[15]Morrison S. Hospital staff nurse for 1 year; critical care for 10 years; pain management for 13 years.

The FNS did indeed survive and the Service's survival was a direct result of women like her who identified themselves with it and its work. Note her repeated use of the word 'we' to describe herself in relation to the FNS. This was particularly remarkable as she had long since retired when she made this statement and had come to the Service from Great Britain in the 1930s. She was also at the Service before, during and after the advent of sweeping governmental change in Appalachia. It is also noteworthy that the crises identified by this nurse were all external to the organization. This stands in stark contrast to the types of comments made by nurses working within health care organizations today. When asked their thoughts on the profession and role of nurses in the future, language used to describe the profession included, 'If *it* [italics added] doesn't change soon, I don't know,' 'I am fearful for the future of nursing, I know that major changes need to take place to adapt and move towards the future, but I don't see anything happening right now' and 'I worry about the future of nursing. It could be fabulous but I don't see that at this time…I continue to eagerly support the work and position of nursing but am dismayed at the thought that the necessary changes may never come and will likely not be seen in my lifetime'.[16] Other comments centred on the fact that things were changing and positive comments were made regarding how 'more technology' was in nursing's future, how ground had been gained via nurses becoming primary healthcare providers with advanced degrees such as Nurse Practitioners and through the continued need for nurses to 'specialize' in order to be competent in the areas where they work (Emergency Room, Operating Room, Coronary Care Units, etc.).[17]

Hope was also expressed regarding nursing's future and the role of nurses in future, in particular that 'nursing would be recognized as a true profession,' while others foresaw the 'nursing shortage getting worse'; 'no change in nursing or nurse roles in future' or worse, that the 'role of nurses has already been reduced to that of technician, pill pusher and recording secretary' coupled with the "fear" that 'with the current trend this would only get worse'.[18] Others expressed "fear" that nurses 'will never be fully respected or (nursing) reach the heights that *it* [italics added] could reach.' Note the use of nouns such as, 'nurses, 'nursing' or 'it' to describe the discipline and not the possessive, relational language consistently used by FNS nurses to describe themselves, fellow nurses or the profession within the FNS. These comments on the surface appear to contradict one another but upon closer examination, there are a few key elements underlying all of them. One was that the language used by some of the nurses currently in practice was bereft of the 'we' descriptor entirely and that the perception of nurses without it were either completely fatalistic in tenor or blissfully optimistic that technology and skill would raise nursing's prospects within the institution where the profession had not been able to do so. Also, all of these responses dealt with the institutional crises experienced by nurses that orig-

---

[16]Deb4, Geriatrics for 12 years; hospital staff nurse for 3 years; emergency room for 4 years; home health for 6 years; part-time psychiatric nurse for 5 years.

[17]Randon L. Hospital neonatal intensive care unit <1 year.

[18]Smarr F. Hospital obstetrics nurse for 5 years.

inated within the organization and not those impacting the profession from outside. This would suggest a professional identity crisis on the part of some of the nurses in practice resulting from a work culture in which their professional identity was either threatened by or competing with that of the institution.

When the descriptor 'we' was used by nurses in practice, the tenor of the comments, though distinctly less positive than those made by former FNS nurses, were decidedly more passionate and optimistic. These included comments such as, 'If we don't change soon, I foresee nursing as a profession that will be drowning… I think unless we make some significant movement in nursing we might be headed towards an even larger shortage'; 'I hope that we will become more autonomous in our profession, that we are seen as our own profession and not simply an extension of doctors'; 'We are going to have to morph, we are going to have to be more educated and independent within our own ranks, we are going to have to prove that we are indeed a professional part of the health care team and as such do more research to help with patient outcomes'; 'My hope is that we learn to use and utilize healthcare more efficiently and wiser, respecting patient, family and health care providers' wishes and expertise.[19] Perhaps one nurse expressed it best when she said:

> We [italics added] have to fight. We [Italics added] have to talk louder and longer. We [Italics added] have to dig deep for the fortitude and resolve that will be required of us in the coming years. The future is bleak but on the horizon, is a shimmer of hope that if we harness and nourish we can make all the difference in the world for our patients and for ourselves. Between the nursing shortage and the dollar watchdogs of companies our backs will bend but we cannot allow these events to break the traditions of nursing. Nursing is on a historical journey, just as it has always been, just as it always will so long as nurses care enough to make it so. I am willing to fight to save our dying profession. (I see the role of nurses in future as) an equal. A body of knowledge and a contender that people will respect and seek out. If we cannot become these things then I fear we will become the handmaidens of long ago with no legs to stand on and all alone.[20]

Aside from the striking use of the word 'we' or lack thereof, what was perhaps the most significant response to the question of nursing's future, was no response at all. Four nurses who are presently in practice all with ten or more years of experience chose not to address the question of the profession or the role of the nurse in future at all.

A nurse with only 5 years of experience made this observation 'Absolutely nurses have changed, I do not know if it is better or worse, I think it is just different'.[21] Yet experienced and novice nurses alike tended to focus on technological, economic, political or ideological rationales for schisms within the disciple and cite them as the causes for its identity crisis. Few consider the role that institutional cultures play in crisis conception and resolution. This is evident in a statement made by a nurse

---

[19] Onster V. Hospital staff nurse for 1 year; telemetry 3.5 years; critical care 2 years; dialysis 1 year; research 2 years.

[20] Miller A. Hospital paediatric nurse for 4 years; educator for <1 year.

[21] Cranford D. Hospital staff nurse for 2 years; critical care for 15 years.

with 5 years of experience regarding her perceptions on the change in nurses enter-ing practice and suggested modes for improvement within the discipline:

> Right now in nursing we have three different generations (baby boomers, gen x, echo/gen y) so with each generation comes a new generational culture and work ethic. I think that as a profession we need to adapt to the people who are in it. The newer generations are more tech savvy and if we want nursing to be more attractive to this generation then we need to be more technologically advanced profession. As the external environment and culture shift, nursing will also need to shift. I do see some movement, but I think nursing needs to pick up the pace (see Footnote 20).

Note the focus on generational culture, work ethic and adaptation by nursing to the culture of wider society. Indeed, a feature in the *Pennsylvania Nurse* echoed the challenges nursing faces with recruitment of mixed generations in the institutional workplace in an article which proposed that today's workplace was increasingly diverse and that for the first time in history four generations are working side-by side in the *business landscape* [Italics added]. Note the use of the terminology to describe the work environment of the nurse as a 'business landscape.' The article also contended that each generation brings with it differing values, attitudes and expectations, and that previous "models of managing the American workforce may no longer work" as a result of this. The major sources of workplace friction between the generational cohorts were identified as differing philosophies on chain of com-mand, clashing values regarding work-life balance and differing levels of techno-logical competency and the reluctance to learn electronic technology [47]. But is this changing philosophy, value and apparent educational resistance associated with generational cohort perspectives within the discipline the cause of crisis or are they merely the result of the institutional rigidity inherent within the 'business landscape?'

It is a common misconception that older workers are unwilling to try new things. Boron et al. (2010) found that older adults reported using a wide variety of technol-ogy items at both home and work and that positive attitudes outnumbered negative ones, suggesting that older adults perceived the benefits of technology use to out-weigh the costs of such use [48]. Becton et al. [49] extended generational effects research by actually examining the differences in workplace behaviors drawing from commonly held generational stereotypes, and it appears the effects of genera-tional membership on workplace behavior are not as strong as suggested by the commonly held stereotypes. Such as, Baby Boomers would exhibit fewer job mobil-ity behaviors and more instances of compliance-related behaviors in comparison with both GenXers and Millennials, while GenXers would be less likely to work overtime in comparison with Baby Boomers and Millennials. Though results pro-vided some support for the job mobility and overtime work and partial support for the compliance related behavioral differences between these generations, the effect sizes for these relationships were small. The existing empirical research provides mixed evidence for significant generational differences in important values and atti-tudes amongst workers [49].

A US nurse with 5 years of experience said that she had noticed a difference in the 'attitudes' of nurses who are 45–50 years of age when compared with those who are 25–40 years of age. She explained, 'newer nurses have less commitment to the profession or the institution and feel that getting another job is no big deal.' Further, she felt that the younger nurses tended to deal with the doctors differently as they 'didn't see a "hierarchy"' (see Footnote 18). Another young nurse stated that older nurses just "followed orders".[22] This would appear to support the attitudes attributed to specific generations, namely, 'Generation X,' who are said to be unimpressed with authority, reluctant to commit and more techno literate than previous generations. Indeed, FNS nurses attributed many of the negative changes at the FNS in its latter years as much to the lack of commitment and dedication on the part of its newer nurses as it did to the advent of hospitalized care delivery in Appalachia.[23]

Yet common experiences should not prescribe common attitudes among all members of a particular generational group thus stereotyping them but rather be used to more closely examine these behaviors and attitudes. It was a recent graduate from a US university school of nursing who made the following statement regarding orientation at her new job in a hospital setting:

> My orientation at my new job was made difficult by senior nurses who were only interested in making their days easier by making mine harder. I was routinely 'dumped' on during that first year and since then have developed a sharper, more cynical attitude toward my co-workers (see Footnote 22).

This nurse stated that she wanted to be a nurse 'since the fourth grade after reading a book about Florence Nightingale.' She reportedly admired her (Nightingale) and wanted to be just like her, carrying this attitude through nursing school. She stated that she wanted to be an asset not only to her patients but to the community as well, feeling that she had a higher purpose to fulfilling her life. This young nurse saw nursing as her 'calling.' She admitted that her attitude had changed since her "naïve nursing school days" and at times to feeling "bitter and angry". In two short years of institutional practice, this enthusiastic, idealistic individual developed what she described as a 'cynical attitude' toward other nurses and viewed herself as 'naïve' to have held such high ideals. This value shift was a direct result of being forced to conform to this organization's culture, something that perhaps the more 'senior' nurses she worked with had already done. Using the generational cohort perspective, this young nurse should have been less dedicated and committed than her more 'senior' co-workers but the direct opposite was in fact true. Her scepticism was born of bitter experience within the institutional culture and not something she brought to either the profession or the institution in which she practiced nursing.

The generational cohort perspective was also challenged by the experiences of a former American FNS nurse who stated her 'first nursing job' was as a staff nurse with the FNS in 1960 (see Footnote 2). She also attributed her desire to come to the FNS to the inspiration provided via a book and admiration for a prominent nursing

---

[22] Sable J. Hospital staff nurse for 2 years.
[23] Molly Lee, British former FNS Nurse-Midwife (1950–1970s).

leader, in this instance it was Mary Breckinridge and not Florence Nightingale whom she wanted to "emulate" after reading Breckinridge's autobiography, *Wide Neighbourhoods*. She stated that as a student nurse in a major, metropolitan teaching hospital in Boston, Massachusetts, she had seen quite a few emergencies and felt prepared as a new graduate to go to the FNS. In training, she had seen disasters like fires, plane crashes, shootings and automobile accidents that brought in victims to the emergency department. She explained that they didn't have 'specialized care units like Intensive Care Units or Cardiac Care Units' in those days so they handled all of these emergencies themselves. Even so, before hiring her, the FNS scheduled a meeting and she went out to the Service with her mother for an interview. She was hired but stayed only 8 months as she ended-up marrying a local man and moving out of the area. This nurse related that she never drove the jeeps as she never desired to do so on the terrain (through the water), and was supervised by another nurse pretty closely throughout her tenure there. What is more, she preferred this as the role and responsibilities of the nurse in the rural setting was much greater than that of the urban setting that she was used to. This nurse also equated the working conditions at the FNS to that of "third world countries" and though she noted and admired the autonomy being demonstrated by the "English Nurses" of longer standing, she did not desire it for herself.

A former long time FNS nurse discoursed on how the idealism exhibited by these younger nurses coming to the Service coupled with the autonomy conflicts being generated by the institutional culture being foisted upon the FNS in its latter years ultimately caused the deterioration of the Service's relationally focused work environment in her response to the question, 'For what reason did you leave the FNS?' She stated:

> Many. There was much frustration with administration. Young, idealistic nurses were given much autonomy and there was a lack of older/wiser guidance. There was conflict about the role of nurses, midwives, doctors and little guidance to sort it out. Frustration boiled over due to long work hours, call days, no chance for escape for diversion or to meet people who were not co-workers (see Footnote 9).

By 1960 the ENOVID birth control study had been underway for a year and the outposts which had been staffed in the past with either one or two nurse midwives with public health experience were now being staffed with one public health nurse and one nurse-midwife as birth rates at the FNS began to decline. It became increasingly difficult for the FNS to find nurses with either public health or midwifery experience due to the rise of specialized care and the technology to deliver it that drove the provision of health care out of the community and into the institutional setting, a move that also created a need for less midwives and a curtailment of the autonomy of the midwives who remained as physicians needed to be present for births [50]. It was also at this time that the clear and explicit philosophy, norms, values and beliefs of the FNS began to disintegrate. The strong sense of identity within the organization and the standing that this identity had among the local community began to collapse.

All of the nurses interviewed who came prior to 1960 or left prior to the advent of governmental interference when asked, 'what were some of the worst things about working for the FNS,' gave vastly different responses. They were much more reluctant to identify anything negative, which would suggest an organizational loyalty born of the FNS's unique reciprocal relational-reward culture. The majority of them stated that they could not think of anything bad about working at the FNS. The negative things these nurses did choose to relate were, having to work without any medical doctor *in emergent situations* [italic added], the lack of appropriate finances to repair the hospital roof or having to do a variety of 'non-nursing' chores; chores that included giving guidelines to the men hired to do repairs or seeing to 'termite control.' It was the nurses who experienced the brunt of the changes in the Service's operation in its latter years who cited 'interpersonal conflict' and 'corporate culture' as the worst things about working for the FNS. Another long time American FNS nurse also used the term 'corporate culture' to describe how the organization's administration operated in its latter years. She went on to state that several of the nurses coined the phrase "perpetual chaos" to describe how solutions were sought from the doctors and staff at this time. As she saw it, it was 'too much flying by the seat of our pants' when it came to necessary planning and organization in the day-to-day activities of the Service (see Footnote 12).

Enculturation is the process whereby an established culture teaches an individual by repetition its accepted norms and values, so that the individual can become an accepted member of the society and find their suitable role [51]. Most importantly, it establishes a context of boundaries and correctness that dictates what is and is not permissible within that society's framework. This process of learning is life-long and affects not only the individual being conformed to it but also wider society. These cultural elements are learned through communication in the form of language and gestures. They are also technological, economic, political, interactive, ideological and world view perpetuating. A world view is a framework of ideas and beliefs through which an individual interprets the world and interacts in it. Our worldview is formed by our education, our upbringing, the culture we live in and the media. For many people, their worldview is simply something they have absorbed by osmosis from their surrounding cultural influences.

For nurses' professional enculturation and subsequent identity formation has proven to be difficult if not impossible to achieve as the established practice environment has never been wholly concerned with professional nursing but rather has perpetuated a conglomeration of the institutional norms and values being generated external to the profession, which unfortunately were often in direct opposition to those that would create characteristics of a strong nursing culture. As a result, nurses have difficulty with cultural and professional identity formation; the fundamental building block upon which shared; conceptual, meaningful symbols and communication are possible for members of a culture [52]. It is this meaning system that is perpetuated by members in order to propagate the culture through learned transmission, which refers to cultural traits and broader cultural patterns inclusive of language, technology, institutions, beliefs and values that are transmitted across generations and continuity is maintained through the nature of the education and training processes both formal and informal. Historically, nurses have perpetuated a somewhat skewed professional identity as a result of the enculturation they have experienced within institutions where they have been educated and practice and within which they have either limited or no decision-making input or control.

An organization's culture is composed of the character of its members. The character of an organization's members is comprised of the assumptions, values, norms and tangible signs (artefacts) of its members and these are demonstrated by their behaviours. Newer members of an organization soon come to sense the particular character of an organization and since a culture is a shared, learned, symbolic system of values, beliefs and attitudes, members of it also bring distinctive sets of spiritual, material, intellectual and emotional features of the wider society to which they belong and this also shapes and influences the perceptions and behaviours of the group. Breckinridge adhered to the progressive and feminist policies that arose from the industrial era in which she lived and valued many of the monastic, militaristic, Victorian and vocational aspects associated with the discipline of nursing as a result of this. She was also reported by those she worked with and people that knew her as innovative, visionary, an exceptional leader and well ahead of her time in many respects.[24] Her personal and professional character set the tone of her organization, and influenced the recruitment, retention and work environment of her Service. Her character also shaped the image of her organization, nurses and the practice of nursing to local, national and international communities for as long as she lived. Even after her death, Breckinridge (and by default her Service) continued to be revered in many respects even when both the nurses and local community recognized that the Service no longer provided the type of care for which it had become renowned. Moreover, hers was a unique institution in two respects. Firstly, it was a *nursing* institution, founded and administrated by and for nurses. Secondly, it was controlled, managed and directed with precious little outside interference in its early days save the philanthropic donations. Hence, it had only one agenda, to meet the health care needs of the local community with an eye toward replicating its success by providing a training field for preparation of nurses as midwives for other isolated areas of the country.

Just how successful her demonstration in Eastern Appalachia proved to be was evident by the fact that other isolated areas of the world came to her Service and replicated her model on an international scale.[25] It also had a singular philosophy, namely that professional nurses and the discipline of nursing needed to be supported in order to achieve this goal.[26] If that meant sending nurses to Britain for nurse-midwifery training or teaching certifications, then that's what needed to be done. If it meant starting a nurse-midwifery school in order to get nurse-midwives during wartime, then that's what happened.[27] If it meant securing the place of nurse-midwives in Kentucky via starting a professional organization, then that is exactly

---

[24]Interview #82OH05FNS148, 1982, Dr. Mary Weiss and Dr. Pauline Fox.

[25]Madonna Buret-Spratt, American FNS Midwifery School Graduate of 1960.

[26]Reprint from FNS Quarterly Bulletin 1948, 85M1: FNS, Box 25, Fol. 21.

[27]Letter of Petition for FNS Graduate School of Midwifery, 1939, 2005M547: FNS, Box 227, Fol. 1.

what she did.[28] This created a very strong cultural identity amongst FNS nurses in the organization's early years. It was also what drew loyalty from the community members it served.

5.5 Institutional Versus Professional Identity or 'Whose Gal Are You?'

The phrase 'Whose are you?' required answering in Appalachia before any further interaction with a community member was possible. A recognized identity to which an individual 'belonged' needed to exist before any potential communication could occur between members within this culture as common relational experiences or familial kinship relations were necessary for any socio-economic transaction to occur [53]. In a larger sense, 'belonging' to a particular organization or profession also became essential to attain the power necessary to change political, economic and social realities in the twentieth century outside of Appalachia as well.

Most scholarship about Appalachia by those both within and without the region also betrays a strong anger against American corporate capitalism and blames it for all of the region's woes [54]. Others cite the perpetuation of denigrating stereotypes associated with Appalachia by outsiders of, in effect, 'stripping the Appalachian soul' [55]. However, most sociologists and anthropologists who have looked into small Appalachian rural communities found the region to be hardly a homogenous one. It is actually divided by family reputation, income differentials and degree of urban sophistication with those closest to the city deemed superior and those in more rural or remote areas being viewed as the poorest and least powerful [56]. Yet this has not stopped romantically inclined intellectuals seeing the entire region as the keeper of the best of traditional, historic America, that is individualistic, self-sufficient and self-sacrificing [57]. Equally, ideologues concerned for the region's or nation's future, see Appalachia as representative of everything negative about America, that is of the gun toting, violent, poor, environment exploiters, welfare-dependent, superstitious and racist ilk [58]. This reality is the invention of mainstream American intellectuals who have made Appalachia into an entity that they believe American society either needs or needs to fix. Parallels could certainly be drawn with the image perpetuated by corporate America about nursing. The historical images and icons of the profession have been caricatured as either monastic, obsequious relics of the past or idealized angels devoid of the need for practicalities such as a living wage, decent hours and a morally habitable work environment. These 'image' distortions and perpetuations by those both without and within the discipline will be discussed more fully in Chap. 9.

---

[28]Frontier Nursing Service Professional Organization Series, 1928, University of Kentucky in Lexington, USA.

The question of 'whose one is' also became a complex one for the FNS and in a larger sense Appalachia in the Service's latter years. This was due primarily to the rise of educational and practice institutions as well as professional and governmental organizations outside of the region, which in a futile attempt at a homogeneity that neither existed inside nor outside of the region permeated Appalachia [59]. These intellectual monocracies, which ruled from a distance, created in the region a paradoxical system that was riddled with irreconcilable ideological differences between these converging cultures. It is through the deconstruction of the ideological underpinnings of shared assumptions, varying interpretations, and a shared sense of progress at the FNS and beyond it that learning or improvements can be revealed [60]. These intellectual traditions when combined with the more pragmatic prevailing social and economic realities (especially regarding power and self-interest) can provide the material emphasis and practical expertise that is necessary to proffer sustained, positive change within the nursing practice environment as well as the discipline itself.

Cultures, by predisposition, both embrace and resist change, depending on culture traits [61]. Unfortunately for Appalachia, the FNS and in a wider sense the discipline of nursing, the colonization of corporate institutional ideology produced the replacement of the traits of one culture with those of another. When this occurs, the related processes of assimilation (adoption of a different culture) and transculturation (conflict when societies encroach upon one another) occur on an individual level [62]. The driving force for conflict and hostility within and between Eastern Appalachia, the FNS and nursing in general was simple proximity. The *frontier* that once separated the Appalachian people and the FNS from encroachment was removed in the Services' latter years. For the Appalachian people, roads and an influx of people as well as a culture that in many ways was alien to them invaded the hills. In a larger sense, the boundary which kept the nurse practice environment outside of the institution for FNS nurses was also severely curtailed and forcefully brought within the walls of the institution by these same forces. This changed the nature, complexion and entire focus of the organization. It meant that a means could no longer be found to co-exist between it and the local population. When this happens between dissimilar cultures the inevitable, conflict and hostility ensues [63].

History shows us that the processes of co-existence, which often begins with hostility and polarization often ends with the passing of polarist individuals and their sentiments, which eventually results in resolution—but at what cost? A case in point was a news brief in the *American Nurse*, the official publication of the American Nurses Association, which reported its support of the striking nurses of Kentucky and West Virginia. More than 800 nurses at nine hospitals owned by Appalachian Regional Healthcare gave their reason for the strike as not relating to salary issues at all but rather the "unsafe staffing" practices and "mandatory overtime" conditions that are impeding their ability to provide "quality patient care" [64]. These issues, normally associated with health care provision outside of Appalachia, unfortunately are hardly 'new' issues to nursing. Nurses' narratives from four time periods, 1934, 1979 and 1995, found that *moral distress* [Italics added] was associated with powerlessness, cultural dissonance and role discrepancy with regard to autonomy by nurses. Moral suffering among nurses was also associated with the 'action' problems created within the institutional work environment and it is nurse researchers, educators, administrators and practitioners who should be leading the work to change these environments and support nurse's efforts to cope within them [65].

The Rockefeller Foundation conducted three research studies over a 30-year period at the start of the twentieth century, which provided irrefutable evidence of not only the consistently dismal education and practice environments of nurses but also illustrated the case for it, namely the foundations reluctance to implement reforms or impose any measures deemed unwelcome to other health care groups, namely the American Medical Association, American Colleges of Surgeons, American Hospital Association and the American Public Health Association. This lack of funding commitment to nursing that was afforded to medicine perpetuated the hard work and poor educational conditions that made nursing an unattractive field for young women.

Nurses have not fared well in institutional environments with centralized power structures that adhere to the business model in the delivery of care. They have struggled to secure adequate hours of work, wages, professional autonomy, respect and a 'voice' on the health care team; all key elements inherent within the cultural value one has inside an organization. The FNS possessed a 'morally inhabitable' work environment compared to those institutional settings outside of Appalachia because it fostered a reciprocal relationship with its internal as well as its external community whereby neither was oppressed, powerless exploited or marginalized. So spiritually *enriching* was this environment that external rewards such as an 8-h work day, competitive salary and even personal comforts were readily endured in order to take on the professional persona and cultural identity of the organization. With the advent of a centralized power structure came institutional rigidity and an environment similar to those of institutional settings outside of Appalachia. This negative change was attributed to mixed generations in the work place by the nurses. The hardships, conflicts and frustrations have been attributed by nurses to other nurses and staff within the system and not enculturalization and subsequent identity formation to the system. The role that gender plays and that corporate-consumer culture value assignation have in regard to humanitarian endeavours within this system is discussed in Chap. 6. The moral distress associated with the powerlessness, cultural dissonance and role discrepancy of nurses within educational and institutional work environments and their efforts to cope can then be more fully examined in the subsequent chapters.

References

1. Cohen J. Minority report: working party on the recruitment and training of nurses, vol. 1. London: Metropolitan Library Archives; 1948. p. 72.
2. Cohen J. Minority report: working party on the recruitment and training of nurses. London: Metropolitan Library Archives; 1948. p. 73.
3. Cohen J. Minority report: working party on the recruitment and training of nurses. London: Metropolitan Library Archives; 1948. p. 71.

4. Frederick W. Values, nature and culture in American corporations. New York: Oxford University Press; 1995. p. 109.
5. Cohen J. Minority report: working party on the recruitment and training of nurses. London: Metropolitan Library Archives; 1948. p. 54.
6. Frederick W. Values, nature and culture in American corporations. New York: Oxford University Press; 1995. p. 125.
7. Palmer C. The nursing shortage: an update for occupational health nurses. AAOHN J. 2003;51(12):510–3.
8. Whelan JC. In: Erwin Levold E, Rose K, editors. Research Reports from the Rockefeller Archives Centre: The Nurse Labour Market and the Rockefeller Foundation 1923–1963. An annual publication of the Rockefeller Archives Centre. New York: Sleepy Hollow; 2000. p. 9–13.
9. Whelan JC. In: Erwin Levold E, Rose K, editors. Research Reports from the Rockefeller Archives Centre: The Nurse Labour Market and the Rockefeller Foundation 1923–1963. An annual publication of the Rockefeller Archives Centre. New York: Sleepy Hollow; 2000. p. 10.
10. Whelan JC. In: Erwin Levold E, Rose K, editors. Research Reports from the Rockefeller Archives Centre: The Nurse Labour Market and the Rockefeller Foundation 1923–1963. An annual publication of the Rockefeller Archives Centre. New York: Sleepy Hollow; 2000. p. 11.
11. Cooter R, Pickstone J. Companion to medicine in the twentieth century. New York: Routledge; 2013.
12. Roux G, Halstead J. Issues and trends in nursing: practice, policy and leadership. Burlington: Jones and Bartlett Learning, LLC; 2018. p. 24.
13. Khamisa N, Oldenburg B, Peltzer K. Work related stress, burnout, job satisfaction and general health of nurses. Int J Environ Res Public Health. 2015;12(1):652–66. https://doi.org/10.3390/ijerph120100652.
14. Khamisa N, Oldenburg B, Peltzer K. Work related stress, burnout, job satisfaction and general health of nurses. Int J Environ Res Public Health. 2015;12(1):662. https://doi.org/10.3390/ijerph120100652.
15. Hong L, Barriball K, Zhanga X, While E. Job satisfaction among hospital nurses revisited: a systematic review. Int J Nurs Stud. 2012;49(8):1017–38. https://doi.org/10.1016/j.ijnurstu.2011.11.009.
16. Wai-Tong C, Sin-Yin Y. An investigation of nurses' job satisfaction in a private hospital and its correlates. Open Nurs J. 2016;10(1):99–112. https://doi.org/10.2174/1874434601610010099.
17. Cohen J. Minority report: working party on the recruitment and training of nurses. London: Metropolitan Library Archives; 1948. p. 70.
18. Olsen T. Historical case study of apprenticeship of nurses at Saint Luke's Training School for Nurses (1892–1937). 1991. Unpublished PhD dissertation, University of Minnesota, Minneapolis.
19. Drake R. History of Appalachia. Lexington: University Press of Kentucky; 2003. p. 223.
20. Diddle G, Denham S. Spirituality and its relationships with the health and illness of Appalachian people. J Transcult Nurs. 2010;21(2):175–82. https://doi.org/10.1177/1043659609357640.
21. Puckett A. Seldom ask, never tell: labour & discourse in Appalachia. New York: Oxford University Press; 2002. p. 130.
22. Shackelford L, Weinberg B. On Appalachia: an oral history. Lexington: The University of Kentucky Press; 2015. p. 295.
23. Reid D. Saddlebags full of memories. Burt Lake Michigan, USA; 1992. p. 340.
24. Andrist C, Nicholas P, Wolf K. A history of nursing ideas. Burlington: Jones and Bartlett Publishers, Inc; 2006. p. 152.
25. Shackelford L, Weinberg B. On Appalachia: an oral history. Lexington: The University of Kentucky Press; 2015. p. 38.
26. Friedman L, McGarvie M. Charity, philanthropy, and civility in American history. New York: Cambridge University Press; 2003. p. 48.
27. Friedman L, McGarvie M. Charity, philanthropy, and civility in American history. New York: Cambridge University Press; 2003.

28. Peter E, Macfarlane A, O'Brien-Pallas L. Analysis of the moral habitability of the nursing work environment. J Adv Nurs. 2004;47(4):356–63.
29. Peter E, Macfarlane A, O'Brien-Pallas L. Analysis of the moral habitability of the nursing work environment. J Adv Nurs. 2004;47(4):359.
30. Paley J. Commentary: the discourse of moral suffering. J Adv Nurs. 2004;47(4):364–7.
31. Dammann N. A social history of the frontier nursing service. Sun City: Social Change Press; 1982. p. 108.
32. Hong-Wei H, Balmer J. Identity studies: multiple perspectives and implications for corporate-level marketing. Eur J Market. 2007;41(7/8):765–85. https://doi.org/10.1108/03090560710752393.
33. Thierry P, Mitroff I. Transforming the crisis-prone organization: preventing individual, organizational and environmental tragedies. San Francisco: Jossey-Bass Inc; 1992. p. 4.
34. Thierry P, Mitroff I. Transforming the crisis-prone organization: preventing individual, organizational and environmental tragedies. San Francisco: Jossey-Bass Inc; 1992. p. 33.
35. Thierry P, Mitroff I. Transforming the crisis-prone organization: preventing individual, organizational and environmental tragedies. San Francisco: Jossey-Bass Inc; 1992. p. 6.
36. Light-Hopson J, Hopson EH, Hagen T. 'Stress puts health care industry in crisis', featured in the 'Living' section (B11), Greensburg, Pennsylvania Tribune Review', Friday, 6 Oct 2006.
37. Andrist C, Nicholas P, Wolf K. A history of nursing ideas. Burlington: Jones and Bartlett Publishers, Inc; 2006.
38. Cherniss C. Beyond burnout, helping teachers, nurses, therapists and lawyers recover from stress and dissillusionment, vol. 17. New York: Routledge/Taylor & Francis Group; 2016. p. 37.
39. Tinsley C, France N. The trajectory of the registered nurse's exodus from the profession: a phenomenological study of the lived experience of oppression. Int J Hum Caring. 2004;8(1):8–12.
40. Smith M, Turkel M, Wolf Z. Caring in nursing practice an essential resource. New York: Springer; 2013. p. 481.
41. Waters A. Hospital sector staffing tool launched at CNO conference. Nurs Manag–UK. 2007;14(7):5.
42. Lancaster J. Nursing issues in leading and managing change. New York: Mosby; 1999.
43. Cartwright F, Biddiss M. Disease and history. 4th ed. London: Thistle Publishing; 2014.
44. Nursing Shortage, American Association of the Colleges of Nursing: Fact Sheet. https://www.ic4n.org/wp-content/uploads/2018/02/Nursing-Shortage-Factsheet-2017.pdf. Accessed 19 Jan 2019.
45. Economic Security Program in 1952. Am J Nurs. 1953;53(4):388.
46. Dammann N. A social history of the frontier nursing service. Sun City: Social Change Press; 1982. p. 152.
47. Snook M. Mixed generations in the workplace. The Pennsylvania Nurse, Official Publication of the Pennsylvania Nurses Association; 2006. p. 31.
48. Boron J, Bailey C, Fausseta A, Adams E, Charness N, Czajad J, Djkstrae K, Fiska A, Rogersa W, Sharitf J. Older adults talk technology: technology usage and attitudes. Comput Hum Behav. 2010;26(6):1710–21. https://doi.org/10.1016/j.chb.2010.06.020.
49. Becton J, Walker H, Jones-Farmer A. Generational differences in workplace behavior. J Appl Psychol. 2014;44(3):175–89. https://doi.org/10.1111/jasp.12208.
50. Dammann N. A social history of the frontier nursing service. Sun City: Social Change Press; 1982. p. 132.
51. Ravasi D. Organizational identity, culture and image. In: Oxford handbook of organizational identity; 2016. https://doi.org/10.1093/oxfordhb/9780199689576.013.25.
52. Bates D, Plog F. Cultural anthropology. 3rd ed. Berkshire: McGraw-Hill College; 1990. p. 7.
53. Puckett A. Seldom ask, never tell: labour & discourse in Appalachia. New York: Oxford University Press; 2002. p. 31.
54. Drake R. History of Appalachia. Lexington: University Press of Kentucky; 2003. p. 190.
55. Branscome J. Annihilating the hillbilly: the Appalachian struggle with American institutions. J Committ Southern Churchmen. Winter 1971;128–30.

56. Drake R. History of Appalachia. Lexington: University Press of Kentucky; 2003. p. 217.
57. Biggers J. The United States of Appalachia: how southern mountaineers brought indepen-dence, culture and enlightenment to America. In: Malloy, Shoemaker and Hoard. An Imprint of Avalon Publishing Group, USA; 2007. p. 1.
58. Drake R. History of Appalachia. Lexington: University Press of Kentucky; 2003. p. 218.
59. Martin J. Cultures in organizations: three perspectives. New York: Oxford University Press; 1992. p. 150.
60. Martin J. Cultures in organizations: three perspectives. New York: Oxford University Press; 1992. p. 161.
61. Rhoads K. The culture variable in the influence equation. In: The Public Diplomacy Handbook. New York: Routledge; 2008.
62. O'Neil D. Process of change. Cultural Anthropology Tutorials, Behavioural Sciences Department, Palomar College, San Marco. http://anthro.palomar.edu/tutorials/cultural.htm. Accessed 25 Jan 2019.
63. Cummins T, Whorley C. Organizational development and change. Boston: Cengage Learning; 2014.
64. Employment section. Am J Nurs. 2007;106(1):84–5.
65. Ulrich C, Grady C. Moral distress in the health professions. New York: Springer; 2018.

Chapter 6
Gender and Role Assignments in the Institutional Hierarchy

6.1 Gender, Role Assignments, Institutional Hierarchy and Their Cultural Value

As stipulated in the previous chapter, with the adoption of the corporate (business) and medical models by hospitals, the moral inhabitability of these institutional settings as both educational as well as work environments for nurses has created an identity crisis amongst its ranks. Yet the adversity, moral distress and dissatisfaction experienced by nurses within institutional settings have been attributed to other nurses and staff within the system and not enculturalization and subsequent identity formation to the system. Male gender role assignments within wider society have long been purported to be a major contributor to nursing's 'handmaiden' status within these establishments as well, due to its mostly female ranks. Historically, female gender role assignments have also been successfully used by nurse leaders to elevate and distinguish both the profession as well as women's contribution to the art and science of healing, at a time when neither was valued in the marketplace. This chapter explores the role that gender plays within health care organizational culture and its relationship to humanitarian endeavours within the system.

During both the First and Second World Wars, American and British women began finding new employment opportunities because of the labour shortages created by so many men enrolling for military service and nursing was forced to compete for recruits [1]. World War Two also created a demand for many more nurses in both Britain and the United States. The US government created the Cadet Nurse Corps in 1943. In this way, the government subsidized nursing education so that thousands of young people (mostly women) were recruited to become military nurses for the duration of the war. The training was intense, brief and graduates were put into the labour force quickly [2]. It should also be mentioned that, in spite of the increased levels of nurse recruits to nursing either as civilians or within the

© Springer Nature Switzerland AG 2019   111
E. West, *Frontier Nursing in Appalachia: History, Organization and the Changing Culture of Care*, https://doi.org/10.1007/978-3-030-20027-5_6

military this type of mass recruitment had little regard for retention, and fast-track education strategy was wasteful. As many as thirty to fifty percent of these students left before completing their 3 years of training.

For women, the choices available to them at this time were factory work, women's services or nursing and the direction of labour for unmarried women was toward nursing.

Nurse candidates for entry into the FNS Graduate Midwifery School as well as nurse employees had to be female. This stipulation was reflected in most nursing schools at this time. A letter addressed to the FNS Executive Secretary, Miss Agnes Lewis from one Orin C. Peters, DVM (Doctor of Veterinary Medicine) revealed a request for information on whether the school accepted men.[1] In response Breckinridge's successor, Helen E. Browne, stated 'at the present time we do not have facilities for admitting male students to the school'.[2] With this letter Browne also included information on the School and stated that any potential nurse candidate to be considered for either employment or Midwifery training had to be a registered nurse and have post-graduate experience in nursing. Browne's use of the verbiage, 'at this time' instead of simply stating that the FNS did not admit men suggested that this could change in future as more men were beginning to consider nursing as a career post WWII, though these men were mostly medics during the war and not veterinarians. The fact that Mr. Peters thought that a veterinarian's degree would be a sufficient substitute for a diploma in nursing reflects either the diminished value placed upon nursing in general and midwifery specifically held by society or the complete ignorance that the general population had regarding the educational requirements necessary to practice both. This ignorance continues today, as is alluded to in unsolicited statements made from nurses in practice lamenting the fact that the general public still does not 'value or understand' nurses and that the general public as well as administration, management and other professions, continue to need "improvement in attitudes toward us as a profession".[3] That Browne sent information from the FNS to Peters along with criteria for entry suggests that she was not dissuading him from a career in nursing or even in midwifery but rather encouraging it, even though he was clearly not eligible for entry into their particular program. Browne, like her mentor, Breckinridge tended to base decisions regarding FNS personnel on what was acceptable to the local community. When a Chinese nurse sought information on the

---

[1] Personal Letter from Orin C. Peters to Agnes Lewis, 19 May 1954, 85M1: FNS, Box 38, Fol. 7. Letter requests information on the FNS and asking whether the FNS Graduate Midwifery School accepted men, University of Kentucky in Lexington, USA.

[2] Helen E. Browne Letter to Orin C. Peters 24 May 1954, 85M1: FNS, Box 38, Fol. 7. Brown states 'at this time' we do not have facilities for admitting male students to the school. She did send him information on the school and explained that nurses had to be registered nurses and had to have some 'post graduate experience in nursing' in order to be admitted to the school. University of Kentucky in Lexington, USA.

[3] Morrison S. Hospital staff nurse for 1 year; critical care for 10 years; pain management for 13 years.

FNS, Browne asked the locals if they thought this nurse could practice there. She was told by the local committee community representatives that if anything bad happened during a delivery to either the mother or child it would be blamed on 'her yellow skin.' Browne wrote to this Chinese nurse and explained this to her. The woman countered that it was the first time she had ever been told the truth as to why she was being turned-down for a nursing position [3].

Several letters of inquiry by Licensed Practical Nurses (LPNs) who sought to either enter the training school or work at the FNS were given a polite refusal by Browne. She explained the 'responsibilities were heavy' and that nurse aides (mostly Red Cross nurse aides who volunteered) were only used during the war due to extreme personnel shortages and paid positions for them were not possible.[4] The language used by Browne suggested that the priority was the professional sophistication of the nurse and not necessarily gender or race, but that if these characteristics proved to be significant to the local population and would preclude meaningful care to the community, the Service would opt in favour of the local culture over any prevailing wider social, political, economic or even institutional culture.[5]

Nurse leaders have long felt that a clean break from its vocational roots is essential for professional advancement and have blamed much of its failure to achieve it on nursing's historically uneasy relationship with feminism, the prevailing gender role stereotypes and institutional oppression [4]. In truth, the contributions that prominent nurses and the profession of nursing have made for equal rights, not only for women but also for humanity have remained hidden from the collective consciousness of the general public. Indeed, it was feminism that abandoned nursing in its zeal to move into male-dominated professions. As one writer noted:

> For in the eagerness of some women to embrace new roles has come a denigration of old ones. No one, these women say, should want to be just a housewife; no one with brains should want to be just a nurse. Have a career! Be a doctor! [5]

---

[4]Browne Correspondence to LPNs 1955–1962. Letters from LPN's (1955–1962). Polite refusal responses from Browne to LPN's seeking admission into the FNS Graduate Midwifery School. Browne states 'the responsibility is heavy' and only registered nurses were admitted with some experience. She further explained that nurse aides were used only during war time and were voluntary, not paid positions. University of Kentucky in Lexington, USA.

[5]FNS 01, 2005. Margaret (Maggie) Willson, British former FNS Nurse-Midwife (1955–1967), Date surveyed: 10/08/2003. Date interviewed: 09/04/2005. Interviewer: Edith A. West.

   FNS 02, 2005. Anne Lorentzen, American former FNS Nurse (1963–1965), Date surveyed: 29/12/2003. Date interviewed: 11/03/2005. Interviewer: Edith A. West.

   FNS 03, 2005. Elizabeth 'Hilly' Hillman, British former FNS Nurse-Midwife (1949–1954), Date interviewed: 04/05/2005. Interviewer: Edith A. West.

   FNS 04, 2005. Molly Lee, British former FNS Nurse-Midwife (1950–1970s), Date interviewed: 05/04/2005. Interviewer: Edith A. West.

   FNS 05, 2005. Jean Corner-Rowan, British former FNS Nurse-Midwife (1964–1966), Date interviewed: 11/03/2005. Interviewer: Edith A. West.

   FNS 06, 2005. Judie Pridie-Halse, British former FNS Nurse-Midwife (1960<>–hcn250@ excite.com, Oncology hospital staff nurse for 2years. Date surveyed: 08/09/2004.

Nursing has long struggled with feminist ideology and the aspects therein which could adversely affect its ability to provide public service, while feminists have grappled with the nurture and care aspects inherent to the work of nursing, which they sought to emancipate themselves from and that modern society continues to devalue. It has been suggested that had nursing joined forces with feminists sooner it would not be in the situation it is in today. It could also be argued that had it done so it would have also had to embrace the values and ideals of one of its oppressors. Equality could hardly be gained by devaluing oneself and one's chosen work. The reality is that nursing was the only bastion for women that offered adventure, freedom, self-sufficiency and significant work well into the 1960s. It is also a reality that modern feminists would prefer to overlook.

The introduction of the medical model in nursing at the turn of the century invariably changed the trajectory of the profession from one of purely vocation, which essentially constituted providing comfort to dying, hopeless cases, to one of a trained, highly skilled professional. The evolution of medicine also brought in its wake a host of ancillary occupations which included therapists, pharmacists, X-ray and lab technicians to name a few. Nursing, which was never really highly prized to begin with as a direct result of being deemed a female vocation, came to be viewed as just another ancillary skill. Yet as medical mastery of technique in the cure and treatment of disease progressed in the burgeoning fields of medical/surgical study, and an ever-increasing array of specialty areas arose, much of what was once considered exclusively medical practice became a routine part of nursing practice. With this increase in clinical responsibility nursing has in turn given up much of the custodial patient care that was once considered exclusively nursing practice by Florence Nightingale to unlicensed nursing assistants, domestic and housekeeping staff. Nurses have attributed the discipline's lack of complete professional emancipation to the prevailing Victorian image of servanthood associated with nursing [6]. Some nurses have attempted an approach to professionalism that challenges and purges all association with humanitarianism in efforts to realign the discipline's focus purely on intellectual and technological savvy. This is much more highly valued by the dominant culture, and in its adoption, lays the hope of securing nursing's rightful place in the health care environment as a true professional. Economists and institutional administrators use the opposing side of this debate to keep nurses from earning the wages they deserve and thereby can lower health care operating costs. Neither extreme is an accurate rendering of nursing's roots nor can fully embracing or eradicating either of them achieve for the discipline the status it desires. When Dr. Beasley replaced Helen E. Browne as Director after her stroke in the 1970s, it was a time when what has commonly been referred to as the 'second wave of feminism' was in full swing as the then Committee Chair and cousin of Breckinridge, Marvin Breckinridge, lamented when attending a health meeting in Washington DC as a representative of the FNS:[6]

---

[6]Interview #7808141FNS01, 1978. Marvin Breckinridge, Cousin of Mary Breckinridge, assisted in committee work outside of Appalachia, Interviewed 13 May 1978, Interviewer: Dale Deaton.

Interview#78OH144FNS04, 1978. Matt Gray, long time resident of Appalachia, Interviewed 21 July, 1978, Interviewer: Dale Deaton.

Interview #78OH145FNS05, 1978. Jailey Zizemore, long time resident of Appalachia, Interviewed 26 July 1978, Interviewer: Dale Deaton.

Interview #78OH146FNS06, 1978. Betty Lester, former long time FNS Nurse (English), Interviewed 3 March 1978, Interviewer: Johathan Fried.

Interview #78OH147FNS07, 1978. Frank Bowling, long time resident of Appalachia/ Community Committee Member, Interviewed 1 July 1978, Interviewer: Dale Deaton.

Interview #78OH148FNS08 1978. Martha Lady, FNS Midwifery School Graduate of 1960, Interviewed 4 August 1978, Interviewer: Johathan Fried.

Interview#78OH149FNS09, 1978. Lawrence Bowling, employed with FNS for twenty years, Interviewed 10 August 1978, Interviewer: Dale Deaton.

Interview#78OH150FNS10, 1982. Mary & Clyde Brewer, long time residents of Appalachia who wrote a book on it called "Of Bolder Me" and later called "Rugged Trails of Appalachia", Interviewed 10 August 1978. Interviewer: Dale Deaton.

Interview #78OH51FNS11, 1978. Georgia Ledford, former Secretary for FNS Community Committee & long time resident of Appalachia, Interviewed 17 August 1978, Interviewer: Carol Crow-Carraco.

Interview #78OH152FNS12, 1978. Glenda Davis, long time resident of Appalachia, interviewed 17 May 1978, Interviewer: Carol Crow-Carraco.

Interview #79OH229FNS121, 1982, Mary Martin & Phoebe Hawkins, former FNS Committee Members outside of Appalachia in the Service's 'latter years', Interviewed 23 May 1979. Interviewer: Anne Campbell Ritchie.

Interview #82OH03FNS146, 1982, Agnes Lewis, former long time FNS Secretary, Interviewed 5 January 1979. Interviewer: Dale Deaton.

Interview #82OH05FNS148, 1982, Dr. Mary Weiss (former FNS Medical Director) & Dr. Pauline Fox (former County Health Officer/Appalachia Regional Health Officer), Interviewed 14 February 1979. Interviewer: Dale Deaton.

Interview #82OH08FNS151, 1982, Kate Ireland, former FNS Courier (1951), Interviewed 1 November 1979. Interviewer: Dale Deaton.

Interview #82OH09FNS 152, 1982, Sherman Wooten, long time resident of Appalachia, Interviewed 7 November 1979. Interviewer: Dale Deaton.

Interview#82OH11FNS154, 1982. Wilma Duvall Whittlesey, FNS Secretary from 1929–1936, Interviewed 30 November 1979, Interviewer: Dale Deaton.

Interview #82OH12FNS155, 1982, Betty Lester, former long time FNS Nurse (English): 2nd. Interview on 27 July 1978. Interviewer: Dale Deaton.

Interview #82OH13FNS156, 1982, Betty Lester, former long time FNS Nurse (English): 3rd. Interview on 3 August 1978. Interviewer: Dale Deaton.

Interview #82OH15FNS158, 1982, Lydia Thompson, Prominent Committee Member outside of the FNS, Interviewed: Unknown. Interviewer: Dale Deaton.

Interview#82OH34FNS177, 1982, Mary Stewart, former FNS Courier.

Interviewed 15 January 1980. Interviewer: Marion Barrett and Nancy Albertson.

Interview#82OH37FNS180. Thurston Morton, former Senator & Grandson of Mrs. Thurston Ballard who was very active in FNS committee work outside of Appalachia, Interviewed 24 October 1978. Interviewer: Carol Crowe-Carraco.

Interview #82OH39FNS182, 1982, Beth B. Jones, former FNS Courier from Cincinnati, Ohio whose Aunt Margaret Rogan was a friend of Mary Breckinridge. She went for six weeks and stayed for two years.

Interviewed: UNKNOWN. Interviewer: Marion Barrett.

The antagonism toward men! And a couple of prominent nurses said to me, "What a pity you've got a man as the head of the FNS." I said, Dr. Beasley is a splendid medical director and has a great respect for nursing. But they were just being horrid about it and I couldn't understand it.[7]

Perhaps the reason this antagonism could not be understood by those within the Appalachia region was due to the fact that in the organization's early years physicians there viewed the nurses as colleagues, neither as menials nor competitors. The prominent nurse leaders at this health meeting could not have known how staunch a supporter Dr. Beasley had proven to be to FNS nurses nor how instrumental he was in the creation of a Nurse Practitioner Program there when other physicians refused to support nurses in this 'expanded' role, preferring instead to create physician assistants that would not threaten their existing sole point of access to the health care system. Indeed, had Dr. Beasley not been committed to it, the program certainly would not have come to fruition. It was due as much to the respect for his long standing within the professional medical community as to the political support of the local and state communities in the face of such overwhelming opposition. The FNS organization, Mary Breckinridge's personal renown and her political connections within the medical, local, state and national communities (which survived her death) also contributed to the opening of the program. This was one of the first in the country and still exists today. It should be noted that when Dr. Kooser resigned in 1943 as the FNS Medical Director after 12 years of service to join the Navy, subsequent medical directors who came to the FNS from the outside seldom stayed more than 2 years. Doctor Beasley jointed the service in 1956 and remained longer than any other doctor since the Second World War.

6.2   Nurse–Physician Relationships

Dr. Annie Veech of the Kentucky Bureau of Maternal and Child Health Association evaluated Breckinridge's health care project proposal in 1923 and her request for public funding under the Sheppard-Towner Maternity and Infancy Act to support her project [7]. Veech accused Breckinridge of 'exploiting and misrepresenting mountain people' and 'not going through proper channels.' She felt Breckinridge was challenging her authority and expertise and told Breckinridge that she would not support her or recommend the Child Health Association to report her findings [8].

Undaunted, Breckinridge wrote to Dr. Veech, thanking her for her attention in the matter and stating that she would not bother the bureau for help again:

It is not unusual, I know for public interests [those outside of the establishment] to take the initiative with new ideas. Private initiatives almost always blazes the trail.[8]

---

[7]Interview #78OH147FNS07, 1978. Frank Bowling.

[8]Breckinridge letter to Dr. Annie Veech, 14 November 1923, Frontier Nursing Service 1789–1985, Mary Breckinridge Series: Correspondence 1925–1970. University of Kentucky in Lexington, USA.

Breckinridge's determination to publish her findings on her own if need be and to move forward her Service through private support if public (governmental) assistance was not forthcoming was interpreted by one researcher as a devious attempt to get the Service established at the expense of the unsophisticated image of Appalachian people presented to those outside of the region [15]. Yet Breckinridge's findings were not disputed by Dr. Veech, nor was the wording of the document deemed unseemly. Veech was concerned only with the possible negative reflection it could have on the state of Kentucky and the potential exploitation of the people that might result from such a report being published outside the remit of the health department channels. But Breckinridge herself consistently shared this concern for the people throughout her tenure at the FNS, as is evidenced by her many letters, for example one written to Dr. Arthur McCormak. In it, she asked him to adhere to her policy of not allowing reporters to attend meetings where she spoke to friends and friends of friends, 'privately,' in the hopes of securing support for the work. It had come to her attention that a 'vulgarly worded and inaccurate description (of the people) had found its way into the press'[9]. The relevant newspaper article had been written as though Breckinridge had been interviewed when she in fact she had not. Breckinridge, however, diverged from Veech in the belief that the suppression of her health care findings was necessary in order to protect the people. If improvement was to occur, then research proving both the need and the worthiness of the people to receive it was vital and Breckinridge laboured to demonstrate both in as positive a manner as possible. Perhaps Veech's concern with 'broadcasting' Breckinridge's report may have had more to do with a challenge to her personal authority as a physician or the threat that such a Service would present to the existing establishment status quo. Breckinridge was told that if she did have her report printed at all, it would be circulated 'only to those few who would understand and know how to help'.[10]

Breckinridge was uniquely placed by her social position within the nation's culture to garner allies. She saw herself within her organization's culture as 'commander-in-chief,' her nurses as 'generals' and the doctors who came into the FNS as either 'relatives or friends'.[11] If she was unable to solicit the friendship of physicians who came in contact with her Service she simply did not engage them in power struggles that she knew she would loose. Dr. Stoddard opposed the FNS in its early days. Breckinridge would send patients to his clinics and ask him to come when they needed a doctor and reluctantly he would. He had come into the county before Breckinridge and thus believed he had precedence. One former FNS secretary stated that 'she (Breckinridge) put up with it because she'd put the patient first'.[12] Dr. Stoddard greatly upset Breckinridge with a 'nasty letter' that she then showed to this

---

[9] Breckinridge letter to Dr. Arthur McCormack, 21 January 1926, Frontier Nursing Service 1789–1985, Mary Breckinridge Series: Correspondence 1925–1970. University of Kentucky in Lexington, USA.

[10] Dr. Annie Veech letter to Breckinridge, 31 October 1923. Frontier Nursing Service 1789–1985, Mary Breckinridge Series: Correspondence 1925–1970, University of Kentucky in Lexington, USA.

[11] Interview #82OH34FNS177, 1982, Mary Stewart.

[12] Interview #82OH03FNS146, 1982, Agnes Lewis.

secretary. After taking 3 days to respond, reported the secretary, Breckenridge produced what 'was the most kind, courteous, sincere letter that one could have written and that this was the way Breckinridge replied to all such things' [19].

Although it is certainly true that many doctors have been vocal in their distain for nurses, there are many who have also been their advocates. Those physicians who contested nursing's professional advancement tended to be the advantaged, political leaders within the medical profession, specialists and academics who practised in more urban environments where nurses were viewed as competitors. Fortunately for Breckinridge, not every physician felt as Dr. Veech and they tended to be those without vested interests in the establishment or were physicians who were personal friends and her social equals. They included Dr. Authro T. McCormack, the State Health Officer and Secretary of the Kentucky State Medical Association in the 1930s. Dr. McCormack was consistently supportive of the work in Leslie County and provided Breckinridge with introductions to others within the medical community with whom she would need to garner support if her efforts for the people of Eastern Appalachia were to be realized.[13] The FNS's greatest supporters within the medical community were the general practitioners who worked in rural communities and saw nurses more as colleagues and less of a threat to their practice.

The FNS's first Medical Director, Dr. John H. Kooser, while addressing members of the Eastern Division of the Kentucky State Association of Registered Nurses, had this to say about the FNS Nurse-Midwives he worked with:

> The relationship of nurse to physician and physician to nurse has been and is a very close one, exemplified particularly well in the motto of 'united we stand, divided we fall'… the viewpoint of the nurse-midwife and doctor is necessarily one of co-operation in a program of prevention and conservatism. Nurse-midwives are completely responsible for the normal obstetrical patient. At first thought this is fine; but I should remind you that they must know the abnormal as well, and for two very good reasons. In the first place by knowing 'what is not,' they will know 'what is' normal. In the second place, they must be able to cope with an emergency until medical aid arrives. This sounds simple, but it takes courage to do a manual removal of the placenta or bimanual uterine compression for a haemorrhage knowing the doctor is 4–6 horse-back hours away… and so you see the emergency is not mine alone but the nurse's as well.[14]

Dr. Beasley, who was Kooser's successor and 30-year veteran of the FNS, wrote a five-page letter to colleagues at Johns Hopkins, the University of North Carolina and the University of Kentucky to argue his case and solicit support for assistance in starting what came to be one of the first Family Nurse Practitioner Programs in the US at the FNS. He stated unequivocally that he felt the 'entire area of normal

---

[13]McCormack letter to Dr. Edward J. Goodwin, M.D., 14 October 1930, Frontier Nursing Service 1789–1985, Mary Breckinridge Series: Correspondence 1925–1970. University of Kentucky in Lexington, USA.

[14]FNS Quarterly Bulletin 1938, 85M1: FNS, Box 15, Fol. 3. 'Mountain Obstetrics (condensed) presented to members of Eastern division of Kentucky State Association of RN's by John H. Kooser, M.D., Medical Director of the FNS', FNS Quarterly Bulletin, winter 1938 (Vol. XIII, No. 3). p. 7.

growth and development in infants and children' was a sphere of practice in which nurses could successfully and safely practise. Though 'terribly important', it was also 'so terribly boring to a paediatrician who gets much more excited about an acute disease process or a chronic disease process and its effect upon the child and their alteration of normal growth and development'. [15]

Beasley's comments underscore the 'cure' versus 'care' focus of medicine and nursing. Yet though he clearly found the 'care' aspect of the work 'boring,' he validated its worth by also stating that it was 'terribly important.' Beasley also felt that nurses were underused in treating sick children in a triage capacity for physicians and quipped that 'he would just love to have a nurse see a baby and have the power to recognize whether or not it was going to drop dead the next 5 min or live until morning.' He stated that the nurses did a better job than he did at keeping growth charts because 'they have the patience to do it accurately' and he credited the nurses for having much more patience than he in dealing with moms who had what he described as 'petty' problems such as toilet-training and the anorexia of 18-month-olds. This admission and language use illustrate both the 'helping' attribute's lack of status in the culture as well as the relational, people-orientation and level of kinship enjoyed by the nurses. Beasley added that he felt quite confident in walking in and doing a complete physical exam in 2 or 3 min and then turning over the entire counselling of the mother's attitude toward the child and vice versa to the nurse, who "can carry on from there and can do a better job than I can do at it" [22]. The culture's emphasis on technology, skill and the status and monetary rewards associated with them is illustrated when in his same letter Beasley quipped:

As you know, there is a great trend in this country right now to over-burden the physician with minutia that really does not amount to much but makes him a lot of money, which eat up a lot of his time, make his brain very dull, make his life very un-colourful and make his pocket book very thick.[16]

The response from all three of his medical colleagues in academia was that their institutions were pursuing 'medical assistant' programs designed to create a 'screening type paramedical personnel' and that they did not support nurses in the role described by Beasley. Their main objections focused on the nurses' 'increased role' in this scheme and their *"serving as a point of first contact in cases of illness"* [italics added], which would essentially cut in on the physician's business. In regard to the former argument, Beasley stated that nurses already had this role in the community setting. In regard to the latter; it could also be argued that it is the nurse's business as much as it is the physicians to *care* for sick people while they are seeking specific treatments designed to *cure* by physicians. An article written on FNS

---

[15] Beasley Letter, et al. 1966, 2005M547: FNS, Box 227, Fol. 10.

[16] Issacs G. 85M1: FNS, Box 38, Fol. 7. 'The FNS: Family Nursing in Rural Areas by Gertrude Isaacs, DNS', The Changing Role Relationship of the Physician and the Nurse (p. 399). Reprint from *Clinical Obstetrics & Gynaecology*, a quarterly book series, medical department of Harper & Row (Vol. 15, No. 2, June 1972). University of Kentucky in Lexington, USA.

Family Nursing by Gertrude Isaacs, DNS, noted the change that had occurred in the role relationship of the physician and the nurse thus:

> The Family Nurse is prepared to assume many functions that have been traditionally per-
> formed by doctors at the same time retaining her former nursing functions, though many
> have been delegated to nurse aides, Licensed Practical Nurses and clerical assistants. This
> is a natural evolution. As technology advances, workers with varying levels of skills become
> necessary to assume efficient operation. Neither the physician with increased specialization
> nor the nurse with increased knowledge can continue to retain all former functions. [17]

Written in 1972, the account had a familiar ring when it argued that nurses have long chafed under practice acts that did not permit them to make use of their knowledge and added that many left the field for these reasons. Most legislative acts stated that nurses were not to make medical diagnoses or prescribe therapeutic treatments, something that they had been doing surreptitiously for years.[18] Issacs argued that both care and cure crossed lines and were intricately interrelated. Attempts to separate them could only result in ever-widening rifts between these two health professions and in-patient neglect.

The obligatory rules for district nurses at the Queens Nurses Institute (QNI), the scheme upon which the FNS was modelled, mirrored the paternalism that existed within organizations at the time, both in institutional as well as community-based health care environments on both sides of the Atlantic. It included the following:

> The general sick nursing of patients shall be carried out under the directions of the
> medical practitioners, the application for services of the nurse may be made direct to
> her or otherwise and that the nurse may attend a patient on application of emergency
> but must not continue to visit without informing a medical man and receiving his
> instructions, if any.[19]

If the nurse should direct a patient to a physician and the patient does not take the physician's advice or if the physician chose not to advise the patient further, the nurse was not permitted to attend this patient except in cases of 'fresh emergency' and she had to report the matter to her secretary (of health). Nurses were not to dispense any drug not prescribed by a 'medical man' and were not permitted in any case to attempt to influence a patient in their choice of doctor. An attending midwife was not to accept an engagement without first asking a patient to state, and herself to register, the name of the doctor to be called should an emergency arise.' These rules existed for midwives at the same time that the 1939 QNI *Report* also found that among cases attended by midwives with no doctor in attendance, there was an

---

[17]85M1: FNS, Box 38, Fol. 7. 'The FNS: Family Nursing in Rural Areas by Gertrude Isaacs, DNS', The Changing Role Relationship of the Physician and the Nurse (p. 399). Reprint from Clinical Obstetrics & Gynaecology, a quarterly book series, medical department of Harper & Row (Vol. 15, No. 2, June 1972). University of Kentucky in Lexington, USA.

[18]QNI Report 1923, SA/QNI/P7/23, Reprinted in a 1926 QNI Report. Royal College of Nursing Archives, Edinburgh, UK.

[19]FNS Quarterly Bulletin 1935, 85M1: FNS, Box 25, Fol. 2.

infant mortality rate of 2.10 per 1000 births. The rate for the rest of the country was 2.97 per 1000 total births.

In 1935, the FNS *Quarterly Bulletin* reported 2400 deliveries with zero loss of life from Obstetric causes [26]. In contrast to QNI nurses, FNS nurses were permitted to dispense medications according to a 'Medical Routines' book that a committee of physicians put together for the nurses to use, though this was a privilege that was lost once more physicians came into Appalachia. FNS nurses functioned under the guidance of a single medical director whom they utilized as a resource in emergency situations that they were not equipped to handle alone and with whom the work was always viewed as a partnership not an autocracy. Indeed, physicians who worked for Breckinridge over the years revered the work, the work's founder and the organization's nurses, and often wrote about them all.

Dr. Kooser described FNS nurses as not only responsible for normal obstetrical patients, but also for abnormal cases and recommended that they reported irregularities "to the mid-wife supervisor *or* me" [italics added]. Kooser said it was the nurse in the cabin who decided when to call for help.[20] By contrast, in Britain, in an address to the annual meeting of the Durham County Nursing Association at Durham on 28 June 1947 by Sir Weldon Dalrymple-Champneys, PhD, Deputy Chief Medical Officer to the Minster of Health, described the work of the QNI Nurse as merely:

> Unspectacular work, the only reward of which is often the conviction of a job well done and the gratitude of your patients and their families, rewards though, which I know you would not wish to exchange for glittering ones.[21]

Dalrymple-Champneys went on to use the following words as descriptors for QNI nurses, 'notoriously modest, missionary spirited, courageous, idealistic, tactful, understanding of human nature and pioneering workers.' He said he believed that the chief agents in securing the future health of the people must be the General Practitioner and the domiciliary nurses, working in close proximity under the 'new' National Health Service (NHS). In this address, he extolled the Christian monastic foundations of nursing, Florence Nightingale's high ideals of devotion and dedication and noted that her teaching was 'out of fashion today' but went on to state that 'her ideals are greater than fashion' and that even if nursing had been 'exploited and its selflessness taken for granted that we should not throw away those priceless ideals that have inspired and sustained her to benefit of community and allow a noble profession to degenerate into a trade' [10]. Dalrymple-Champneys went on to suggest that if the NHS succeeded in giving the family doctor his 'proper status,' then it would naturally follow that the role of the family nurse would also be 'adjusted', adding that 'she is his (the doctor's) chief and trusted *helper* [Italics added] without whose aid his best efforts would be in vain' [10].

---

[20] FNS Quarterly Bulletin 1938, 85M1: FNS, Box 15, Fol. 3.

[21] Sir Weldon Dalrymple-Champneys, Address to QNI Meeting 1947, SA/QNI/PG12. 'Address to the Annual Meeting of the Durham County Nursing Association at Durham by Sir Weldon Dalrymple-Champneys on 28, June 1947.' Royal College of Nursing Archives in Edinburgh, UK, 2.

Dalrymple-Champneys saw the efforts of the nurses he worked with as 'aids' to 'his' best efforts and not as colleagues who not only had 'his' best efforts in mind but also those of the patients.' He clearly felt that the role for the nurse in the 'new' health scheme (NHS) was that of help-mate. His other statements intimated that the role of the family nurse would continue to be 'revered' by both the patient and the world only if nurses did not choose to make or fulfil 'bargains with employers.' In other words, vocation dictated that the nurse should remain subordinate, poor and invisible in comparison to the doctor. He used nursing founder, Florence Nightingale, to sustain his argument, which is something that continues today. It should also be considered that the obvious posturing on the part of this physician probably had more to do with the uncertain 'status' within the 'new' health care scheme for the general practitioner than with nurses or nursing.

This same argument has been used 65 years later by Barigozzi and Turati (2012) and by Heyes (2005) who stated that increasing wages, "might attract the 'wrong sort' of people into the (nursing) profession" [11]. Heyes argued that lower wages, "attract better 'vocationally called' nurses," hence implying that lower-paid nurses make better nurses. He goes on to identify nurses as being in a 'vocation-based sector', along with teaching, another mostly female profession, that is considered a 'helping' or humanitarian service oriented discipline by the general public [12]. Nelson & Folbre (2006) were quick to rebut this view. They have argued that a lack of wage incentive in the US is one factor contributing to the nursing shortage and that wages actually retain 'good' nurses. They have emphasized the positive impact of pay on employee morale and retention and that a 'calling' to nursing does not necessarily guarantee skill [13]. Though it might be true that 'the wrong sort' could well be attracted into nursing, based solely on the material rewards on offer, they would be likely to opt to either leave when the work load would begin to take its toll. Pay would no longer be compensation. Alternatively, they might stay and approach the job as less a service and more a business venture. It has been equally true that nurses who enter the profession viewing it as more of a service vocation are, on finding that the existing system does not attach any value to this ideology, equally apt to make the same decision to either leave the profession entirely or find a way to live with the inherent job dissatisfaction. In each case the nurse would be adversely affected and the decision to stay or go negatively affect patient care and the profession. According to many experts, substantial variation across states in the US is observed for registered nurses (RNs) in 2030 through the large differences between their projected supply and demand. "While the projections presented here are directionally consistent with findings in recent studies on RN supply, historical experience demonstrates how sensitive enrollment in training programs and the resulting labor supply of nurses are to the job market and economic conditions" [14]. Unfortunately, these variables have never been either reconciled or particularly stable within the profession of nursing, not even by its own leadership.

The truth is that neither the vocational nor the professional perspectives alone are correct or realistic. People enter professions to which they feel they are adequately suited physically, mentally, emotionally and spiritually. They also expect to be adequately compensated for their time, energy and talents within this environment.

This 'either-or' mentality has created a paradoxical approach to what is fundamentally a very complex problem. It has also forced nurses to take sides on whether good nursing care is the result of superior clinical and technical knowledge alone or is a 'calling' (people-focused or driving internal humanitarian impulse) for the profession, when both are not essential for good nursing care but are also necessary to draw and keep good nurses in practice. Yet nurses continue to feel the need to take a position on the care versus intellect (scientific skill) debate.

The comments of a former President of the North Carolina Nurses Association, Dennis Sherrod, EdD, RN who was also faculty at Forsyth Medical Centre and Endowed Chair of Recruitment and Retention at Winston-Salem State University, North Carolina in regard to his choice of nursing as a career. *The American Nurse* is a superlative illustration of exactly how deeply the fragmentation of care in our society has affected the disciplines cultural roots:

> I'm always looking for new knowledge and ideas. Nursing has never been what I felt was a "calling," but it's the "people purpose" that drives my passion to make a difference in people's lives. It's what causes me to live and breathe nursing each day. Nursing is not just a part of my life-it's who I am! [15]

The statement was an oxymoron. He stated he felt he was not 'called' into the profession and then proceeded to describe exactly what such a calling would 'feel' like, citing it as the reason he became a nurse as well as stayed in nursing. One has to wonder if gender and role-identification played a part in the wording of his response as his choice of nursing as a career was also motivated by his desire to 'get off the farm.' He also mentioned that 'funding was available for nursing education in the 1970s,' and went on to state that he had an interest in 'science and health care.' Clearly all of these elements are essential in making and keeping a 'good' nurse, yet they are clearly viewed as not only separate entities by those within the discipline but also as entities that require either a particular priority or allegiance to in order to advance the profession.

6.3 Gender Role: Myth?

The traditional doctor-nurse relationship described by Stein in 1967 captured the hierarchical structure of authority in health care and the subordinate role of women nurses to physicians [16]. However, nursing literature also suggested that the nurse-physician relationship was changing, a situation that Svensson (1996) attributed to the feminization of medicine, changing ideas about nursing and nurses' autonomy and nursing students being socialized to assume a more independent professional role [17]. The fact that Sirota (2007) is still asking if "Nurse/Physician Relationships are Improving or Not?" and citing that nurses are still reporting "that the same negative issues between nurses and physicians that have existed for years persist, that these issues continue to make nurses dissatisfied with the nurse/physician relationship, contribute to poor job satisfaction among nurses and hamper nurse retention" indicates that progress has been slow, very slow to say the least [18]. Each factor attributed the change (or lack of change) in the nurse-physician relationship to the transformations in traditional gender-power relations but the impact of institutional power structures on the degree, rapidity or sustainment of these changes are very rarely if ever considered.

Some studies have found that males and older students placed less value on working with people than females and younger students. Other studies support this finding and note that male nurses experience greater satisfaction than females, advanced more rapidly and have found the monetary rewards as the most influential aspect of their job satisfaction compared with managerial support, free expression and professional development [19]. Male nurses have also been found to be more likely to leave a job due to a lack of money and poor career prospects [20]. These studies have traditionally been used to suggest that males entering the nursing profession damaged its 'vocational' image and made it a 'trade.' Others used these same studies to argue that in order to increase nurses' salaries and the disciplines' acceptance as a profession, more males were needed in nursing. Both schools of thought are biased. The former suggests that men are not capable of humanitarian urges when the fact that they chose to enter nursing out of the myriad of other possible professions open to them indicates that some desire for human service had to be evident in their choice, even if it was not ranked as highly as that of their female counterparts. The latter suggests that women are neither capable of garnering wage increases for themselves nor have the drive to be promoted to positions of leadership, both of which have been proven to be false assumptions as women in nursing have done so long before men began to join their ranks in significant numbers [21].

An American and a British former FNS nurse volunteered their views on men in nursing in response to a general question on their perceptions regarding how the profession has advanced or changed over the years. A British nurse stated, 'It was the beginning of the end when they started admitting men into nursing'.[22] An American former FNS nurse said that 'men helped to curb a lot of the back-biting and squabbling within nursing. They helped the profession, at least those who didn't use it as a stepping stone to administration'.[23] This prompted her British nurse colleague to respond in kind that 'men could be as 'malicious' as females!' see Footnote 22.

Another FNS nurse recounted her frustration with a male nurse who became the director of nursing at the hospital and supervisor over the district nurses in the Services latter years. She explained that a new "Motorola radio system for communication when the phones didn't work" was put in place but the district outpost that she was at had very poor reception. This new male supervisor decided to institute an 8 a.m. radio check very day at every district winter or summer. The district nurses could not call from inside the cabin but had to go out on the edge of the driveway where they could get radio reception. She tried to explain to him that they would

---

[22] Jean Corner-Rowan, British former FNS Nurse-Midwife (1964–1966).

[23] Anne Lorentzen, American former FNS Nurse (1963–1965).

often be working till nine or ten o'clock at night and running the evening clinic till well past 8 p.m., which meant they would be seeing patients till 10 p.m. and following that with paperwork, yet, this supervisor insisted on squawking the radio at eight o'clock in the morning and she'd have to go out in her bathrobe to respond. She finally stormed into his office and yelled, "Quit calling me at eight o'clock in the morning! You know the reception at Red Bird is lousy and half the time, the weather inversion, the clouds are not right and you can't hear me responding anyway!".[24] Though this nurse mentioned in her discourse the fact that her supervisor was male, her major objection was to the enforcement on his part of a rather poorly thought out institutional policy and not the fact that he was male.

A 2003 American nurse graduate expressed that 'more men in nursing was a positive change' for the profession and another stated that "she did not like working in a 'predominantly female workplace.'"[25] None of these nurses was asked specifically about men or gender issues in nursing, yet they all chose to volunteer it while expressing their thoughts regarding professional change. Their ambivalence resonates throughout nursing's history. Their comments reinforced stereotypes about men as well as women, which would indicate that the prevailing 'us and them' mentality coupled with an 'either-or' approach to the humanitarian and professional aims of nursing has not served to advance the discipline. Relying on stereotypical gender roles and class status assignments have not provided the cultural transformation necessary to create the sustained positive change needed to either draw more men into practice or keep more women from leaving it.

The argument has also been made that the reason men advanced more quickly was more to do with the fact that more men were in positions of power within hospital institutions and most other corporate settings and that a social bias still existed regarding placing women in positions of authority. To understand this phenomenon, one must understand the gender-based class regime of the healthcare system that has been sustained by class and race relations within broader society. Traditionally, nurses (mostly female) have been from working or middle-class families and thereby represent a 'lower-class relative to (mostly male) physicians'[22]. Physicians, regardless of gender race or ethnicity, have traditionally come from the ranks of the upper middle or upper classes [23]. An additional plausible cultural explanation, supported by many studies, theorizes that women value monetary rewards and professional advancement less than they do the 'working with people' aspects of the job [24]. At first glance, this would appear to be confirmed by the statements of at least one former long serving British FNS nurse who began as a nurse-midwife in 1958 and later became an administrator in the Service. When asked what she enjoyed most and least about her tenure in the Service, she stated that the most enjoyable feature was the 'triple worker' job of district nurse, midwife and health visitor' that no longer exists in professional practice

---

[24] Judy Haralson-Rafson, American former FNS Nurse (1971–1976; 1971 Graduate of FNS Family Nurse Practitioner Program).

[25] Sable J. Hospital staff nurse for 2 years and Jean A., Hospital oncology nurse <1 year.

today.[26] The least enjoyable feature was the work she did when she went into "management and administration" there. She expressed her frustration with the increase in paperwork, governmental and professional regulatory enforcements and the lack of connectedness with patients that the institutionalisation of health care brought in its wake. She also felt she never had enough money, not so much her personal salary but rather the funds necessary to properly equip the nurses and support work in the community. She valued more making an impact toward improving her patients' quality of life and supporting her fellow nurses than she could as a manager. What made the administrative job less valuable was the institutional constraints placed upon her within that role not felt as acutely while a 'triple worker.'

Five nurses currently in practice mirrored the enjoyment of the 'collaborating,' 'working together,' and 'being a member of the health care team' aspects of working with their peers to either the autonomy or status facets of the job.[27] Four of these nurses, as well as eleven others presently in practice, also cited 'working with patients,' 'interacting with people,' 'connecting,' 'learning from them,' 'making a real difference,' 'affecting their patients,' 'abilities to live and cope,' and 'empowering' them as the most enjoyable aspects of nursing, wistfully acknowledging that the current health care system did not support or value these elements highly enough to provide the space within the institutional setting to foster this work. Both FNS and non-FNS nurses currently in practice cite the relational elements of the work as being both the draw and major reason for continued practice, even in the face of some pretty overwhelming obstacles within their work environments. They also acknowledge both the team and empowering aspects of the work between staff and patients as positives. But what is perhaps most intriguing about the discourse of younger nurses is the fact that they also cite the monetary rewards, opportunities and "flexibility" of the profession as positives; things that the FNS nurses did not. This challenges conventional ideology, which asserts that women's value of monetary rewards and professional advancement is less than that of men.[28]

---

[26]Margaret (Maggie) Willson, British former FNS Nurse-Midwife (1955–1967).

[27]Sloan M., Hospital operating room staff nurse for 2.5 years; research .5 years; Onster V., Hospital staff nurse for 1 year, telemetry 3.5 years, critical care 2 years, dialysis 1 year, research 2 years; Jean A., Hospital oncology nurse <1 year; Miller A., Hospital paediatric nurse for 4 years, educator for <1 year.

[28]SWN 02, 2004, Richard@neckar.us, Hospital emergency room staff nurse for 5 years; home health nurse for 4 years. Date surveyed: 31/12/2004.

SWN 03, 2005, msloan1109@hotmail.com, Hospital operating room staff nurse for 2.5years; research .5 years. Date surveyed: 21/01/2005.

SWN 04, 2005, judy.conedera@childrens.com, Hospital paediatric nurse for20 years. Date surveyed: 15/02/2005.

SWN 05, 2005, j.sable@sbcglobal.net, Hospital staff nurse for 2 years. Date surveyed: 10/04/2005.

SWN 06, 2005, suemorrison@doveworks.ca, Hospital staff nurse for 1 year; critical care for 10 years; pain management for 13 years. Date surveyed: 17/06/2005.

SWN 07, 2006, vernonster@adelphia.net, Hospital staff nurse for 1 year; telemetry 3.5 years; critical care 2 years; dialysis 1 year; research 2 years. Date surveyed: 07/02/2006.

SWN 08, 2004, duron.cranford@mwsu.edu, Hospital staff nurse for 2 years; critical care for 15 years. Date surveyed: 15/08/2004.

Research has also purported to show that male nurses have significantly changed the physician-nurse dynamic in the practice setting, citing that men are less sympathetic to the dominant role of the physician and do not tolerate it. Hence, they are treated with more respect, listened to and taken more seriously by male physicians [25]. Male nurse are also said to be more likely than their women colleagues to be on a first-name basis with physicians, engage in on-the-job banter and socialize with them outside of work [26]. This may be true in some cases but whether it has positively benefited their female nurse colleagues or raised the status of the profession as a whole remains far less certain. A male emergency room nurse, in practice since 1998 and with a bachelor's degree, in interview, has stated that he, too, would like to see the profession "treated with more respect from physicians".[29] He adds that nurses who are good nurses do have the respect of physicians who work with them regularly; bad nurses bring the opposite response to the overall profession. He has enjoyed the "respect" shown emergency room nurses. The least enjoyable aspect has been working with patients and their families who "think you are a servant," though simultaneously citing his desire to "help people" as one of the reasons he entered the profession see Footnote 29. This nurse's responses indicated that though

---

SWN 09, 2005, deb40253@earthlink.net, Geriatrics for 12 years; hospital staff nurse for 3 years; emergency room for 4 years; home health for 6years; part-time psychiatric nurse for 5 years. Date surveyed: 11/10/2005.

SWN 10, 2005, lauraann@slampnet.com, Hospital staff nurse for 2.75 years. Date surveyed: 08/10/2005.

SWN 11, 2007, nursetipper@gmail.com, Hospital telemetry nurse for 3 years. Date surveyed: 05/11/2007.

SWN 12, 2007, tctopcat423@hotmail.com, Primarily hospital staff nurse for 5 years; brief stints in newborn nursery, occupational nursing, physicians' office (family practice) and as a campus nurse. Date surveyed 24/11/2007.

SWN 13, 2007, mrssconway@yahoo.com, Hospital paediatric nurse for 3 years; neonatal for 4 years. Date surveyed: 29/09/2007.

SWN 14, 2006, annjean47@hotmail.com, Hospital oncology nurse <1 year. Date surveyed: 05/09/2006.

SWN 15, 2006, lisarandon@yahoo.com, Hospital neonatal intensive care unit <1 year. Date surveyed: 11/11/2006.

SWN 16, 2006, smarrfive@comcast.net, Hospital obstetrics nurse for 5 years. Date surveyed: 19/11/2006.

SWN 17, 2006, bethscarfe@aol.com, Hospital staff nurse for 6 years; critical care 2 years. Date surveyed: 9/10/2006.

SWN 18, 2007, andreanmiller@eastlink.ca, Hospital paediatric nurse for 4 years; educator for <1 year. Date surveyed: 18/04/2007.

SWN 19, 2007, shelleywc@gmail.com, Hospital telemetry nurse for 1 year; internal medicine & obstetrics-gynaecology office nurse for 5 years; labour & delivery room nurse for 9 years. Date surveyed 8/06/2007.

SWN 20, 2006, fightingheart@hotmail.com, Hospital staff nurse & telemetry for 10 years; critical care & telemetry step-down for 1 year; nursing education & staff development for 2 years. Date surveyed: 07/07/2006.

[29] Neckar R. Hospital emergency room staff nurse for 5 years; home health nurse for 4 years.

he enjoyed the "respect" of physicians this reality did not extend to the profession in general. He, like his female nurse counterparts, parcelled out some of the blame for this on 'bad' nurses, though what constituted a 'bad' nurse was not elaborated upon. It was of particular interest to note that he, as well as his female nurse colleagues, felt more respected in the specialty areas within the institution, where the patient to nurse ratio as well as the team approach by staff was more pronounced. This male nurse also echoed the humanitarian impulse cited by all the female nurses as a virtue which he too valued highly while, like them, rejecting the servant mentality often associated with this impulse. He also stated that he most enjoyed feeling 'comfortable' and 'confident' in a "high stress" job, the "technical aspect" of the work, the "opportunities" and "above average pay" nursing afforded him. These are all statements that female nurses also made about nursing. Indeed, female nurses both welcomed the change associated with more technology while also fearing that it could continue to shift the focus away from patient care.[30] Regardless of their perceptions regarding where it would take the profession in the future, they all recognized that it was here to stay. The male nurse's statements in no way uphold the stereotype that men value less the 'working with people' aspects of the job than do women, anymore than do the statements made by the female nurses in practice uphold the stereotype that women are less interested in professional advancement or do not value as highly monetary rewards. Indeed, the most that can be construed from any of these statements is that the institutional setting has done a better job of meeting the monetary needs of its nurses and the technological needs of both the general population and its nurses than in meeting their human value needs. The statements of all the nurses (young and old) and former FNS nurses do not in any obvious way uphold the stereotype that nursing resists or is intimidated by change and technological advancement. Rather nurses recognize the secondary status that they share with their patients in relation to technology within the institutional setting.

In the years prior to World War Two the choice of career for women was limited. Yet even with these limitations and a World War nursing struggled to retain nurses in the profession while refusing to accept men into it. The discipline has historically had an uneasy relationship with feminism due to the prevailing gender role stereotypes and lack of value attributed to the service, to the 'helping,' care and nurture roles associated with both women and nursing (which remains a predominately female profession). The institutional hierarchy that existed outside Appalachia in hospitals had physicians (a mostly male dominated profession) in positions of authority who viewed nurses as 'helpers.' By contrast, the FNS had physicians who viewed nurses as colleagues, equal partners in the provision of care to the local community. At a time when physicians within the establishment's urban, centralized power settings, such as hospitals and academia, were opposing nurse practitioner programs, FNS physicians were not only supporting them but

---

[30]Shelley WC. Hospital telemetry nurse for 1 year; internal medicine & obstetrics-gynaecology office nurse for 5 years; labour & delivery room nurse for 9 years.

were actively lobbying for their creation. As a result of this support, one of the first family nurse practitioner programs was established at the FNS that is still in existence today. In contrast to this and more generally, physicians and hospital administrators have used and continue to use nursing's vocational and charitable roots to make a case for their continued subordinate role within the establishment. In an attempt to circumvent this reality and garner full professional status and recognition, nurses have tried to distance themselves from those humanitarian impulses most associated with feminine traits that are undervalued by the culture. This attitude has caused dissonance within the discipline and has also created an equal amount of ambivalence regarding men entering the profession. Yet both male and female nurses value the intellectual and technical challenges coupled with the 'people purpose' of the work that make it more than just a job to them. Chapter 7 explores further the identity confusion experienced at the FNS with the adoption of the corporate health care model being utilized outside of the region, the crisis this system created in education and practice environments for nurses, the moral distress associated with the powerlessness, cultural conflict and role incongruity of nurses within institutional settings and nurse's efforts to survive within them.

References

1. Davies C, Beach A. Regulating professional self-regulation: a history of the United Kingdom Central Council for Nursing. London: Routledge; 2000.
2. Brown M. American Women and the Military. 2001. http://www.gendergap.com/military/usmil4.htm. Accessed 25 Oct 2004.
3. Dammann N. A social history of the frontier nursing service. Sun City: Social Change Press; 1982.
4. Andrist C, Nicholas P, Wolf K. A history of nursing ideas. Burlington: Jones and Bartlett Publishers, Inc; 2006.
5. Muff J. Why doesn't a smart girl like you go to medical school? The women's movement takes a slap at nursing. In: Muff J, editor. Women's issues in nursing: socialization, sexism and stereotyping. Prospect Heights: Waveland Press; 1988. p. 178.
6. Abel-Smith B. A history of the nursing profession. London: Heinemann; 1960.
7. Alitzer A. The establishment of the FNS: a resource mobilization approach. Unpublished Master's dissertation, University of Kentucky, Lexington, Kentucky; 1990. p. 8.
8. Alitzer A. The establishment of the FNS: a resource mobilization approach. Unpublished Master's dissertation, University of Kentucky, Lexington, Kentucky; 1990. p .17.
9. Alitzer A. The establishment of the FNS: a resource mobilization approach. Unpublished Master's dissertation, University of Kentucky, Lexington, Kentucky; 1990. p. 31.
10. Dalrymple-Champneys, et al. Sir Weldon Dalrymple-Champneys, Address to QNI Meeting 1947, SA/QNI/PG12.
11. Barigozzi F, Turati G. Human health care and selection effects. Understanding labor supply in the market for nursing. Health Econ. 21(4):477–83. https://doi.org/10.1002/hec.1713.
12. Heyes A. The economics of vocation or why is a badly paid nurse a good nurse? J Health Econ. 2005;51(12):56–9.
13. Nelson J, Folbre N. Why a well-paid nurse is a better nurse. Nurs Econ. 2006;24(3):127–30.

14. US Department of Health & Human Services, Health Resources & Service Administration [HRSA]. Supply and Demand Projections of the Nursing Workforce 2014-2030 (July 21, 2017) Department of Health and Human Services Health Resources and Services Administration Bureau of Health Workforce, National Center for Health Workforce Analysis. https://bhw.hrsa.gov/sites/default/files/bhw/nchwa/projections/NCHWA_HRSA_Nursing_Report.pdf. Accessed 26 Jan 2019.
15. The American Nurse, Official Publication of the American Nurses Association. In Brief, ANA Supports Striking Appalachian Nurses. September/October 2007. p. 5–10.
16. Stein L. The doctor-nurse game. Arch Gen Psychiatry. 1967;16(6):699–703.
17. Svensson R. The interplay between doctors and nurses—a negotiated order perspective. Sociol Health Illness. 1996;18(3):379–98.
18. Sirota T. Nurse/physician relationships: improving or not? Nursing. 2007;37(1):52–6.
19. Zangaro G, Soeken K. A meta-analysis of studies of nurses' job satisfaction. Res Nurs Health. 2007;30(4):445–58. https://doi.org/10.1002/nur.20202.
20. Sochalski J. Men leaving nursing faster than women? Nursing2002. 2002;33(11):33.
21. Andrist C, Nicholas P, Wolf K. A history of nursing ideas. Burlington: Jones and Bartlett Publishers, Inc; 2006. p. 5–19.
22. Boughn S. Why women and men choose nursing. Nurs Health Care Perspect. 2001;22(1):14–9.
23. More E. Restoring the balance: women physicians and the profession of medicine (1850–1995). Cambridge, MA: Cambridge University Press; 1999.
24. Beagan R. Everyday classism in medical school: experiencing marginality and resistance. Med Educ. 2005;39(8):777–84. https://doi.org/10.1111/j.1365-2929.2005.02225.x.
25. Murray M, Chambers M. Characteristics of students entering different forms of nurse training. J Adv Nurs. 1990;15(9):1099–105.
26. Evans J, Frank B. Contradictions and tensions: exploring relations of masculinities in the numerically female-dominated nursing profession. J Mens Stud. 2003;11(3):277–92.

Chapter 7
Moral Inhabitability and Educational Environments

7.1 Moral Inhabitability and Educational Environments

By the beginning of the twentieth century, urbanization, industrialization and immigration contributed to the rapid rise in the number of hospitals in America and Britain, a change that continued well into the twentieth century [1]. Nightingale's strategy of nurse education which in effect meant the staffing of hospitals with a strictly disciplined labour force of probationers (women) who practised under the watchful eye of physicians (men) was one which was based on the existing culture as much as it was the institutional framework of the hospital. In Nightingale's effort to make the profession 'respectable' within the culture, it had to be tied to the prevailing Victorian idea of womanhood and subordinate to medicine [2]. This inherently created a system that was too strict to yield enough nurses to meet the demand, even at a time when women were not given a choice of 'vocation' outside of teaching or nursing. The system of nurse education conceived in this fashion made political and economic sense for its time and the model existed in both America and Great Britain with some variations. Hospital nurse training schools opened in both countries because of a need for nurses to staff them. It was an exploitative system whereby a cheap labour force of female nurses worked 12-h days, 6 days a week, 50 weeks per year in a strict, paternalistic, demanding, physically, emotionally and mentally draining environment, a system free from any contractual agreement with the hospital or the school at the completion of their training [3]. These schools developed due to a social need, and their growth was fuelled by the advent of two World Wars [4].

The prevailing ideology was that nursing was an occupation that required a specific temperament or nature best suited to a woman and required no skill or intellect. It was perpetuated by the few women within the profession in a position of authority who, for whatever reason (either personal or professional), became the profession's gatekeepers [5]. It should also be stressed that the institution's administrators chose the women given these positions of authority with input from the physicians on

© Springer Nature Switzerland AG 2019

E. West, *Frontier Nursing in Appalachia: History, Organization and the Changing Culture of Care*, https://doi.org/10.1007/978-3-030-20027-5_7

staff. The larger general hospitals in both Britain and America adhered to a policy of relatively lax entry requirements for training, coupled with strict regulations (contracts) of service by which nurses agreed to serve the hospital and abide by its rules, were penalized for resigning prematurely while also being liable to be dismissed at any time for misconduct or neglect of duty. This misconduct and neglect was rarely more clearly defined as anything but 'wilful disobedience or gross insolence, habitual neglect of duties and great incapacity', which together with or without more serious offences were grounds for instant dismissal and forfeiture of wages [6]. For nursing, the expectation of the institutional environment was that individuals should fall in line with a culture which was organized for the purposes of the institution, administrators, physicians and even prominent nurses within the existing structural hierarchies, while having little influence therein [7].

Breckinridge, conversely, adopted an opposite strategy, which had stricter entry requirements for nurses into her organization and was much less punitive in approach once the nurse was a part of the organizational family. In other words, instead of taking in nurses and trying to force them to adopt the organization's culture, she selected people (women) who came to the organization with the qualities most conducive for them to want to become a part of the culture of the organization and community. Her focus was on having her nurses make the organization and not the organization shape the nurse. This philosophy held true in both the community and hospital setting. The FNS, its supporters and local community united to accomplish the community health goals of the organization and built a 12-bed hospital in Leslie County in 1928, the only one in over 1000 square miles.[1]

In its long history, there was only one instance at the FNS where a nurse was fired for breaking one of these rules and even then, it was for the nurses' benefit that she was sent home and quickly. An FNS nurse took it upon herself to turn-in one of her patients because he was making moonshine (home-made whiskey) and selling it, which was illegal. Once Breckinridge was made aware of this breach of confidence, she quickly summoned the nurse, dismissed her immediately and paid for her to be sent back to England that same day for her own safety. Moonshine making was one of the very few ways that the local inhabitants made enough money to keep from starving to death, and anyone who took it upon themselves to turn-in a neighbour was likely to be shot dead for their efforts. The nurse sent out to fill the resultant vacancy reported that she had been 'shot at' on the night of her arrival and at the clinic the following morning she made a point of making her presence known amongst the locals as 'the replacement nurse'. She also made it known that she had a firearm and knew how to use it.[2] Along with the nurse's safety, Breckinridge had to be concerned with maintaining the trust of the people in order to continue to meet their health care needs. Therefore, any adverse discourse regarding the local community's socio-economic or political environment which could impinge upon the provision of service was circumvented entirely. The focus must firmly remain upon the community.

---

[1]FNS *Quarterly Bulletin* 1935, 85M1: FNS, Box 25, Fol. 2.
[2]Alice Herman, American former FNS Nurse (1956–1978).

The only other instance reported of an FNS nurse being dismissed from service was a case of one who came to the service in its later years and was found to be stealing money paid for care rendered by the clinic. As the nurses were paired-up at district clinic centres it was the companion nurse at the centre who noted a discrepancy between the books and the amount of money being counted. Breckinridge insisted it must be an accounting error on the nurse's part but when it was proved to be true, she promptly dismissed her. The nurse relating this story stated that 'Mrs. B.' simply could not believe that a nurse could be capable of doing such a thing if she hadn't seen it with her own two eyes (see Footnote 2). The idea that money could be valued more highly than the trust or care of other human beings was a concept foreign to Breckenridge.

7.2 Nursing Educational Cultures: QNI Versus FNS

The standard curriculum for schools of nursing in institutional settings in the profession's early years was based on the hours of duty and what few classes there were, were arranged around these long hours of work. Nurse leaders from the bastions of their newly formed professional organizations at this time began to push for educational and practice reforms. A debate ensued about where students should be trained and many felt that this should be at institutions of higher education and not the hospitals, citing the necessity for nurses to be 'students' and not 'staff' [8]. Outside of the institutional environment in Great Britain and America there existed other volunteer organizations designed to provide health care to patients in the community. These organizations also trained nurses with the traditional mentorship system of a nursing diploma education. In the context of this study, the Queen's District Nurses organization (Scottish branch) in Great Britain provided the model which Frontier Nursing Service founder, Mary Breckinridge adapted to the Eastern Appalachian Mountain population in her home state of Kentucky.

The Queen Victoria's Jubilee Institute for Nurses, later to become the Queen's Nurses Institute (QNI), was founded via a £70,000 gift from Queen Victoria, as part of an offering to her from the Women of Great Britain at her Jubilee in 1887, to be applied to providing better means of nursing for the sick poor [9]. In 1889 the service trained eight nurses. By 1920 there were 402 Queen's Nurses employed and an additional 33 in training.[3] The function of the Institute was to provide trained nurses in district work, supply nurses to local district nursing associations and arrange for the inspection of each nurse's work. If a nurse had been hospital trained and wished to undergo QNI training, they had completed the full course of training with the Institute. These nurses had to make practical use of utensils found in the community, tolerate limited space, carry out duties despite interruptions, offer simple instructions on cleanliness, ventilation, cooking, etc. to patients in the home and their families. Because of the nature of the setting in which QNI nurses were to

---

[3] QNI Report 1920, QNI Reports for the Years 1920–1946, 5.

work, they were taught District (or Home Health Visitation), Public Health (including School Nursing) and Midwifery. The training course lasted 6 months (or longer if doing midwifery and qualifying for that certification). A QNI nurse was qualified to work for a local association, perhaps in a crowded industrial mining centre or a remote, sparsely populated district of the Highlands. The types of clients they saw varied in age, situation and condition. The type of woman the QNI looked for was described as 'Physically vigorous with something of the hero and something of the saint in her composition'.[4] QNI nurses were generalist practitioners and before Breckinridge began her midwifery school in 1939 she actively sought recruits from the area she once visited when envisioning a similar health care scheme for Eastern Appalachia. It would be fair to state that Breckinridge adopted a similar view of the 'type of nurse' she wanted from the QNI based; witness the similarity of her adverts. She also relied on the QNI to supply her with Nurse-midwives before she had to develop a Graduate School of Midwifery of her own, out of necessity when her mostly British-nurse-midwives left the service in 1939 to serve their country during World War Two.

An address by Miss M. Wilmshurst, the General Supervisor of the Queen's Institute of District Nursing on 3 December 1936, 'The Silent Service of District Nursing,' commented on the tremendous growth in the past 49 years made by the QNI for the public 'in silence and largely unobserved' by the QNI.[5] She alluded to the service's difficulty in promoting and giving sufficient publicity to the notion that much of the work was done in private homes. In another lecture by Miss Wilmshurst, this time to QNI Nursing candidates, entitled 'Not Barriers But Guides', she stressed that patients must be under the care of a 'medical man' and that 'though the nurse can teach patients, she must never allow her work to be such as to make the doctor feel she is taking his work.' She further advised her students to 'Be professional with the doctor, even if you become friendly with him when off duty and keep your position as nurse when working with him.' Hence, the problem with promoting the Service and securing the recognition these women earned was due not solely to the nature of the work, in patients' 'private homes,' but also to a reluctance on the part of the organization's leadership to appear to rival the authority of physicians within the existing organizational structure. Wilmshurst's acquiescence to the status quo could be due to the power afforded to her as a reward within this hierarchy. It could also be due to the cultural norms held by society or even the belief that to not be 'self-effacing' would in some way negates the altruistic elements inherent in the work. Wilmshurst went on to tell the students 'Difficult doctors are manageable, as are other workers' and 'Be loyal to doctors and supervisors and look on the Institute as a mother, even if she has to scold or correct. She is always ready to help you in every way'.[6]

---

[4] QNI Report 1920, QNI Reports for the Years 1920–1946, 4.

[5] Wilmshurst MM. Address to QNI 1936, SA/QNI/PG/10-11. Public Address entitled 'The Silent Service of District Nursing' by General Supervisor of the QNI, Miss Wilmshurst on 3, December 1936. Edinburgh: Royal College of Nursing Archives in Edinburgh. p. 10.

[6] Miss M. Wilmshurst et al., 11.

These remarks reveal the institutional loyalties that nurse leaders of the day had and even the subordinate role that such loyalties supported within this hierarchy but it also suggests a team approach to patient care in which the nurse was not only instrumental in patient care but was also the central manager of the said care, viewing herself as 'matriarchal' and functioning in conjunction with the 'patriarchal' system therein. Perhaps a more forceful stance on the part of the leadership within this organizational culture would have curtailed the vital position of the nurse supervisor (or matron) and this also contributed to the leadership's reluctance to change it.[7] Breckinridge, on the other hand, had no such barrier. As founder and Director of the FNS the 'buck' began and ended with her and she took every opportunity to let her nurses have either an equal accolade with her attending physician or full recognition for a job well done in his absence. This was done via the FNS *Quarterly Bulletin* put out by the service and in the re-telling of many of the nurses' stories, often written by the nurses themselves, for the *Bulletin*, physicians or guests visiting the FNS who wrote of its founder, organization and nurses and also had publications run in the popular national and international magazines of the day.

The QNI was different from the hospital institutional setting in that it provided payment to student in training, in addition to board, laundry and uniform. It also guaranteed its nurses a minimum salary with rooms, fire, light and attendance and an annual increment for five years. If they were a certificated midwife, they also received an additional £5 to their minimum salary. The Institute kept in touch with nurses via reports and visits of inspection at least once a year and provided a 'home of rest' which was located on an estate for nurses to go to for 6 weeks' residence free of charge during periods of convalescence, unfitness to work or holiday, provided they supported it by paying £1 per year. If QNI nurses worked for 2 years they received a certification badge and after 6 years of service a pension fund. The QNI offered comparable salary and conditions with the other women's professions of the time, a priority in order to attract the 'best type of nurse.' Similarly, they offered an 8-h working day and an annual holiday. Though the nature of the work did not allow for absolutely regular working hours, they did compensate for this by spells of leisure where necessary for the nurse. General funds were also used to raise the standard, social position and status of the whole body of trained nurses.[8]

Yet while the efforts of the QNI in raising the situation of the nurses within their organization was laudable, it also circulated fliers on the Queen's Nurses, entitled 'Queen's Nurses & What They Do' to districts which would hire them that undermined these very efforts by suggesting that 'One Queen's Nurse was sufficient for a town with 8000 inhabitants and could be had at a cost of 240–250 British Pounds Sterling per year.' For a county district, a QNI nurse trained in midwifery, general nursing and public health, it was suggested a population of 3000 per nurse was reasonable. At the FNS, where the terrain was similar to the Outer Hebrides, which

---

[7] Williams K. Nurse Training in the Carnarfon and Anglesey Hospital 1935–1949.

[8] QNI *Reports* 1920–1950, Royal College of Nursing Archives in Edinburgh, UK.

the QNI serviced, the nurse to population ratio was eight (including supervision and relief) for 10,500.[9]

Breckinridge' FNS *Quarterly Bulletins* also went out to mostly supporters, staff and former staff who were already aware of the work in much the same way that the QNI's reports did. She used excerpts from these bulletins on the finances, number of cases or nurses' features on their experiences and had them run in local, national or international magazines and nursing journals, but much of the work's recognition was as a direct result of visitors who came out and saw first hand what the service was doing and then wrote or spoke about it. Breckinridge also had a circle of prominent, wealthy, and in some cases famous, friends who aided and abetted her work, which, like the QNI, relied heavily upon outside financial assistance to maintain operations. She often 'played up' the nurse on horseback angle, using tiny leather saddlebags that she sent out in letters to supporters and extras for 'one or two of their friends' to be filled. She detailed the nurses' needs, '$150 dollars will support a nurse-midwives service for 1 month, seven dollars will nurse a sick baby in the hospital, five dollars will send a crippled child to the city for treatment and one dollar will feed two horses for 1 day.[10] In the Service's latter years its philanthropic roots were grafted to the prevailing national, state and local health care system and as such, became less and less visible to those beyond the hills, though the *Quarterly Bulletin*, which functions more as a newsletter today, still goes out to staff, former staff and foundation contributors.

The relationship between doctors and nurses, and the value placed upon nursing by both physicians and the general public reflected the prevailing cultural norms. The *Times* for October of 1926 featured an article entitled 'District Nursing A Great Social Service' wherein the work was described as 'real, practical, unobtrusive and little heard of,' and that 'readers have a vague notion of.' It was further described as 'not vaineth in itself, not puffed up and that official record of it scanty, though the official authorities make great use of it and would be in difficulty without its assistance'.[11] This article went on to call the sick nurse 'the doctor's assistant and ally, universally recognized today as indispensable.' It is interesting to note the equating of any form of recognition with 'vanity' on the part of the discipline. There is a conscious effort on the part of the writer to equate the virtuous aspects of humanitarianism with self-effacing and unassuming behaviour as a matter of course. Although Breckinridge certainly sought selfless, dedicated nurses, she never devalued their achievements and any cross-training that was to be done in the organization's early years was done by the nurse in an expansion of her role. One FNS

[9] QNI *Report* 1940, Reprint from FNS *Quarterly Bulletin*, February 1928, Royal College of Nursing Archives in Edinburgh, UK.

[10] FNS *Circular* 1930, 85M1: FNS, Box 25, Fol. 2. 'Will You Fill Her Saddlebags?', FNS Circular sent out to supporters that asks and answers the question, 'Do you know the Frontier Nurses? It includes an itemized operating cost per nurse. University of Kentucky in Lexington, USA.

[11] QNI Report 1926, SA/QNI/P7/23. 'District Nursing A Great Social Service,' *Times* (October of 1926). Portions of which are reprinted in a 1926 QNI Report. Edinburgh: Royal College of Nursing Archives. p. 7.

nurse stated that when Mary Breckinridge was ill and bedridden toward the end of her life, it was she who type-matched, crossed and administered her blood transfusions. This is something that was, and is, done exclusively by laboratory technicians outside of Appalachia. FNS nurses were also X-ray and laboratory technicians when this technology was introduced to Leslie County.[12]

The Queen's gift that formed the nucleus of the seed fund given to the QNI, although it had grown steadily since its inception, was never sufficient to keep pace with the demands upon it. By 1921, the Institute had a £6000 plus deficit, which curtailed the number of nurses trained. A report to the executive committee of the Queens Fund in 1923 stated that it was essential that there should be more Queens' nurses and in order to secure this end two things seemed necessary. The conditions of the service had to be made as attractive as possible and the opportunities offered for public service be made more widely known. According to the QNI *Reports* for the years 1923–1947, it is not surprising then that the number of QNI district nurses leaving always outnumbered the number of new QNI nurses in training by as much as three or four to one, with most leaving at or before the second year, with the most acute nurse shortages occurring in the early 1920s and during the World War Two. This persisted even with the addition of 'motor cars' instead of cycles and £30 up keep for each recruit and an effort by established nurses to reduce resignations. Among the reasons for resignation from district nursing in 1923 were (in order of frequency): marriage, private nursing, prolonged holiday or health reasons, a return to hospital nursing, home duties, midwifery course, health visiting, school or TB nursing, or 'other' work not specified. Other reasons included retiring from nursing altogether, working with unaffiliated district nursing associations, taking up posts in schools or starting a nursing home, practising as independent midwives or working as daily visiting nurses, affiliating to mission work or entering religious sisterhoods.[13]

In comparison with this, the majority of Breckinridge's nurses also left the Service when they became married or when their contract (usually for a two-year term) was completed. A majority stayed longer than their contracted years of service and not a few midwifery students stayed once their training was completed for a contracted period of time or before going to the mission field. The reasons cited for leaving had more to do with the isolation of living in the Appalachian Mountains, where modern conveniences often did not exist, than with the actual work, organization or local culture. Increasingly, this became a problem for the FNS as technology advanced and the socio-economic climate changed both outside and as inside Appalachia. For some, the loss of autonomy in practice was a cause, for others the disparity between the growing popular culture from which they had come compared with the rural culture which they found too alien to embrace. The 'relatedness' that was crucial to the socio-cultural communicative repertoire in Appalachia became obscured by this ever-increasing divide. Some FNS nurses departed to equally challenging practice environments, such

---

[12] Elizabeth 'Hilly' Hillman, British former FNS Nurse-Midwife (1949–1954).

[13] QNI *Report* 1921–1939, Royal College of Nursing Archives, Edinburgh, UK.

as the Canadian Out-Back or mission fields abroad (see Footnote 12). Many FNS Graduate Midwifery School nurses were predestined for the mission field prior to coming to the FNS to be educated. Some FNS nurses went on to take higher degrees in nursing and stayed at the FNS to use their qualifications in an administrative or supervisory capacity for a number of years before they too finally left the Service or retired. These nurses also often cited the cultural change within the organization as the cause, lamenting that it had become too much like 'every other practice environment elsewhere in the US'.[14]

By 1941, in the context of the QNI's financial struggle, the number of applicants for district nursing was again dwindling to an alarming degree, exacerbated in large part by the Second World War. A £5 'war bonus' was given to nurses who stayed on working for the QNI but retention was also hampered by the lack of suitable accommodation, which added to the already arduous work of the nurses. By 1947 in the *55th Annual Report* to the executive committee of the Queen's Fund, the future of the service was stated to be in question with the Institute's transfer to the local health authorities upon the eve of the National Health Service (NHS), and the place of the QNI in future training of nurses remaining to be determined.[15]

The Institute did survive into the 1950s but recruitment remained a problem. To help, a projector and film of district nursing was purchased for recruitment tours. By this time the number of resignations (139), the highest on record, was partly attributable to so many younger nurses seeking experience abroad, some of whom came to the FNS. The final date for examination for the Queen's roll was 16 January 1969. Thereafter, nurses trained for the national certificate and the work of the QNI passed into oblivion with no one outside the executive committee, the clients the nurses had served faithfully and the medical personnel with whom they worked ever knowing of the contributions by the Institute to improving the provision of health care and quality of life to the communities. This is a fate only narrowly escaped by the FNS with the influx of the national health system into Appalachia. It was also a fate that forever changed the quality of care the FNS provided.

7.3   Professional Versus Institutional Conformity: What Makes a 'Good' Nurse?

The Chippewa County War Memorial Hospital Training School of Nursing's supervisor in the US used strikingly similar language to that of QNI supervisors in the UK to describe students, comments that suggest appearance, interest, speed and ability to adhere to the rigid rules, regulations and power structure of the institution were the priority. The identifiable negative qualities included being 'untidy in appearance,' 'does not dress quietly,' 'too familiar with maids,' 'careless of details,' 'very slow at times,' 'interest questionable,' and 'mentally and physically able to

---

[14] Anne Lorentzen, American former FNS Nurse (1963–1965).

[15] QNI *Report* 1949, Royal College of Nursing Archives, Edinburgh, UK, 10.

take up training'.[16] One is left to ponder, however, exactly what the institutional supervisor meant by 'mentally and physically able.' No pre-requisites were placed on the potential nurse candidates that specifically outlined what the hospital was looking for in a trainee. Assessment comments made by a QNI nurse supervisor about district nursing students aptly illustrate where the nurse manager's preconceptions lay regarding what constituted a 'good' nurse:

> She is a conscientious nurse but rather stolid and stupid until she has grasped what is required. Nurse has required much in instruction but has grasped a good district routine, which she will faithfully carry out. Midwifery may smarten her up a bit, but she will always belong to the rank and file.[17]

> First class type of nurse with refined, educated, pleasant manner. Her patients are devoted to her. She has high ideals and a real interest in her patients. She has their welfare at heart. She will have a good educational influence over her patients.[18]

The best that seemingly could be hoped for with the 'rank and file' nurse was to grasp the district routine and 'faithfully carry it out,' whereas a 'first class type' of nurse needed only to be 'refined,' 'educated' and 'pleasant' with high ideals to have a positive influence over her patients. Much of the documentation by both the QNI and War Memorial Hospital supervisors dealt with the individual character traits of the nurse, highly subjective in their descriptions and emphasizing the perceived social standing of the students. One QNI supervisor recorded that a student was 'the right type for district nursing' but did not stipulate what constituted a 'right type.' Descriptors used by QNI Supervisors when evaluating student nurses for district also echo class snobbery and focused on the physical strength, the nurse's 'interest' and appearance in uniform. Though 'interest' in the records of both British and American supervisors superficially seemed to be a reference to the practice of nursing, when examined more closely and with reference to student accounts, they suggest that the real 'interest' being sought for was institutional conformity. Such loaded comments placed the blame for dismissal or resignations squarely on the student. They were not limited to US hospital based training institutions. For example, matrons' comments on probationers at the Caernarvon and Anglesey hospital in Bangor, Wales in the 1930s and 1940s also included the following negative descriptors, "bad influence," and "resented correction." The power wielded by these supervisors and matrons within the institutional setting was demonstrated by the fact that both US and Welsh trainees could be "called" back to the floor or office at any time to be reprimanded, put back to work or sacked on the spot.[19]

---

[16] Chippewa County War Memorial Hospital Training School of Nursing Students Records 1929–1934, Sault Ste. Marie Hospital Training School of Nursing. Surviving Student Records for the Years 1926–1934. War Memorial Hospital, Sault Ste. Marie, Michigan, USA.

[17] QNI Student Record 1950, QNI Nursing Student Records 1920–1950. Queen's Nursing Institute, Surviving Student Records Spanning the Years 1920–1950. Royal College of Nursing Archives in Edinburgh, UK.

[18] QNI Student Record 1950, QNI Nursing Student Records 1920–1950.

[19] Williams K. Nurse Training in the Carnarfon and Anglesey Hospital 1935–1949, 175.

In marked contrast to this, FNS records were more positive and listed their student nurse's educational progress as either 'good' or 'excellent.' Student class grades were also deployed.[20] Breckinridge's records, instead of evaluating the students' personal character strengths or weaknesses, focused on measuring demographic and statistical data dealing with the number of nurses in each class, degrees held at time of admission, the average grade received on the state board of nursing examination and the tracking of the professional lives of the graduates upon graduation, particularly where they worked and if they procured further education in nursing. Thus, the focus of evaluation at the FNS was the educational ability of the student to meet professional nursing standards, not subjective personal or institutional benchmarks. Indeed, the expectation of education beyond the FNS Graduate Midwifery School must have been a goal, for why else did it track post-graduation? While undoubtedly these students were needed to do the work of the Service, they were never merely working for it but rather were working toward a career as professional nurses. Perhaps the dissatisfaction expressed by student nurses within the other institutional settings and the fact that so many left training prior to completion had more to do with the fact that their training was focused on institutional instead of professional goals, growth and development.

Though Breckinridge did not wholly concur with the reigning ideology of a homogenous approach to nurses' training opting instead for a decentralized power structure, she did believe in generalization (not specialization) and a practical (clinical focus) approach to education best served the community. She wanted to open her school of midwifery at the University of Kentucky and not in a hospital setting so that students could be students first and not staff. The University approved but she was unable to secure the finances necessary for a school based so far away, in Lexington, Kentucky; so, she set up the school at the Service, at Wendover. There, the mentoring of junior by more senior nurses, coupled with classroom instruction, worked well because nurses ran all aspects of the district, public health and hospital environments, administratively, educationally and in practice. This was not the case outside Appalachia. Her curriculum followed the Central Midwives' Board of England and Scotland which required student nurses to deliver 20 cases, five of which were to be done in the hospital and five on district. The emphasis was on teaching and almost at once the school began preparing Nurse-Midwives for other agencies [10]. FNS nurses, both British and American, when asked what they remembered about their nurses training, offered responses that underscored the harsh work environment and difficult training conditions by using descriptors, such as, 'pretty grim,' 'stressful,' and 'hard work with long hours' (see Footnote 12). One FNS nurse highlighted the militaristic, matriarchal and exacting task priority-setting inherent in the institutional training setting with the following response:

> You would work 8–12 h a day and we went to school when we weren't working... I had one head nurse that if I worked on her unit, and we did a lot of split shifts at that stage of my training, and I never got out of uniform because I knew she'd call me back.... She would

---

[20] FNS Graduate School of Midwifery Admissions 1939–1968, 2005M547: FNS, Box 228, Fol. 1, University of Kentucky in Lexington, USA.

find something little and call me back… It was no big deal, I mean, you know, but it was just she was just that type (see Footnote 14).

Another former FNS nurse added that in addition to the long work hours and the class time scheduled when off duty, 'we had to spend our time at night when we should have been going to bed writing up our lectures'.[21] These comments support those made by UK nursing students in a London hospital who left training prior to completion in 1948 explaining their reasons variously as being the 'unnecessarily strict discipline,' 'constant, harsh and unfair treatment meted out by the Matron,' 'long work hours and short leisure periods with interruption of these periods to attend lectures when off duty,' 'reprimand and humiliation in the presence of patients for several of the minor offences due to lack of experience and knowledge,' 'many domestic duties and not sufficient teaching of the science of nursing,' and 'iron-rod discipline which seems to be thought necessary but should be replaced by understanding and leadership.' One student went on to state that those who did not willingly agree to be "puppets in the superior's hands" were then classed as "unruly" and put on chronic wards for long spells of duty while the superior's "pets" were put on wards where they got a good all–round training' [11]. Probationers in the Caernarvon and Anglesey hospital during the 1930s and 1940s mirrored these sorts of complaints, stating that they were often treated as if they were "naughty children." Clearly, nurses in positions of authority within the institutional setting wielded what little power they were allotted over students and nurses, to propagate the status quo within the establishment. What was perhaps most troubling were the comments made by more than one student, which suggested they were taught 'not to think' but rather 'just do as they were told' by either the physicians or the nurse administrators within the institutional setting.[22] Great emphasis was placed in US, English and Welsh nurse training schools on socializing the students to endure hardships, be obedient and above all to be subservient. They were 3-year apprenticeship systems that relied heavily on providing instruction through precept and example, and great emphasis was placed on manual skills, obedience and discipline.

In the US, the national move from hospital based training schools to college or university education for nurses was designed to eliminate the 'staff' component and maximize the 'student' status of the nurse, hence creating an educational environment that was more concerned with producing professional nurses than hospital staff. Yet it also served to obliterate the contributions made by trainee nurses to the health care offered in hospitals during the 1930s and 1940s, and the nursing profession has often failed to appreciate what was achieved during this period. The discipline has consistently deprecated its own worth because it was counted as 'routine care,' 'mundane' and therefore 'less worthy' by the institution. The move within nursing to higher education and away from 'traditional and ritualistic' care, to a more 'evidence-based care system', has served to exaggerate the lack of value placed upon the discipline's past by nurses and non-nurses alike. Ostensibly

---

[21] Molly Lee, British former FNS Nurse-Midwife (1950–1970s).
[22] Williams K. Nurse Training in the Carnarfon and Anglesey Hospital 1935–1949, 176.

this move was also made to negate at least some of the power being wielded by those whom the students called 'petty and tyrannical' ward sisters (matrons or supervisors) thus 'humanizing' their work experience. However, comments volunteered by nurses in practice today challenge that assumption and reinforce the fact that their work is still viewed by those within institutional settings as of less worth when compared with that of other health care providers. The fact that very similar comments continue to be made by nurses in practice today are evident in the following responses from nurses who were asked what they did not like about nursing; 'I do not like *not* being treated as a professional by the doctors,' 'I don't like the fact that nurses are not respected as the true professionals we are,' and 'you receive no respect for the knowledge and responsibilities we have from administration, management and other professions, the thought still being that we should just do what the doctor says.[23]

Further evidence that this corporate trend continues is made by a 1997 US graduate nurse. As a new graduate, she was told by her director of nursing, 'tough, suck it up, this is the way it is,' when she complained about not being able to provide a 'safe' care environment for her patients when, on her first night working in an institutional setting, she was assigned 11 patients, five of whom were preoperative patients.[24] A 2004 US graduate nurse alleged, 'nothing could have prepared me for the way doctors treat nurses and the fact that administration backs up the doctors over the nurse.' She also lamented that 'real life was so much different than school'.[25] A US master's prepared nurse echoed these sentiments from a different perspective when she stated that the reason she left nursing education was that she didn't feel she was adequately preparing her students to practice 'in the real world'.[26]

Former British and American FNS nurses who were at the Service in its early years stated emphatically that they had the 'respect' and trust of the physicians they worked with and always felt they were 'colleagues.' But their practice area was decidedly within the community and not the hospital setting. It was in the Service's latter years, after the provision of care was moved out of the community and into the hospital setting that things changed. The accompanying curtailment of the nurses' autonomy required them to now provide patient care under the watchful eye of physicians, something they had never had to do before:

> We had done with one doctor for so long but then they gradually got a surgeon in and a medical man and then paediatrics. And you know when we started in the new hospital, you had to realize that we had to have these things because they wouldn't have been accredited for one thing, and they were needed. We… we did our own necessitation on the babies unless we… until we had the paediatrician and he came for all our… ones that we expected to have trouble (see Footnote 26).

---

[23] H.C.N. Oncology hospital staff nurse for 2 years. Date surveyed: 08/09/2004; Sable, J., Hospital staff nurse for 2 years; Slampnet, L., Hospital staff nurse for 2.75 years, Date surveyed: 08/10/2005.

[24] Onster V, Hospital staff nurse for 1 year, telemetry 3.5 years, critical care 2 years, dialysis 1 year, research 2 years.

[25] Cranford D, Hospital staff nurse for 2 years, critical care for 15 years.

[26] Conedera J, Hospital paediatric nurse for 20 years. Date surveyed: 15/02/2005.

This was indeed ironic as it was the administrative staff at the FNS after Breckinridge's death who, with the support of the local people, worked to get a hospital built there. The then FNS Director, Helen Brown asked the local people on the district committees if they wanted the FNS to stay even when it became apparent that they would not be able to do so unless they could offer comparable services that rivalled those offered by institutions outside of the region, which the people were more readily able to access in the Service's latter years. Yet the new government health regionalization regulations prohibited the construction of a hospital for small populations of approximately 18,000, which the FNS serviced. They were able to get the hospital through the advocacy of Doctor Beasley who told the regional government that the hospital was needed for "the teaching of primary health care personnel" [12].

Twenty-first century research has shown that unhealthy work environments continue to contribute to medical errors, ineffective patient care, conflict, and stress among health professionals [13]. This is so much so that the American Association of Critical Care Nurses and the Nursing Organization Alliance, a coalition of 72 different nursing organizations, have created specific criteria designed to foster patients' safety, enhance staff recruitment and retention, and maintain an organization's financial viability. These include a call for 'culture change within the institutional setting' via the creation of collaborative practice cultures, communication rich cultures, cultures of accountability, shared decision-making at all levels and recognition on the part of organizations as meaningful and valuable those contributions made by nursing. They also call for authentic, present, expert, competent and visible leadership [14].

Yet how effective these calls for 'cultural change' really are is debatable. It is the prevailing culture that continues to produce seemingly inconceivable errors, such as the one reported in the Pittsburgh, Pennsylvania *Tribune Review*, which cited that brain surgeons at a Rhode Island hospital cut into the wrong side of the head of not one, but three patients. Ironically, the reason cited for nurses not stopping surgeons from doing this, even after an explicit set of required operating-room precautions had been recently adopted by the medical profession to prevent 'wrong-site-surgery' mistakes, was "a culture of fear." It should be mentioned that in one of the cases, it was reported that the surgeon insisted to a nurse who had challenged him that he knew what side of the head to operate on but got it wrong. The fact that the language used by the reporter to describe the nurses was "timid," whereas the physicians were described as "overconfident" aptly illustrated just how ingrained within institutional settings these patterns really are; and that they are created by humans, in accordance with the inclinations of wider society regarding values, language and thought.[27] These patterns have been mutually constructed through a constant process of social interaction, becoming habitual, perceived as 'natural' and taken for granted [15].

---

[27] *Tribune Review*, Greensburg, Pennsylvania, 'Brain surgeons cut wrong side: At Rode Island Hospital, safety checks thwarted by overconfident doctors, timid nurses', The Associated Press, Sunday, 16 December, 2007.

The assistant director of the division of health policy at the Minnesota Health Department, who incidentally is female, was quoted as saying:

> There's a big cultural issue in most operating rooms where there's a hierarchical culture there. A surgeon is used to being the captain of the ship, and his *or her* [italics added] word goes.[28]

Note the status of female doctors within this culture. These acts carried out by physicians at a prestigious medical centre and teaching hospital for the Ivy League's Brown University would have been considered criminally negligent had they been done by anyone else, anywhere else. Yet the terminology used to describe them was not criminally negligent but rather 'overconfident.' The aforesaid assistant director also stated, "Surgeons need that. You don't want an *under*confident [italics added] surgeon operating on you. But that's the downside." Cutting into the wrong side of a person's brain was considered a "downside" to what was viewed by the health care establishment as a valued and necessary cultural trait in surgeons. The Chief Quality Officer for the hospital, who was also female and had apparently bought into the dominant ethos, added that, "The institution was encouraging the staff to report mistakes" and that the only way to "fix" this problem was to "bring it forward." Apparently, simply following existing policy or instituting legal ramifications or policy additions designed to discipline or remediate offending physicians, or even the outright dismissal of offenders was not considered appropriate methods by the institution to "fix" the problem. As long as such a culture is not only permitted to exist within health care institutions but also tolerated by both organizational and wider societies, it does not matter how many principles or standards for sustaining healthy work practice environments nursing organizations create or even how many professional medical protocols are put into place by physician organizations, there can be no sustained, positive change within the culture.

In the previous century at the FNS, disruptions to the nurse-physician relationship had less to do with gender role assignments or even any prevailing patriarchal social mores and much more to do with this move to institutionalized care, its accompanying hierarchy and ingrained cultural patterns. With this came a curtailment of autonomy that was due in large part to the government, which linked payment for services within these walls to physician (male or female) dominance. For example, FNS's long established physician, Doctor Beasley, trained the nurses on the use of a vacuum extractor when it became available for use instead of forceps to aid in difficult deliveries and he permitted the nurses to use them when necessary. Later, newer doctors coming into the FNS would not permit the nurses to use the device. A long established British FNS nurse, who later became an instructor for the midwifery school, related that one night when she was on her own for a delivery she called the physician to use the device and she (the doctor) wouldn't allow her to use it. She called the physician several times in the night and she wouldn't come or give her permission to use the vacuum extractor. This nurse knew it was the right thing to

---

[28] *Tribune Review*, 'Brain surgeons cut wrong side: At Rode Island Hospital, safety checks thwarted by overconfident doctors, timid nurses.'

use. Indeed, she had used it successfully numerous times in the past, without having to contact a physician for permission to do so. This nurse expressed her frustration and sense of failure because as a result of the delay, the patient was in the second stage of labour for a long time and when the doctor eventually did come, the patient had a fourth-degree laceration that needed sutured. The doctor then had to suture the patient, which was also something that this nurse had been taught to do by Dr. Beasley and had done many times without his supervision in the past but was now, no longer permitted to do. She recognized immediately that this physician was "stitching it wrong." because "She'd stitched quite a loom herself when she'd had tears,... bad tears" (see Footnote 21). This nurse's inability to care for her client competently or advocate for her safety was a direct result of this cultural shift. It also could be said to have made her 'timid' about challenging the physician as well as "foolish" in her own eyes for her powerlessness. She added, "Doctors do not trust nurses who have had many years of experience." The physician in this nurse's discourse was female, which raises some intriguing questions concerning gender role and institutional culture perceptions. Her predecessor was a male physician who was a staunch supporter of nurses and was instrumental in launching a Nurse Practitioner Program at the FNS when his contemporaries were opposed to it as a to their 'legal responsibility' as sole providers of 'medical care'[29]. This particular nurse left the FNS shortly after the move toward institutionalized care citing the decline in professional practice as well as patient care as the driving force behind her final decision to leave. She was also documented as asking for clarification from administration regarding "suturing on district" in the 18 March 1965, FNS Staff Meeting minutes. Nursing staff were told at this meeting that "numbing" done on district had always been discouraged because of the danger of a "reaction." Minor cuts could be sutured without "numbing" and more serious cuts should come in to the physician. Therefore, the meeting concluded that "No district nurse was to use numbing without first checking with the physician".[30] So, the female administrator who replaced Breckinridge also began backing the physicians over the nurse's due solely to the regulatory and consequent cultural changes imposed upon the organization in its latter years.

Apparently, it was not only the nursing staff who was dissatisfied with the changes wrought in the advent of institutionalized care at the FNS. In the September 1966 FNS Staff Meeting Minutes, the then Director, Miss Browne stated in answer to her staff's question, 'why can't more patients be seen since we now have two doctors,' that Dr. Beasley had become "very discouraged" because he felt he was practicing "first aid medicine only." Browne also stated that Doctor Wise was an "able physician" but that the FNS didn't want to swamp her with so many patients that she too would feel she was only doing "first aid medicine".[31] It was shortly after this that Dr. Beasley left the FNS. One could certainly argue that he became just as frustrated

[29] Letter from Robert R. Huntley, M.D. to W.B Rogers Beasley, M.D. 26 April 1966, 2005M547: FNS, Box 227, Fol. 9.

[30] FNS Staff Meeting Minutes, 18 March 1965, 85M1: FNS, Box 70, Fol. 9. University of Kentucky in Lexington, USA.

[31] FNS Staff Meeting Minutes, 1 September 1966, 85M1: FNS, Box 220, Fol. 9.

with the increase in his responsibilities as the nurses were with the decrease in theirs. By this time, legislative regulations had disrupted the original way of doing business at the FNS and the nurse-midwives were removed from district and placed within the walls of the hospital.[32] It should be noted that it was not until the British Nurse-Midwives were forced to move into the institutional setting that they, who once had worked so closely with physicians, began to be perceived as enemies of "progress" and "foreigners," and that had little to do with gender as the physicians who made these comments were also female.[33]

The battle between nurse autonomy and physician authority continues, albeit where one is working tends to be the barometer regarding exactly how far and to what degree that obtains. The US nurse graduate who stated that she 'did not like *not* [italics added] being treated like a professional by doctors' went n to explain that this did not happen often but when it did she was "quick to stand up for herself".[34] A 1992 master's prepared Canadian nurse who began her 24-year career as a hospital diploma graduate stated that she didn't like the 'assistant/handmaiden role that was so prevalent where she trained,' explaining:

> As students, we had to stand when the doctor entered the nursing station and stop whatever we were doing if he needed the chart. The head nurse or charge nurse was about the only one who could even talk to the doctor'.[35]

It should be noted that this nurse got her diploma as recently as 1981. She conceded that the sort of royal treatment that doctors were given when she was in training was indeed a thing of the past, but lamented that physicians still didn't understand advanced (nursing) practice and realized that she was now living in a "medical backwater" in many ways with a strong "old boys" network despite her advanced degree. A US nurse who graduated 25 years later also stated that she too disliked the fact that she had to "clear things with the medical doctor, that most medical doctors do not care about or have the same level of knowledge that many nurses have." She explained, "One incident would be a patient's activity ability, restraints or at times even diets".[36] Three US nurses, all of whom graduated within the last 25 years, had the following to say about physicians they worked with, 'they can be ungrateful and I am disappointed by that fact. I am disappointed that there seems to be an "us" against "them" attitude with the doctors,' and that they (the nurses) would like more "respect" from them.

Midwifery training was universally described by former FNS nurses who graduated in the 1950s and 60s as a vastly different experience, whether the training was taken up at the FNS or in the UK prior to coming to work for the Service. This

---

[32] Judy Haralson-Rafson, American former FNS Nurse (1971–1976; 1971 Graduate of FNS Family Nurse Practitioner Program).

[33] Interview #82OH05FNS148, 1982, Dr. Mary Weiss & Dr. Pauline Fox.

[34] Sable J, Hospital staff nurse for 2 years.

[35] Morrison S, Hospital staff nurse for 1 year, critical care for 10 years, pain management for 13 years.

[36] Scarfe B, Hospital staff nurse for 6 years, critical care 2 years.

should not be surprising as the FNS based its program on that which was the norm in the UK. One long time former FNS nurse stated it most succinctly when she compared her midwifery training with that of her general nurses training:

> Midwifery training…. I had gotten so much more from, and quite a lot of that was to do with having a tutor, Margaret F. Myles, who was the first person to actually write a textbook for midwives. Before that we didn't have any Obstetricians. And she…. She was very dynamic, and I don't know how she managed to do everything she had to do but there were new students coming in all the time and I worked it out that she had about 180 students under her care at any one time, with no… no assistance. So, she did the clinical teaching and the…. the theoretical teaching, and all the rest of it. Yeah, I was enthused by that, it was good training, I'm sure. But things are different now. It was hard working on the… on the wards. There were a lot of people stayed in bed and shortage of stock supplies and so forth…. But it was good training (see Footnote 12).

Note the pupil-midwife's description of training where the teacher- midwife has 'no Obstetricians' and the practice setting, though within a hospital setting, was arduous, completely autonomous and described as 'good' even in an over-worked and under supplied institutional environment. In addition, the fact that the student was mentored by a positive role model was also significant in both the student's satisfaction with the training and the quality of the training. The only other really positive comment on training was made by another British former FNS nurse who trained for her midwifery certificate at the same hospital as Mary Breckinridge in London. She stated that she was 'surprised how much she enjoyed it (midwifery training) and how kind all the top-notch staff were to us pupil midwives' when compared with the general training. A British former FNS nurse highlighted the status distinction made between University and Hospital-based education when she commented in her discourse that the headmaster at her school was "disappointed" to learn that she was choosing to go into nursing and not on to University.[37]

The moving of nursing education from hospital based to college or university settings was conceived of to emphasize the status of the student as scholar-apprentice and not merely as staff-employee. It was also designed to eradicate enculturation on the part of the student to a specific institution in favour of developing a professional identity within the discipline of nursing. Yet responses from nurses demonstrated that this conflict has not been fully eradicated but rather deferred. Only four of the 20 nurses in practice responded wholly in the affirmative that their education to practice transition was all they thought it would be. A US nurse with fourteen years' experience stated, 'I had great and inspiring registered nurses from instructors to preceptors but those that instilled the pride and honor of nursing in me earlier on were my Vietnam veteran registered nurses'.[38] This nurse shared in her discourse that she was working in a 'Magnet Hospital' in California, the only state in the country that has a law governing the patient to nurse ratio in institutional settings. 'Magnet' status has been given by the American Nurses' Credentialing Centre (ANCC), an affiliate of

---

[37] Margaret (Maggie) Willson, British former FNS Nurse-Midwife (1955–1967).

[38] Fighting H, Hospital staff nurse & telemetry for 10 years; critical care & telemetry step-down for 1 year; nursing education & staff development for 2 years. Date surveyed: 07/07/2006.

the American Nurses Association, since the 1980s, to hospitals that satisfy a set of criteria designed to measure the strength and quality of nursing. A Magnet hospital indicates nursing involvement in data collection and decision-making in patient care delivery, rewards nurses accordingly and delivers excellent patient outcomes as a result. It is also where nurses purportedly have a high level of job satisfaction, and where there is a low staff nurse turnover rate and appropriate grievance resolution. Magnet hospitals are supposed to have open communication between nurses and other members of the health care team and an appropriate personnel mix to attain the best patient outcomes and staff work environment [16].

However, though some nurses are enthusiastic about the Magnet program, others have been highly critical of the way the program has been implemented and have asserted that there is little evidence that nurses at Magnet hospitals are really much better off than nurses elsewhere, suggesting that many of its voluntary guidelines may offer only the illusion of nurse empowerment. Critics including the California Nurses Association and the Massachusetts Nurses Association have argued that the Magnet program is primarily a hospital promotion tool that resembles the Joint Commission on Accreditation of Healthcare Organizations in its seemingly incestuous relations with hospital management [17]. The Centre for Nursing Advocacy has heard many first-hand reports of some hospitals trumpeting their new Magnet status even as they proceed to betray some of the program's key principles. This reality was reinforced by a nurse who volunteered the following information about her Magnet Hospital while addressing how she felt that the profession, nurses and the professional role of nurses had changed:

> I find the rushed atmosphere in the academic hospital to be counter-productive to meaningful patient care. It is truly a factory with very little consideration for individuals (patient and practitioner alike). I am even sorrier to say that I practice at a "Magnet Hospital." If this is the pinnacle of nursing practice, I am truly concerned.[39]

This observation by a 1992 US nurse with 14 years' experience was also expressed, practically word-for-word, by a 1990 US nurse graduate, a 1952 UK Hospital Diploma graduate, a 1957 US Hospital Diploma graduate and several student nurses who left training prematurely in 1948 who had participated in Dr. Cohen's survey for a UK Report that called for 'change' and the 'humanizing' of hospital conditions and improved salaries for nurses.[40] The use by these nurses of the term 'factory' to describe the work environment was significant as it is language usually reserved to describe industrial or manufacturing work. The lack of consideration for individuals (patient and practitioner alike) was also evident in a statement made by a student nurse in a London Hospital in 1948 when she commented that, "priority was given to tidying of lockers and straightening of beds before the care of the patients".[41] Institutional tasks may have changed since

---

[39] Sloan MS, Hospital operating room staff nurse for 2.5years, research .5 years.

[40] Cohen J. Minority report: working party on the recruitment and training of nurses. London: Metropolitan Library Archives. p. 56.

[41] Cohen J. Minority report: working party on the recruitment and training of nurses: Metropolitan Library Archives. p. 71.

1948, but the frustration was still clearly evident in a comment made by a nurse in practice who stated, "Healthcare in general has too many regulations and much of the work is paperwork." Another also used the term "factory-like experience" to describe the work of a nurse (i.e., getting patients into their rooms, assessed quickly, providing treatment, charting and shipping them out again)," in response to what aspects of the work they didn't like.[42]

It was of particular interest to note that the nurse respondents in their discourse concerning work environment were not asked about Magnet status but rather spontaneously volunteered the fact that the hospital at which they were employed had this status. It should also be mentioned that two other nurses responded affirmatively regarding their work environments within a Magnet designated hospital. One had less than 1 year's experience and was working in a specialty, neonatal intensive care unit in California where she said, 'the pay isn't bad' either.[43] Another, with only 1 year's experience, working in an Oncology specialty area, also mentioned that her job satisfaction was in part due to the facility in which she worked, had realistic nurse to patient ratios and was a Magnet Hospital.[44] All the positive experiences expressed here regarding the move from education to practice environments for new nurses occurred within specialty units in the institutional setting with either appropriate patient to nurse ratios, or where nurses were adequately compensated or felt they had some level of autonomy in practice. Yet despite the fact that professionalism, autonomy and patient advocacy is certainly taught in nursing education environments, are nurses really in a position within health care institutions to accomplish these aims when they enter practice?

The following by a nurse illustrated how wide the gap between education and practice cultures really was and the disillusionment experienced by nurses attempting to bridge it:

> My greatest disappointment is the lack of respect from all facets of healthcare providers (medical doctors, physical therapists, occupational therapists, nutrition and other registered nurses). I find a great deal of the blame placed on nursing, questionable cooperation, and dismissal of nursing concerns. I find my education is not honored. Those moments when you connect with a patient and make a difference for them, those situations where you are considered part of the team and your input about the patient is valued in a functional dynamic, it is the most rewarding thing I have ever experienced. I am hopeful that there will be a time where these moments are the rule and not the exception (see Footnote 39).

Embedded within this nurse's statement regarding objective versus subjective rewards are issues concerning the lack of autonomy and professional value experienced by nurses within the existing culture. Unfortunately, it is a perspective shared by many nurses. Note the vivid language used by this nurse who described her dislike of having her opinions about patient care "discarded like yesterday's trash." She goes on to stipulate that she also doesn't like when nurses are not more professional within their own ranks citing, 'accountability, responsibility and keeping up

---

[42] Neckar R, Hospital emergency room staff nurse for 5 years, home health nurse for 4 years.

[43] Randon L, Hospital neonatal intensive care unit <1 year.

[44] H.C.N., Oncology hospital staff nurse for 2 years.

with advances like evidenced based practice' are not embraced by all nurses (see Footnote 24). A US nurse with fourteen years' experience stated that she felt the "culture of nursing" was encouraging confidence in knowledge and skills to advocate for patients' amongst new nurses but also stated that she had found her "niche" as a fitness and labour and delivery *specialist* [italics added] where she was able to "merge" her veteran fitness expert status with her career in pre-and post-natal labour and delivery. It was in this 'specialist' capacity that she could "empower women" within the institutional culture in which she worked.[45] Indeed, the evolution of nurse specialist roles is increasing and the general public as well as nurses have expressed increased satisfaction when these nurse's follow-up on patient care in the community as well as the institutional setting [18].

Like many problems and schisms associated with the discipline of nursing, the concept of education is fraught with ambivalence among nurses. The lack of 'academic' requirement associated with nursing and the distinctly 'hands-on,' 'working with people' (relational) element to the work was strongly evidenced as a motivation to choose nursing by the American and British FNS nurses. Of the seven American and five British FNS nurses interviewed or surveyed, ten stayed in nursing in some capacity until they retired; with three of the American nurses still in practice. Half of these FNS nurses also furthered their education in nursing by taking advanced certifications, a bachelors, masters or PhD. All of these diploma nurses felt that their hospital based education was valuable, despite the harsh conditions, due to the amount of clinical exposure it afforded. This has been lost with the move to colleges or university settings, though none advocated a return to diploma schools and all agreed that the move had decreased the severity of the environment for students, which was more conducive to their overall education.

Nurses in practice are less cohesive as a group than their FNS colleagues on this issue. One nurse found nursing more "technical" than she thought of when she went into nursing because she "wanted to help people", advocated bachelors' level (a 4-year degree) as the entry level to practice: "not because they are better nurses but because it gains more respect from other professions" (see Footnote 42). This would appear to contradict the reality expressed by other nurses who felt disrespected regardless of their education level. A bachelor prepared nurse felt that multiple entry levels (varied academic preparation) to practice (i.e., Licensed Practical Nursing Certificate, Hospital Diploma, Associate and Bachelors Degrees) contributed to the overall lack of respect for nurses as educated, thinking, caring individuals and kept them out of important choices for patients (see Footnote 39). The Canadian nurse who began her career with a diploma held an opposing view. She felt the educational process doesn't often give nurses a realistic idea of what nursing is before or during their education. Additionally, she questioned the worth of taking a 4 or 5-year degree in order to work 12-h shifts, nights, weekends and holidays when for that same investment of time, energy and money one could get a degree in a subject with good pay and better hours. This nurse stated that one should

[45] Shelley W, Hospital telemetry nurse for 1 year, internal medicine & obstetrics-gynaecology office nurse for 5 years, labour & delivery room nurse for 9 years.

not require a bachelor's degree as entry to practice in order to legitimize and boost nurses' standing among other health care professionals, with degrees like physical therapy, et cetera. Instead, she called for nursing to value, recognize and support the various roles nursing can play from bedside care to community and outpatient work to advanced practice nursing that included, *but was not limited to* [italics added] advanced practice areas, such as Nurse Practitioners (see Footnote 35).

The FNS Graduate School of Midwifery listed the following criteria for entry in addition to having a diploma from an accredited nurse training school: state registration or foreign country with equivalent standards, good health, good professional and character references. There was no age limit and college credits were allowed but on an individual basis.[46] The School incorporated hospital and home care pre-natal visits, deliveries and post-natal follow-up for the students, which was not the standard program of study outside of Eastern Appalachia. It was a well-rounded education that focused on teaching the students how to be nurse-midwifes and not employees. Students were paid $40 per day in addition to receiving free room, board, uniforms and laundry services. They did pay for some of their own food but were able to save quite a bit of their wages, which for both students and employees admittedly were never comparable to what they could have made outside of Appalachia. The sole reason for expulsion was a breach in nursing ethics and records from inception of the school in 1939–25 July 1957 reveal that no one was ever expelled from the school.[47]

In stark contrast to FNS policy concerning criteria for dismissal, the dismissal of hospital based student nurses, who were in effect the 'employees' of the institution in all but wage and name, were much more the norm outside of the Service. In addition to nursing ethics, illness, disobedience and any manner of a number of institutional rules and regulations or what was deemed by hospital administrators as 'character' breaches were also considered valid reasons for dismissal. A student was dismissed from the Chippewa County War Memorial Hospital Training School by a supervisor for the following:

> Continuing to disobey after having been warned several times and promising that if she was allowed to stay, she would do what was right. That same night she again disobeyed.[48]

Of the surviving student records for this US hospital based school of nursing, four to ten students from 1920 to 1928 were admitted and on average less than half of the class graduated. Some of the other reasons for dismissal documented included 'easily distracted by things external to work,' 'angry outburst,' 'ill health,' 'intoxication' and 'being too young' (see Footnote 48). One student who was docu-

---

[46] Letter of Petition for Approval of the FNS Graduate School of Midwifery 1939, 2005M547: FNS, Box 227, Fol. 1. 'Letter of Petition for Approval of the FNS Graduate School of Midwifery to Immigration and National Service Department, 1939', University of Kentucky in Lexington, USA.

[47] FNS Graduate School of Midwifery Admission Documents 1939–1957, 2005M547: FNS, Box 228, Fol. 1.

[48] Chippewa County War Memorial Hospital Training School of Nursing Students Records 1929–1934.

mented as having done good work 'resigned' but for the majority of those who were either dismissed or did not finish the program there was no substantiating documentation. Indeed, even when there was documentation giving a reason for dismissal for disobedience on the part of the student, there was no record as to what that entailed.

A former American FNS nurse who received her diploma from a hospital based school of nursing, Geisinger Medical Centre, and later a Bachelors of Science and Public Health Nursing degree from the University of Pennsylvania, and Case Western Reserve, a Master's degree from the University of Kentucky and a PhD from London University stated, with a sly grin, that when she graduated from nurses' training in 1939 she was given an award for 'best bedside nurse' while simultaneously having accumulated 299 'demerits' for breaking many of the rigid hospital rules that existed for nursing students at the time. She stated that she was 'always in trouble' but that to be 'in trouble' all one need do was be 'out late' to receive 'demerits.' She also said that if a student received 300 demerits at her nurses' training school they were automatically expelled from the program. She reported that 'lights out' was at 10 p.m. and when the house mother would make rounds she was sure to have a dummy in her bed when she was out past curfew (see Footnote 2). She also admitted to liking to wear 'bright red socks' because they were prohibited. This nurse was at the FNS from 1956 to 1972, with occasional leaves of absence to further her education in nursing. She has just become one of the first five inductees into the University of Kentucky College Of Nursing's Hall of Fame on 1 June, 2007.[49] Yet this nurse was considered undesirable and disobedient in 1939. Not only did she stay in nursing but she had a very diverse career that included procuring a PhD, teaching nursing, doing a 4-year stint with the US Army Nurse Corps from 1960 to 1964 during the Vietnam war and working as a pioneer nurse in Alaska where she ran a team of 23 dogs and 409 pounds of equipment in a basket on her sled to visit villagers and travel to others by bush plane (see Footnote 2). The rigidity she experience in 1939 at a US hospital diploma school was mirrored in the comments made a decade later by student nurses in a UK hospital diploma school who cited one of the many reasons for leaving the program prior to completion as being, "the 10:30 p.m. time limit with one late pass a week and the fuss to get it," and 'the "boarding school" element, which the modern girl will not take' [19]. These nurses should perhaps have been grateful for the half hour of extra time away from the institution that post-war progress had afforded the discipline. The fact that the former FNS nurse was given leave to pursue advanced degrees attests to the FNS's desire to provide for the professional development and personal needs of the staff as well as the needs of the community. This approach not only benefited the nurse but it also benefited the organization as retention of the nurse was much more likely to be maintained. It also benefited the community as the skill level, confidence and educational level of the nurse increased upon her return. Also, the advantage that a mentally and emotionally revitalized nurse would be to her patients could not be

---

[49] *Harrodsburg Herald*, Kentucky. 'Local woman to be honored for years of service: Dr. Herman will be one of first five inductees into nursing hall of fame' by Debbie Jenkins-Cook (2007), 1A & 14A.

over emphasized, particularly in rural Appalachia. In fact, a nurse did not need to be ill, have an accident or wish to further her education in order to get leave. Often, all she had to do was ask for it. A former British FNS nurse who was at the Service from 1949 to 1954 requested 6 months leave "to travel" and was given the time off (see Footnote 14).

The following was a vivid illustration of just how dissociate the FNS was from other organizational cultures regarding the approach taken by administrators in the treatment of their nursing staff. A report about a nursing student in 1929 by a supervisor at the Chippewa County War Memorial Hospital Training School, 'Does not seem very strong, moves as though very tired.' This student also had copies of letters written to her mother by the supervisor in her student file. They revealed that the girl was thought to have Typhoid fever but was later diagnosed as having influenza, was being treated and urging the mother 'not to be alarmed.' This student was later dismissed due to 'illness' (see Footnote 48).

When Breckinridge was faced with productivity problems due to nurses being physically or emotionally ill as a direct or even indirect result of the work environment, she never dismissed them. She made sure that they received the same quality of health care that the Service provided to the community and the time off necessary to enable them to eventually return to work. Leaves of absence were common amongst FNS nurse employees who, due to the rigorous work environment and the relative isolation from friends, family and the amenities of modern life in Appalachia, found themselves in need of a respite, some for as long as 6 months or a year.

Three long time employees who had cancer were treated at the Service at no cost to the nurses. Breckinridge herself was treated at the hospital prior to her death, as were nurses who were injured or simply fell ill, whether or not it occurred on duty [20]. Over the Service's long history, only a few FNS nurses were either hurt or fell ill while employed there. Accidents tended to involve mishaps with horses or jeeps, river or bridge crossings and snake bites [21]. However, by far the most horrific example of a physical injury sustained by an FNS nurse was when an explosive device meant for a law enforcement officer who halted the moonshine production of a local man inadvertently blew-up an FNS jeep carrying a nurse and her sister who was visiting the area (see Footnote 21). The nurse, who was British, was not on duty at the time, yet the FNS made sure that both she and her sister who were seriously injured in the blast were stabilized at the local hospital and received specialized care at a larger, more urban hospital in the US free of charge prior to returning to Great Britain. All the costs of their hospitalization as well as their journey back to England were paid for by the Service.

Then FNS director, Helen E. Browne also secured district nursing services through the QNI and a rehabilitation facility for them once they arrived back in the UK.[50] This British nurse eventually returned to the FNS after a few years absence, finally officially retiring in 1978 (see Footnote 21). Nurses who received this type of

---

[50] Helen E. Brown Letter to QNI Director, Miss Grey 1965, SA/QNI/'Correspondence between QNI Director, Miss Grey and FNS Director, Helen E. Browne', 24 October 1965.

consideration from their employer were more apt to stay with the organization due to a reciprocated loyalty. Therefore, it is not surprising that of the eight former FNS nurses who did not go to the Service for a midwifery certification, four chose to stay well beyond their contracted two-year commitment. Of these four, two when they did leave the Service opted to come back for lengthy periods (one of these to attend the Nurse Practitioner Program as well as work) before retiring from the Service altogether. Thus, a comment made by a nurse regarding the education and practice environment at the FNS:

> As there were only three students in my class we were on call night and day for home deliveries—plus working in prenatal and postnatal visits (mostly on horseback) with only emergencies on Sundays. I was the only driver in my class so I got the calls which were where there were roads, one of which I noted was my 38th. delivery and my first without a supervisor![51]

Note the fact that this student had done 37 deliveries before she was permitted to do one on her own. The FNS had a 1 month 'mentoring' program when short staffed. The preference was for a 6-week preceptorship with an experienced nurse.[52] New nurses were not to be given a district but act as a 'floater' instead to relieve district nurses where necessary; and in this way become familiar with the centres. Overall, the FNS nurses interviewed tended to downplay the negative aspects of the general training, and focused instead on the camaraderie with fellow nurses, the nurses over them who inspired them and the use of training to better them selves or enhance their lives in future. These records from British and American schools of nursing, as well as the comments made by former British and American FNS nurses, illustrate an oppressive environment created as much by conformity to the institution on the part of nurse educators and administrators as on the existing socio-economic power structures external to the profession. They also reveal the class prejudice and precedence being placed on institutional tasks over and above either the care of the patient or the personal growth and professional education of the nurse. Clearly, the ability of student nurses to exhibit the strength, speed and the unquestioning obedience necessary to complete the exacting work of the institution was imperative. All of these comments suggest nursing's gate-keepers, namely its leaders (educators and administrators), helped to create generations of disenfranchised nurses through enculturation to the institutional culture.

7.4 Enculturation: Am *I* 'Just a Nurse' or Is *It* 'Just a Job?'

An ex-army nurse preceded Dr. Cohen's call in 1948 for UK nurse training school reform in an October 1946 issue of *The Trained Nurse and Hospital Review*, a US publication. Though the article focused on the 'public perception' or image of

---

[51] Madonna Buret-Spratt, American FNS Midwifery School Graduate of 1960.
[52] Reprint of FNS *Quarterly Bulletin* 1935, 85M1: FNS, Box 25, Fol. 2. 'Organization & Supervision of the Filed Work of the FNS', University of Kentucky in Lexington, USA.

nursing and not the work environment, it mentioned the need for salary increases and blamed hospital supervisors and principals of schools of nursing as part of the establishment for contributing to nursing's problems, as did Dr. Cohen. She accused nursing administrators and educators of allowing the public perception of nursing to 'slip' by admitting and graduating women who hurt the reputation of nursing, stating 'standards are not high enough' in training schools,' morally low classed women should be weeded-out and rules should be enforced.' She mentioned that though hospitals were 'desperate for nurses,' they were turning down women in the interview process who 'talked pay raises or unions' in favour of women who were 'second rate' in 'intelligence, maturity and moral fibre'.[53] Clearly, salary (economic power) and nursing solidarity (political clout) would threaten the existing power disparity within the institutional setting and this nurse felt a conscious effort had been made on the part of nurses within the establishment to maintain the institutional socio-economic and political status quo at the expense of the profession.

This same criticism was repeated 59 years later by a 13-year veteran nurse presently in practice who observed, 'nursing accepts quantity not quality' and stated 'they should have higher criteria for entering the nursing profession' (see Footnote 39). Yet in this nurse's interpretation it was the socio-economic advantage sought in 1946 to increase the quality of nurse applicants that was cited as the reason for a lack of quality nurses entering practice today. This nurse stated that many nurses were choosing the profession for the wrong reason, namely 'money' and 'job security'; that they viewed the profession as 'just a job.' Indeed, the exact language, 'just a job,' was also used by another nurse who was a licensed practical nurse for 16 years and then an associate degree nurse for 9 years. She also stated that younger nurses 'do not take ownership in their positions as a nurse' preferring instead to, 'come in, do your time and go home'.[54] Further, she stated that she was currently a preceptor for registered nursing students in an institutional setting where she made the following observation:

> Out of those 20 (students) maybe, just maybe, two to four of them really are in it because they want to be a nurse and the rest are in it for the money and that's it. They have no initiative to do anything except watch. It saddens me because you can get back much more than you give to your patients. They just see it as a job. I give 100% to all of my patients and have no regrets. I love what I do.

The nurse with the most experience who began as a diploma graduate and now holds a master's degree lamented that too many 'new' nurses, especially those with bachelor's degrees do not want to do basic care, work shifts or work in hospitals, she said, 'they want to, "start at the top" and are unwilling to "pay their dues" (see Footnote 35).

---

[53] *The Trained Nurse and Hospital Review*, 85M1: FNS, Box 36, Fol. 6. 'Nursing Ethics by Frances O'Reilly, RN, an ex-army nurse who writes on the public perception of nurses slipping and blaming it on educators and administrators not maintaining high enough standards, (October 1946). University of Kentucky in Lexington, USA.

[54] Deb40253, Geriatrics for 12 years, hospital staff nurse for 3 years, emergency room for 4 years, home health for 6 year, part-time psychiatric nurse for 5 years.

This attitude from older, more established nurses was underscored by a nurse who had been in practice for only 5 years. She volunteered that as a young nurse, very eager to move her career from a clinical focus to more of an education/research focus was not feeling very supported from 'the larger nursing community' to do so. She stated:

> The saying that nurses eat their young has been very true for me. I have found that you are not taken seriously in nursing unless you have "put in your time".[55]

Former FNS nurses made remarkably similar observations of students and nurses coming into the Service in the mid-1960s and 1970s. A former FNS Nurse-Midwife turned Midwifery instructor whose tenure at the Service spanned over 30 years volunteered with distaste that 'They put a Jacuzzi or something in Hyden after I left', in reference to changes made to accommodate students at the Service in its latter years (see Footnote 21). FNS staff meeting minutes also reflected the need for then director, Helen E. Browne to coach the 'younger nurses' to reassure patients as to why they refuse to see them. She told them that they are often 'too quick to say "it's too late" or "I can't come until tomorrow".[56] Prior to this, patients were seen at home and at a time more convenient for them. With the advent of Medicaid and Medicare payment for services, the government decided that the clinic or hospital was where patients should be seen, within set hours that were either more convenient or cost effective for the institution. Further, FNS nurses had never refused to see patients for any reason in the past and this created friction not only with the community but also with nurses of longer standing. At first glance, this schism between 'older' and 'younger' nurses would appear to focus on the level of humanitarian values held by them but closer examination reveals a more complex problem that also deals with governmental, professional, educational and practice institution enculturation and the rigidity inherent within these environments than any specific age group.

This is evidenced by the fact that younger nurse respondents in practice with less than 6 years of experience also stated their dissatisfaction with how 'nurses' have changed. One said, 'The American Nurses Association Code of Ethics no longer seemed to matter to many nurses'.[57] She explained that though some nurses 'take a stand and unite for the common good of patients,' others 'feel that they can undermine the entire process and sell themselves to the highest bidder.' In reference to how this was a problem not only for 'new' nurses but also for those long enough in the profession to enter positions of leadership, she cited an instance where nurse educators tried to teach students the 'values of the profession' while simultaneously forcing them to cross the picket lines of hospital nurses on strike to uphold those very same values. Newer nurses proved to be as ambivalent about the profession and the work as the older ones though their reasons varied. Some admitted they had 'less commitment to the profession or the facilities as they felt that getting

---

[55] Miller A, Hospital paediatric nurse for 4 years, educator for <1 year.

[56] FNS Staff Meeting Minutes 18 March 1965, 85M1: FNS, Box 220, Fol. 9. 'FNS Staff Meeting Minutes (1965–1966)', University of Kentucky in Lexington, USA.

[57] Slampnet L, Hospital staff nurse for 2.75 years.

another job was no big deal' while others expressed concern that, 'we (nurses) were still more worried about what the other nurse was doing than what the government and American Medical Association was doing to us' (see Footnote 36). The former comment reinforces the perception made by more experienced nurses that nursing was 'just a job' to these newer nurses but perhaps this phenomenon should be expected as, historically, professional, educational and practice institutions have not demonstrated their fidelity to nurses. So, to expect the same sort of reciprocal loyalty from these nurses that the FNS enjoyed from its nursing staff in its early years proved to be an unrealistic expectation. The latter comment suggested a desire for more professional solidarity amongst nurses but less from identification with one's profession and from a perceived need to unite against those external forces deemed to be more powerful. Here we see multiple generations of nurses identifying a problem and solution only to have the solution not only create another problem but more often than not prove to be merely another facet of the same problem.

Economic advantages (higher wages) and political power (unions or even professional organizations) are perceived by nurses to attract quality applicants into institutional settings and create solidarity amongst nurses. Yet those 'above average' wages have also been blamed for drawing nurses into practice 'for the wrong reasons [22]. Furthermore, nurses have crossed the picket lines of nurses who were seeking to increase wages, improve patient to nurse ratios (patient safety) and increase nursing's 'say in patient care,' a reality which hardly evokes an image of solidarity, professional or otherwise [23]. A 17-year nurse veteran who is still working in an Intensive Care Unit (ICU) in the US, illustrated the harsh reality of many institutions where nurses continue to feel trapped and disillusioned within the culture regardless of salary considerations:

> My attitude changed when I reached the top of the pay scale and realized I couldn't make anymore. At the same time I felt I was more knowledgeable and a good resource, but the hospital didn't recognize that. Hospitals are caught up in the paperwork to satisfy the Joint Commission on Accreditation for Hospital Organizations (JCAHO) and budgets, the essence and spirit of what a nurse brings to the patients has been lost… Nursing needs a major overhaul. We need to get back to respect ourselves and the profession. Nursing needs to have some control over the patient environment and the way nursing functions (see Footnote 25).

Note the language used here imitated that by nursing students in 1948 to describe institutional drudgery and the preference given to it over and above that of the patients' needs or care. Moreover, this nurse stated that the 'essence' and 'spirit' of what a nurse brings to the patient had been lost. The realization that knowledge and experience do not equate with either status or pecuniary reward and the obvious humanitarian loss associated with the business model was also highlighted. This nurse in no way indicated that any of these key elements; respect, knowledge, experience, professional control, essence or spirit of nursing care, were either mutually exclusive or of greater or lesser value. What was perhaps most illuminating in this nurse's discourse was the call not for institutional change but 'nursing' to change. She stated emphatically that it was 'nursing' that needed a major overhaul and 'nursing' that needed to gain control. She still saw herself as a part of a wider organizational culture, 'we need to get back to respect ourselves and the profession.'

A Canadian nurse stated that she had, many times, seriously considered leaving nursing but could not get a job with anywhere near the income she could make as a nurse. In addition, her many years of education were all in nursing and thus did not leave many options when coupled with the personal and financial barriers which existed for her (see Footnote 35).

She had hoped to enter medical school but was not able to do so, ending-up instead with a long career in nursing. She began her career with a diploma, earned a master's degree and had over 24 years of experience but admitted that if she had it to do over again she might not choose nursing as a career, stating that if she did do nursing again, she would go for a 'clinical doctorate' in nursing so that she could 'at least get some of the recognition as a serious clinician.' She went on to state that she hugely supported nursing's ability to provide top notch, individualized, holistic care but felt the "environment both inside nursing as well as without is too far from valuing nurses appropriately." Remarkably, this nurse also used possessive descriptors when relating her view of what ailed the profession when she stated twice in the same paragraph, 'nursing doesn't know who nursing is. We don't value ourselves or our contributions to care so it was no wonder other professions and the public often don't value or understand nurses and nurses work.' Perhaps the most significant and abysmal reality was uncovered when she admitted, 'I'm 'too old' to go back to school to become a 'Nurse Practitioner' only to finish when 'almost ready to retire,' I am 'frustrated,' 'angry' and 'trapped' by the institution as well as 'a very good salary.'

On the surface, this would appear to support the claims made by Heyes who has argued that a high income "attracted the 'wrong sort' of person into nursing" [24]. Except for the fact that this nurse didn't cite a 'high wage' as a reason for entering nursing at all but rather as the sole reason for not leaving it so close to retirement. This nurse's obvious cultural identification with the profession as evidenced by the possessive language used, her desire for personal 'recognition' and her 'support' of the overall profession's abilities, coupled with the negative statements made in reference to the 'value' placed upon both from nurses and non-nurses alike, indicated that she fully grasped the limitations inherent within the existing system for the humanitarian and professional rewards that she valued regardless of the economic advantages.

At the FNS in its early years, this value system was reversed, even in its hospital. This was because the function of the FNS hospital was the opposite of how hospitals were being utilized outside of the region. The hospital in Eastern Appalachia was only to be utilized for emergent, serious cases that required closer monitoring of the patient than could be done by the nurse out in the community. The FNS organization, hospital and outposts were nurse founded, nurse controlled and not dependent upon the government or any institutional entity for survival in its early years. This was not the norm outside of the Service where hospitals, clinics and public health organizations were primarily either directly or indirectly controlled by third party reimbursement systems (mainly government, insurance company and employers).

When asked what affected change the most at the FNS, it was not the great depression, drought, the advent of World War Two or any other external force cited as having the most negative impact on the Service but the government sponsored health insurance plans introduced into the region and which subsequently dictated practice by what it would pay for. Hence, the change shifted the main focus of care from more than just a social standpoint. The move was not merely from a social (home to hospital) but also from an economic perspective (from individual patient or community to institution). Births at home became the exception and not the norm as one nurse could oversee more than one patient and less time was required to get to the patient.[58] As with most of the changes made at the FNS in its latter years, they gave the organization as the priority and not the patient. One nurse for more patients certainly reduced costs and increased productivity but only when productivity was measured by the amount of output created (in terms of goods produced or services rendered) per unit input used. As Henry Hazlitt (1946) explains in *Economics in One Lesson*, increasing production reduces prices and therefore goods become more widely available [25]. This focus may work for automobiles, which were initially hand made and only available to the wealthy. As productivity increased in the advent of automation and assembly lines, the price of automobiles fell making them more widely available to the general population. Yet these business principles of automation and assembly line production applied to health care delivery have proven to do little to improve individualized patient care, the work environment of the nurse or ultimately to decrease the cost of health care delivery in the long term [26].

Former American and British FNS nurses who worked as district nurses together at the inception of these changes at the FNS reluctantly admitted that pregnant mothers were transported to the hospital while in labour solely to secure payment for services as home deliveries became no longer reimbursable services.[59]

This was purportedly done not only to satisfy the stipulations placed upon the FNS by outside regulatory bodies but also to keep from having to bill patients too poor to pay for the service themselves (see Footnote 14). A British FNS Nurse-Midwife also admitted that she had been "more comfortable" with a mother delivering her baby at the hospital than she was when doing home deliveries (see Footnote 59). This change in the comfort level of the nurse was considered by many of the older nurses as a decline in the calibre of nurse coming to the FNS. A more disinterested analysis was offered by former FNS courier and long time financial supporter, who attributed the need for the creation of the Family Nurse Practitioner Program to these nurses' coming into the hills "feeling inadequate" due to the establishment of more sophisticated drug and treatment regimes at the Service being done outside of Appalachia. These incoming nurses had been used to having physicians "behind them," and not having enough physicians at the FNS.[60]

Technological advances in prenatal as well as medical and surgical treatments drove levels of care to meet these standards ever higher and the skill and equipment necessary for provision of care quickly became something that could only provided

---

[58] Phyllis Long, American former FNS Nurse (1964–1967; 1973–1976; 1993–1996).

[59] Jean Corner-Rowan, British former FNS Nurse-Midwife (1964–1966).

[60] Kate Ireland, Former FNS Courier (1951).

within the walls of the institution. This increasingly required the FNS nursing staff to be transferred from the community to these facilities, which was costly for the FNS and disruptive for their families, while simultaneously being cost containing and convenient for the institutions they were being sent to (see Footnote 58). In the FNS's early years, specialists and the services they provided were available to the Mountain people periodically as they would come out to the Service and either do district visits or the nurses arrange to get the people within their districts to go to the clinics when they were offered [27]. A nurse who graduated and worked at the FNS in its latter years as a Family Nurse Practitioner stated that the Service was 'behind in many ways' when compared with the technological and medical advances occurring outside of the hills in larger urban facilities in Cincinnati and at the University of Kentucky. Yet at the same time nursing education had expanded at the Service and was "ahead of the pack" (see Footnote 32).

FNS nurses were sent to many different, large, urban US facilities for additional education paid for by the Service and as far away as the UK for midwifery training. One nurse stated that she spent two days at the University of Kentucky Medical Centre to learn "Emergency Medical Technician stuff" while Cincinnati physician residents and Orthopaedic physicians came to the hills every few months (see Footnote 32). She further stated that it was at the FNS that the advanced practice model for nurses had its start, "going out beyond Dr. Loretta Ford in Colorado." Dr. Ford was a PhD prepared nurse who found paediatric health care in America woefully lacking in the 1960s and created a model that combined clinical care and research to give Public Health Nurses the preparation necessary for them to help children and their families. Individuals who participated in this training became known as Paediatric Nurse Practitioners.

Although the Service was perceived as behind the times technologically speaking when compared with those institutions outside of Appalachia, another former nurse graduate from the FNS Midwifery School in 1945 commented that she was impressed by the fact that postpartum infections were very rare at the Service in spite of the lack of sterile sheets, bedpans, etcetera (the boiling of scissors and clamps being the only precaution that she remembered being done). This was in great contrast to all the sterile techniques and frequent use of Sulpha drugs that were being introduced during her training days in Chicago in 1944.[61] Since sulphanilamide first came into use in the 1940s, more than 150 different derivatives appeared on the market, chemically modified to achieve more effective antibacterial activity. Because of their low cost they are still used in many parts of the world. However, resistance to sulpha drugs emerged among many micro organisms, especially streptococci, meningococci, and shigella, making them less effective and causing a recent surge in reconsidering their prolific use [28]. It was the combination of best practice, good nursing care and the patient's response to normal flora within the home as opposed to the foreign flora of the institutional setting that contributed to the absence of postpartum infection at the Service.

---

[61] Elizabeth C. Walton, American FNS Midwifery School Graduate of 1945.

A Graduate from the FNS School of Midwifery in 1960 described herself as being 'intrigued' by the similarities between the people in Africa (whence she was furloughed) and the people of Appalachia. When asked to expand upon this, she stated that the people were 'not complicated with a lot of civilization,' not that they were *un*civilized [italics added] but rather that they were 'uncomplicated;' there was a "basic oneness with nature," a 'close connection that made it easy to really become attached to people'.[62] This was true not only of the nurse-patient relationships but also the nurse-nurse relationships at the FNS in its early years. All the nurses identified themselves primarily as FNS nurses and had a firm grasp of what that identity entailed. They were women from all social strata, personal backgrounds and nationalities. Yet they reportedly often maintained friendships and ties to the community long after they had left the Service. Perhaps the schism within the nursing discipline stems from the break between the social and economic components of care and the value placed upon specific facets of care within the wider culture. Neither of these scenarios existed for the FNS until it became dependent upon government reimbursement for services that required it to conform to the established rules and regulations regarding physician oversight, institutional hierarchy and the medical/business model of health care delivery. When these changes came, they created an 'either-or' focus by society at various levels. Either focus on the well/ill person/community to keep them well/heal them or focus on the lowest possible expenditure necessary to keep them well/heal them. Indeed, it is this paradox between what nurse's feel they 'ought' to do and what the overstressed health care system will actually 'allow' them to do that creates the morally uninhabitable environment inherent in their practice and educational settings [29]. The characteristics that are said to put nurses at risk of developing moral distress include human resource constraints, competing value systems, the nurses' role as advocate, the lack of administrative and managerial support and the lack of nurse-physician collaboration. This, in turn, contributes to staff 'burnout,' 'turnover' and cyclic nursing shortages [30. Further, technology and specialization skills are highly prized by society, are thought to be the best way to optimize or maintain health and are traditionally housed within institutional settings. In regard to the discipline's cultural identity, the 'either-or' mentality asks am I 'just a nurse' (vocationally or 'humanitarian' inclined) or is it 'just a job' (am I in it for the money)? In the first instance, the nurse is impeded by the lack of value as well as the lack of financial reward placed upon humanitarian aims within the wider culture while simultaneously being frustrated by the obvious lack of both within the institutional setting. In the second, the nurse must, by definition, be only concerned with herself and not the patient, facility or the profession. Yet is either of these judgements accurate concerning nurses or are they rather spawned by compulsory conformity and a subsequent allegiance to a particular institution or establishmentarian identity? This concept, often confused by nurses as choosing between a humanitarian/vocation (people) *or* business/professional (object) focus is further explored in relation to recruitment, retention and its contribution to the moral inhabitability of the work place in Chap. 8.

---

[62] Interview #78OH148FNS08 1978. Martha Lady, FNS Midwifery School Graduate of 1960.

Historically, nursing within the culture has had to be subordinate to medicine in order to make the profession 'respectable.' It has also served to staff the repositories of medical care, namely hospitals, which harboured an equally subservient environment in which nurses were trained. This institutional environment required that nurses conform to the culture's hierarchy, while having little influence therein. Breckinridge's school of nurse-midwifery adopted an opposing strategy to that of the typical hospital schools of nursing, which had lax entry requirements but very rigid rules, regulations, routines and evaluation criteria and a punitive approach towards students who did not conform. Instead, Breckinridge had stricter entry requirements and a much less punitive approach toward staff and students. Her model, based upon the QNI (Scottish branch) in Great Britain sought to train generalist public health, district nurses and nurse-midwives. These nurses would be able to function in a variety of settings outside of the FNS.

The cultural characteristics inherent in education environments outside of the FNS that created morally uninhabitable environments were human resource constraints, competing value systems, the nurses' role as advocate, lack of administrative and managerial support and lack of physician collaboration. These were characteristics foreign to the FNS until after its adoption of the prevailing health care system (medical and business models). The move from hospital to college or University education settings for nurses, though serving to eliminate some of the 'student as staff' or 'slave labour' mentality of institutions has not eradicated it. Indeed, many of the comments made by nurses in practice today regarding the cultural characteristics of institutional settings remains remarkably similar to those made by hospital diploma school graduates and mirrors the dissatisfaction experienced by FNS nurses with the hospital practice environment of the Service in its latter years. The cultural paradox experienced by professional nurses between the humanitarian impulses and demands for institutional conformity has created the risk of moral distress as well as the lack of morally inhabitable environments. The degree to which outside forces played a role in maintaining this cultural status quo and those internal forces (within the discipline) also contributed are explored more fully in Chap. 8.

References

1. Connolly CA. Hampton, Nutting and rival gospels at the John Hopkins Hospital and training school for nurses 1889–1906. Image J Nurs Sch. 1997;30(1):23–9.
2. Leathard A. Health care provision: past, present and into the twenty-first century. 2nd ed. Cheltenham: Stanley Thornes Ltd; 2000.
3. Sirota T. Nurse/physician relationships: improving or not? Nursing. 2007;37(1):52–6.
4. Baly M. Nursing and social change. 3rd ed. London: Routledge; 1995. p. 56.
5. Williams K. Nurse Training in the Carnarfon and Anglesey Hospital 1935–1949. Unpublished M. Phil. thesis, University of Wales Bangor, N. Wales, UK; 2000.
6. Burdett H. The nursing profession: how and where to train. 4th ed. London: The Scientific Press; 1927. p. 5.

7. Van Maanen J, Kunda G. Real feelings; emotional expression and organizational culture. In: Cummings LL, Staw BM, editors. Research in organizational behaviour, vol. 11. Greenwich, CT: JAI Press; 1989. p. 43–103.
8. Lancaster J. Nursing issues in leading and managing change. New York: Mosby; 1999.
9. QNI. Queen Victoria's Jubilee Institute for Nurses, Scottish Branch, The Story of the Queen's Nurses in Scotland, 1887. Edinburgh: Lindsay and Company Printers, Royal College of Nursing Archives; 1887.
10. Dammann N. A social history of the frontier nursing service. Sun City, AZ: Social Change Press; 1982. p. 28.
11. Cohen J. Minority report: working party on the recruitment and training of nurses. London: Metropolitan Library Archives. p. 70, 72, 73.
12. Dammann N. A social history of the frontier nursing service. Sun City, AZ: Social Change Press; 1982. p. 12s, 123.
13. Meir-Hamilton J. Creating healthy workplaces: what every nurse can do. Pa Nurse. 2007;62(2):25–7.
14. Grindel C. A healthful work environment: a call to action. Medsurg Nurs. 2005;15(2):58–9.
15. Bates D, Plog F. Cultural anthropology. 3rd ed. Berkshire: McGraw-Hill College; 1990. p. 10.
16. Hess R, DesRoches C, Donelan K, Norman L. Perceptions of nurses in Magnet® hospitals, non-magnet hospitals, and hospitals pursuing magnet status. J Nurs Adm. 2010;41(7/8):315–23.
17. Hess R, Desroches C, Donelan K, Norman L, Buerhaus P. Perceptions of nurses in Magnet® hospitals, non-magnet hospitals, and hospitals pursuing magnet status. J Nurs Adm. 2011;41(7–8):315–23. https://doi.org/10.1097/NNA.0b013e31822509e2.
18. Naylor MD, Kurtzman ET. The role of nurse practitioners in reinventing primary care. Health Aff. 2010;29(5):893–9. https://www.aanp.org/advocacy/advocacy-resource/position-statements/quality-of-nurse-practitioner-practice. Accessed 2 Feb 2019.
19. Cohen J. Minority report: working party on the recruitment and training of nurses. London: Metropolitan Library Archives. p. 72.
20. Breckinridge M. Wide neighborhoods: a story of the frontier nursing service. p. 323.
21. Reid D. Saddlebags full of memories. Burt Lake, MI. p. 31, 57, 62.
22. Heyes A. The economics of vocation or why is a badly paid nurse a good nurse? J Health Econ. 2005;24(3):561–9.
23. Briskin L. Resistance, mobilization and militancy: nurses on strike. Nurs Inq. 2011;19(4):285–96. https://doi.org/10.1111/j.1440-1800.2011.00585.x.
24. Heyes A. The economics of vocation or why is a badly paid nurse a good nurse? J Health Econ. 2005;51(12):51.
25. Haslett H. Economics in one lesson: the shortest and surest way to understand basic economics. New York: Random House; 1988. p. 203.
26. Kamal R, Cox C. How has U.S. spending on healthcare changed over time? Kaiser Family Foundation, Posted: December 10, 2018. Chart Collections: Health Spending. https://www.healthsystemtracker.org/chart-collection/u-s-spending-healthcare-changed-time/#item-start. Accessed 2 Feb 2019.
27. West E. History, organization and the changing culture of care: an historical analysis of the frontier nursing service. Unpublished PhD dissertation, Bangor University, Bangor, Wales, UK.
28. Brackett CC. Likelihood and mechanisms of cross-allergenicity between sulfonamide antibiotics and other drugs containing a sulfonamide functional group. Pharmacotherapy. 2004;24(7):856–70.
29. Jameton A. What moral distress in nursing history could suggest about the future of health care. AMA J Ethics. 2017;19(6):617–28. https://doi.org/10.1001/journalofethics.2017.19.6.mhst1-1706.
30. Paillé P. Stressful work, citizenship behaviour and intention to leave the organization in a high turnover environment: examining the mediating role of job satisfaction. J Manage Res. 2011;3(1):1–14. ISSN 1941-899X.

Chapter 8
Recruitment, Retention and Morally Inhabitable Environments

8.1 The FNS Environment: Recruitment and Retention

The FNS expected much of its nurses. The work was difficult, demanding and the hours long, even when compared to the equally dismal hospital standards which existed at the time outside of the region. In addition to this, the physical environment was isolated, rough, rustic and rural and the culture alien to all those outside of Appalachia, even to other Americans coming into the area. Yet Breckinridge managed to keep her staff at a time when other organizations and institutions outside of Appalachia with less physically and emotionally demanding work environments could not. Breckinridge's personal background, education and professional employment history prior to founding the FNS equipped her to understand the challenges she would face in decreasing her nurses' responses to 'burnout' in such an environment. It also helped her to develop a health care delivery system that promoted positive adaptation and facilitated quality care. These personal qualities as well as professional expertise are characteristics that set the tone of any organization's culture [1].

Importance was given at the FNS to ethical aspects, not just the physical or administrative aspects, of patient care and FNS personnel's morale was refreshed by social gatherings in the hills with one another and the community, as well as time off, in some cases for 1, 3 or 6-month leaves and even as long as a year when necessary for the mental, physical or emotional well-being of the nurse. These benefits were not 'set' by the organization. Nurses did not come in with an understanding that they had 2 weeks of paid vacation leave per year and could not receive any more than this or take this leave if the organization needed them to stay on the weeks they wanted 'off.' Nurses requested leave time for family emergencies, personal reasons or due to 'burnout' and were never refused the time off. Often Breckinridge insisted the nurses take the time off if she felt they were becoming too stressed. She and the other staff would 'cover' for the absent nurse or she would find another nurse (often former or retired FNS personnel who welcomed the opportunity to

© Springer Nature Switzerland AG 2019
E. West, *Frontier Nursing in Appalachia: History, Organization and the Changing Culture of Care*, https://doi.org/10.1007/978-3-030-20027-5_8

provide short term relief work that would afford them a visit 'home') and bring her in. Breckinridge knew this about her staff because she worked to maintain a relationship with them as well as the population and her financial 'networks' outside of Appalachia, in other words, Breckinridge saw her workers as individual human beings, not cogs in the wheel of industry. She saw them as human beings who had the same wants and needs as the people they were caring for and in order for the organization to be successful she understood the need to attempt to meet both the personal and professional expectations of her nurses as well as the health needs of the population. What was perhaps the key to her early success is the fact that she was both founder and manager of the FNS's organizational and institutional environments. She was not a leader who was external to either her nurses or their practice area. For her, the work was personal and emotional. She understood the experiences of the individuals involved in it from more than one angle. She was a woman and a practicing nurse-midwife. She had also suffered the personal tragedy of losing two children, one in childbirth. This helped forge her relationship between personnel and with the people within the local community [2].

Breckinridge did not self consciously engineer loyalty or commitment on the part of her nurses or from the community. However, more than one nurse commented of her that you never dared say 'no' to Mrs. Breckinridge. Some expressed the perception of intimidation from her forceful personality but most followed-up these statements with the view that you always felt that you never 'wanted' to say no or 'couldn't possibly' say no to her due to the respect she inspired. Her nurses report that she would often ask them to tea and afterward take a walk outside with them and ask them about themselves while she fed the chickens.[1] Breckinridge took a personal interest in her staff. They were people first and employees second. She took the same view of the recipients of her brand of health care. They were people first and 'patients' second. They were never just 'consumers' or 'clients.' This belief was confirmed by the fact that alongside all of the honorary certifications, licenses and degrees she had either earned or been given in honorarium throughout her life she also held an equal number of awards and citations given to her for her humanitarian efforts and distinguished service to humanity. So, though she may not have sought to create a culture cast in her own image, due to the fact that her image was such a forceful one, in the end she did perpetuate just that and achieved an organizational form of immortality [3]. This was evidenced by the fact that her organization had been replicated in many rural third-world countries, with similar health care needs, environments and problems. It was further proved by the fact that many of these organizations still have FNS Nurse-Midwife graduates working as missionaries in them today.[2] Also, testament to this was the fact that quite a few of the nurses who came out to the service in the late 1940s and 1950s opted to stay and eventually moved into managerial roles because they believed in and valued the work being done and enjoyed the organizational and wider-environmental culture afforded them at the FNS.

---

[1] Margaret (Maggie) Willson, British former FNS Nurse-Midwife (1955–1967).
[2] Madonna Buret-Spratt, American FNS Midwifery School Graduate of 1960.

Nurses who knew her called Breckinridge's replacement, Helen Browne who began her long career at the FNS in 1938, 'The lady that I would have liked to have been'.[3] Though Breckinridge inspired replication of her style of management within her organisation, many of the former FNS nurses who were there in the 1950s and beyond made a distinction in the service's administrators before and after the mid-1960s. Administration prior to this time got very high marks by the staff. Most voiced the following in some form or another:

Administrative… I had a great respect for all the people that were there. I mean it was really a great respect for all of them… They believed in what was being done, and what they were giving to the people. It was not a… it was not a business as it is or it seemed to us when we were back (visiting) the last time (see Footnote 1).

A former FNS nurse who began in the service as a Nurse-Midwife when she went out to Eastern Kentucky in November of 1958 and left the service in March of 1967 due to her parents' ill health stated that she enjoyed least the work she did when she went into management and administration there. She expressed her frustration with the increase in paperwork, governmental and professional regulatory enforcements and a lack of connectedness with patients that the institutionalisation of health care brought in its wake. She also stated that she never felt she had enough money, not referring to her personal salary but rather the funds necessary to properly equip the nurses and support work they were doing with and for the people (see Footnote 1).

Dr. Wiss and Dr. Fox attributed what they saw as the Service's decline in its latter years to Breckinridge's successor and not the organization's founder, who was 'old, ill, didn't keep her finger on everything that was going on and received bad advice'.[4] Dr. Fox viewed the problems at the FNS as having to do things 'the British way' after Breckinridge's death, referring to the fact that the new director was a British Nurse-Midwife and that the nurses began to be called 'sisters' after this administration took over. Also, Breckinridge's successor, Helen E. Browne said of herself that she was not as 'at ease' with Leslie 'Countians,' as Breckinridge had been. Browne stated she was used to government meetings and health planning councils where there was 'always a smart-aleck who would come forth with an answer almost before questions were out of one's mouth' whereas the local council members didn't speak until they had thought about what you said [4]. Betty Lester, a long-time FNS nurse, loved the local meetings where she would stimulate participants to express their ideas. She was a great help to Browne there and as a result Browne had a better relationship with the locals than she did the physicians on staff. Neither Dr. Fox nor Dr. Wiss were included in fund raising, decision-making and purportedly got 'grief' from administration (Browne) for trying to 'improve' and 'upgrade' the hospital. They both felt that the 'camaraderie' and 'mystique' of the organization was dying-out and that this was due to the 'bureaucracy' of the existing establishment coming into the area in 1979 that didn't exist there in 1929.

---

[3] Anne Lorentzen, American former FNS Nurse (1963–1965).
[4] Interview #82OH05FNS148, 1982, Dr. Mary Weiss and Dr. Pauline Fox.

Both physicians attributed this to 'progress' and felt that this was what had to happen if the care was to continue. They both also felt that though the Service had always attracted first rate nurses, they were not as readily accepted by the local community in the organization's later years because they came from a culture that didn't value the traditions of the hills or the organization. The physicians reported that some of the young women coming into the area at that time 'lived with' local men, wore jeans instead of the standard FNS uniform (the exact descriptor used by the one doctor to describe the nurses' appearance was 'sloppy') and the traditional four o'clock teas and six o'clock suppers were 'made fun of' by many of them because 'they didn't understand.' The physicians interviewed were quick to point out that some of the local women also lived with men and had children outside of marriage even before the 1960s and 1970s but that the standard for the nurses was higher, which created a double standard where moral behaviour was concerned (see Footnote 4).

The FNS's founding resolutions included specifics on how committees would be formed and operated, identified the role of the nurse-midwives would play in Breckinridge's demonstration project and integrated a commitment to research, record keeping and cooperation with the medical, local and state communities. The expressed purpose of the organization was, 'To safeguard the lives and health of mothers and young children by providing nurse-midwives for rural areas where there was no resident physicians'.[5] By 1928, the name of the organization had changed from the 'Committee for Mothers and Babies' to the 'Frontier Nursing Service.' In 1932, article number three changed to include the addition of all of the following organizational purposes: to provide and prepare trained nurse-midwives for rural areas where there is inadequate medical services; to give skilled care to women in childbirth and to give nursing care to the sick of both sexes and all ages; to establish, own, maintain and operate hospitals, clinics, nursing centres and mid-wife training schools for graduate nurses; to carry out preventative public health measures; to educate the rural population in laws of health and parents in baby hygiene and child care; to provide expert social services; to obtain medical, dental and surgical services for those who need them at a price they can afford to pay; to ameliorate economic conditions inimical to health and growth and to conduct research toward that end; to do any and all other things in any way incident to or connected with these objects and in pursuit of them; to cooperate with individuals and with organizations, private, state or federal and through the fulfilment of these aims to advance the cause of health, social welfare and economic independence in rural districts with the help of their own leading citizens. What began as a service to mothers and babies had grown to include a more comprehensive rural community health approach to care that one former FNS Nurse succinctly described as 'from cradle to grave' (see Footnote 1). This was happening at a time when elsewhere in the US the tide of public health was ebbing and the rise of the medical model and modern hospital based care was flowing.

---

[5]FNS Resolutions 1925. 5M1: FNS, Box 2, Fol. 2. 'FNS Summary of Executive Committee Meeting Minutes (1925–1935).

The Service had always struggled to make ends meet financially since its inception. Breckinridge most had to curtail services in the 1930s during the Great Depression. She cut the staff of 30 trained nurses down to 22 and necessarily had to increase the remaining nurses' workloads, including that of the administrative staff. The depression also made it impossible to reach their goal of increasing their service area from 700 to 1000 square miles by 1935.[6] Even so, the hospital never turned away patients and was often over capacity, greatly straining the Service's resources. A former lifetime FNS nurse related this story regarding the hardship the staff faced when having to institute these changes. She had a woman come to her who had lost her first-born, a son. She lived five miles outside of this nurse's district limit. The woman begged her to deliver the baby and she could not refuse. She took her predicament directly to Mrs. Breckinridge who said that she mustn't neglect her own work, but if that she could do that it was acceptable to deliver the woman. She did help the woman with the necessary prenatal care and delivered her daughter to her in the woman's home.[7] Rules that existed within the organizational culture that related to human beings that were 'bent' were supported by administration. This retired nurse remembered and related this story as an old woman in answer to the question, 'Does anything standout in your memory?' It had clearly meant a lot to her to be able to help this woman. Had this nurse not been supported in her desire to provide this care she could not have looked so fondly upon it as a positive, meaningful aspect of her work.

Breckinridge was frugal with the money she received for the service and shrewd in ways to get the most for it. She wrote in a letter to her secretary on one of her many fund-raising trips that she had engaged a 'perfectly marvellous woman who is married' who was one of the best stenographers in a law firm. Breckinridge had engaged her for $18.00 per week when the going rate was $15.00 per week explaining, 'She does twice as much work than one less experienced who I could get for $15.00'.[8] When nurses who were hired that were coming in to the service from out of state had a problem due to reciprocity laws in Kentucky regarding registration she obviated the needless expense of eight days off per nurse at an expense of $300.00 by arranging for them to register in Arkansas, which had reciprocity with Kentucky and then had them register with Kentucky at very small expense.[9] She was reportedly prudent with the money coming into the service both during the depression years and beyond. One former FNS nurse who eventually became the administrator of the hospital in the late 1960s related that the hospital roof began leaking and that '…it came to the stage where we had thirteen receptacles catching the rain that was coming through the roof and Mrs. B. said we hadn't got enough money to repair the

---

[6]Reprint from the FNS *Quarterly Bulletin* 1935, 85M1: FNS, Box 25, Fol. 2.

[7]Betty Lester, Former long-time FNS Nurse (English).

[8]Breckinridge Letter to Knechtly. 5 January 1932. 85M1: FNS, Box 329, Fol. 2. Breckinridge Letter to FNS Secretary, Lucille 'Thompy' Knechtly, 5 January 1932. University of Kentucky in Lexington, USA.

[9]Breckinridge Letter to Lexington Committee. 7 August 1926. 85M1: FNS, Box 2, Fol. 15. University of Kentucky in Lexington, USA.

roof or put a new roof on until she came and saw the receptacles.' Then '… we had the roof pretty quickly!' (see Footnote 1). So, though frugal, Breckinridge was also swift to meet the work environment needs of her nurses and the community. She took requests, recommendations and comments seriously enough to verify and act upon them swiftly when necessary.

Breckinridge had forged relationships with people in health organizations both in the US and abroad that she later relied upon to create and maintain operation of the FNS politically and financially. Breckinridge also became well-connected politically with the organizational heads of such prominent associations as the American Red Cross, the Queens Jubilee Institute for Nurses in Edinburgh, the British Hospital for Mothers and Babies in London and the Highlands and Islands Medical and Nursing Service in Edinburgh, Scotland [5]. Breckinridge established a nursing service that provided a unique blend of district, public health and midwifery nursing care. It was her approach to the development and execution of the organization, which allowed her to pioneer her idea into a successful health organization. Breckinridge sought solutions to problems by making contact with and soliciting the ideas of contemporaries who had had some measure of success in tackling similar problems elsewhere. The only difference between her local partners and those outside of Appalachia in the Service's 'early years' was that local partnership rarely relied on monetary assistance, instead relying on the people's existing economic system of volunteer reciprocity which often times included pigs, chickens or manual labour assistance as a form of payment for services rendered by FNS nurses if the small nominal monetary fee could not be managed. The local committees also had a voice in managing the health service provided through the FNS. Anyone associated with the FNS as a partner, and they were as prolific as they were diverse, received a personal correspondence from Breckinridge thanking them for whatever they could give toward the Service's work. If it was one dollar or five thousand dollars, they received the same personal note of gratitude.[10]

Beyond the mere 'thank you' notes, Breckinridge honored those who were as tireless as she in the support of her organization. An example of this is her invitation to Dr. MacKenzie and his wife to come from Edinburgh, Scotland to attend the dedication ceremony for the FNS. It was his Highland & Island Scheme that she explored fully and modelled her organisation upon and Dr. MacKenzie was invited to speak at the ceremony.[11] She was also a tireless campaigner for the constant funding that was needed to run the FNS and was frequently travelling to speak personally at fund-raisers, committee meetings, board meetings and the like. So much so that she requested some time off after the first 4 years of the organization's existence from her executive board as she'd not had a day off in all that time.[12]

---

[10]Breckinridge Correspondence 1926–1961. Mary Breckinridge Series: Correspondence 1925–1970. University of Kentucky in Lexington, USA.

[11]FNS Summary of Executive Meeting Minutes. 10 March 1928. 85M1: FNS, Box 2, Fol. 1.

[12]FNS Executive Committee Meeting Minutes. 14 November 1930. 85M1: FNS, Box 2, Fol. 1.

Breckinridge wrote in her spring appeal promotional material that the FNS employs no publicity agent, pays no large salaries and gifts are deductible from your income tax. She also urged continuous supporters throughout the years to: 'Please DON'T send extra money your self, please DO use the attached letter, booklet and saddlebag to win interest of another friend'.[13] Promotional materials included a summary of the major costs associated for the support of the Nurses as well as the basic services the FNS nurses provided the community. The material also included a tiny leather saddlebag, which she asked people to fill and for $2.00 to secure annual membership. She often urged her supporters to find two more supporters and told them that with just two more sponsors per member pledging financial assistance of $2.00 per annum the work could continue free of financial crises. Breckinridge often invited her supporters to come out and see the work and what their money was doing for the work first hand.

Breckinridge kept all of her supporters abreast of the financial situation at the service over the years, down to the last penny, through an annual financial report to all of her supporters via the FNS *Quarterly Bulletin* that began in 1926 and continues today. This 'corporate transparency' was something innovative, even by today's standards. This bulletin also includes the personal experiences of the FNS nurses and residents of the community, research endeavours that the service was conducting and any news regarding virtually anyone associated with the service. It was unique in that it functioned as a medical and nursing journal, corporate financial quarterly and featured section of a local newspaper. It also went out to all of the staff, nurses, former staff and nurses, as well as the services many financial supporters both in the US and abroad. She was truthful in her reports citing not only what the FNS had achieved but also where it had failed to meet its goals and its aims to rectify this.[14] This, as well as the personal notes, letters, appearances and invitations to come out and see the work, brought all of the vast and varied cultural environments outside of the organization and within the local community together in a common purpose.

By the 1940s, American hospital institutions outside of Appalachia also began to see the necessity of decreasing work hours and providing other incentives to entice nurses into employ that were already being done in other businesses. The *Trained Nurse and Hospital Review* of October 1946 had many advertisements for nurses touting an 8-h working day, 48 h working week with 2 weeks of paid vacation and 2 weeks of paid sick leave.[15] The advertisements for hospital employment centred on the business model being used nationally, focused on monetary wage competitiveness, benefit packages and even the location of the institution in reference to climate and proximity to outdoor or intellectual activities. Incidentally, these are all

---

[13]FNS Spring Appeal 1942. 85M1: FNS, Box 29, Fol. 13.

[14]Breckinridge Report 1940. 85M1: FNS, Box 25, Fol. 11. Breckinridge Report, What has FNS failed to do (1940)? University of Kentucky in Lexington, USA.

[15]The Trained Nurse and Hospital Review. 85M1: FNS, Box 36, Fol. 6., 275.

incentives that one can find in advertisements designed to recruit nurses today.[16] The problem was, and remains, that the core cultural issue, namely the humanization of the work environment and system of care delivery, have never been adequately or fully addressed.

In stark contrast to the existing ambivalence that existed and continues to exist today between the benefits promised to nurses coming into the organizational culture and the realities therein, the FNS chose to run the following advertisement to recruit nurse-midwives from England, Scotland, Wales and Ireland to the Eastern Appalachia's:

> Attention! Nurse graduates with a sense of adventure! Your own horse, your own dog, and a thousand miles of Kentucky Mountains to serve. Join my nurses' brigade and help save children's lives. Write to: M. Breckinridge, Hyden, KY, U.S.A.[17]

The issues of objective and subjective rewards, professional autonomy and value were all successfully addressed by the FNS in its early years. Breckinridge was realistic, honest and wise to advertise for nurses who would value the subjective appeal of the work in Appalachia over the objective rewards because she knew that it wouldn't matter how much money she offered a prospective nurse to come into such a practice environment who did not have the correct value orientation. She must have realized that any nurse requesting more information about the FNS after reading such an advert would at the very least have some idea of what type of work environment they were getting themselves into. Though the FNS did not advertise the objective rewards associated with the work, such as salary and benefits, efforts were made by Breckinridge to be competitive or at least to compensate nurses for any lack of comparable benefits that living and working in isolated, rural Appalachia would entail.

Breckinridge looked at salaries outside of Leslie County, specifically at the existing salaries of the Public Health Nursing service, the American Red Cross, the National Organization for Public Health Nursing, the Maternity Health Association and the Henry Street Association in New York City prior to determining what salary she would offer to prospective FNS Nurses. In addition, she used information attained by a Miss Bertram, former Director of the Community Health Association in Boston, who made a special investigation of Midwifery in selected parts of Europe for the Rockefeller Foundation and found there that $150 per month with yearly increases to a maximum salary of $2000–$2500 per annum was the norm. Breckinridge decided after reviewing all of this information to offer her first British Nurse-Midwife $3000 per annum, minus the estimated living expenses in New York at a rate of $20.00 per week, plus fare to and from Leslie County and New York, plus living expenses in Leslie County and the expense of a horse.[18]

[16]Employment section. Am J Nurs, 84.

[17]Glasgow times 1928, newspaper clipping of FNS advertisement. Mary Breckinridge Series: Correspondence 1925–1970, University of Kentucky in Lexington, USA.

[18]FNS Kentucky Committee for Mothers and Babies Meeting Minutes 1925. 85M1: FNS, Box 2, Fol. 2.

Later, when experienced American Public Health Nurses were taking Midwifery courses in London to be hired upon completion of this training by the FNS, she offered them $150 per month including their horse upkeep and place to live with 1 month of vacation annually with salary, plus an increase in salary after 1 year of $10 per month. In addition, she paid the travel expenses for all of her British nurses coming into the US [25]. Breckinridge also commissioned a study to be conducted by Ella Woodyard, PhD examining the average visits per nurse and costs associated with these visits after her first year of operation, from 1926 to 1927. She then compared these findings to the Visiting Nurses Association (VNA) in New York. She found that her organization's total cost for all purposes of the organization, including publicity, scholarship funds for midwifery education for her nurses in Europe and all administrative as well as field work costs to be $25, 907.37. The VNA's total operating costs was found to be $436,167.03. The FNS nurse averaged 3286 visits per year or 11½ calls per working day at a cost of $1.45, in comparison with the VNA nurse who made approximately 2115 visits or 7½ visits per nurse per day at a cost of $1.25. The VNA had a total staff of 253,164 nurses who made 346,810 visits upon 49,120 patients in the city, whereas the FNS had eight nurses, including supervisors and relief nurses who covered bedside nursing, midwifery, baby hygiene and intensive work as well as public health over approximately a 373-square mile radius for a population of 10,500 people.[19]

In the 1950s Breckinridge made comparison studies to what nurses in the most similar work environments outside of the hills were making and increased her nurses' salaries accordingly.[20] Though it can certainly not be said that FNS salaries were ever exceptional and particularly not in the organization's lean years (during the Depression and World War Two) it can be said that they were both adequate and acceptable to the nurses choosing to come who sought the professional and personal experience being offered at the FNS that was not being offered elsewhere. Breckinridge relied more on external sources of revenue to balance the budget than on any financial sacrifices on her nurses' part. She realized the sacrifices they were making to be there and to meet their patients' needs and strove to not make any further demands upon them than that. Her fundraising endeavours were an enormous undertaking that she worked at and reported on tirelessly to her benefactors as well as her staff.[21] Even as late as the 1950s and early 1960s, the nurses interviewed appear to have been satisfied with their salaries due to a prevailing communal mentality between administration, staff, nurses and the community that was lacking in other institutional cultures at the time. One nurse summed it up nicely with the statement, 'Money wasn't that important as they (the people) didn't have much more than the necessities. We all dressed out of the mission barrel. It was a step back for me but made me realize what was important' (see Footnote 3).

---

[19] Reprint from FNS Quarterly Bulletin 1928, Frontier Nursing Service Professional Organization Series (1928). University of Kentucky in Lexington, USA.

[20] FNS comparative reports from 1950–1959. 85M1: FNS, Box 11, Fol. 22.

[21] FNS Quarterly Bulletins 1925–1958. University of Kentucky in Lexington, USA.

Later, the wording was different but the spirit of the call was the same in an advertisement for the FNS that ran in the *Trained Nurse and Hospital Review's* (1946), which requested the following sort of nurses: '...the kind our army and navy nurses were, as good sports, as ready for adventure, as fond of people. No others need apply. Requesting those adventurous nurses who seek a field of endeavour where service to the community will pay off in values infinitely more permanent than a weekly salary check.' These advertisements ran alongside those placed by hospitals in various states that at the time, which were touting the new 8-h work day, paid sick days and 2 weeks paid vacation for qualified nurses. The wording in the FNS advertisement capitalized on the pre-war sentiment associated with a higher calling, service, adventure and humanitarian endeavours over merely monetary remuneration.

If viewed through the eyes of the dominant culture, one would expect that such idealism would surely disappoint and consequently far more nurses would leave a practice culture that touted such rewards than those who entered the institutional culture knowing up-front what tangible benefits and remuneration awaited them for their work. In fact, the exact opposite has proven to be the case. Of the former British and American FNS nurses interviewed two left the profession entirely when they married, the rest stayed in nursing, many stayed at the FNS longer than they had intended to, a majority of them went on to advanced practice degrees and a few on to managerial or teaching roles within the FNS. When asked their reasons for going to the FNS, they all cited humanitarian impulses and a majority also cited the desire for adventure and travel. The FNS was able to deliver on its promises, whereas the vast majority of hospital institutional settings have never been able to make the same claim though there are certainly exceptions. One former British FNS nurse spoke very highly of the British Hospital for Mothers and Babies stating that unlike other institutions, there, the doctors, nurses and administrators were 'gentle, loving and really got through to you.' She described it as a very good atmosphere in which to learn (see Footnote 1). It is interesting to note that this hospital is the one that FNS founder, Mary Breckinridge also attended while studying in England over 40 years before.

The tradition of humanitarianism that is essential to quality nursing has been steadily devalued over time. Its value to the health care system usurped by technological advancement and commercial enterprise. This, in turn, has generated an ever-widening schism within the profession between those who are deemed to be 'in it for the money' or as a 'stepping stone' on to administrative aspirations and those who are grieving the continuing loss of connectedness to their patient's due to the ever-progressive fragmentation of care within the existing institutional culture [6]. In either instance, no amount of money is enough to compensate for the lack of recognition, prestige and the long, difficult hours inherent to work with ailing human beings or the inability to meet their needs within such a system. As one former FNS nurse phrased it:

> You have the opportunity to develop relationships with people, which is what we had the opportunity to do when we were in Kentucky. And I don't think in most jobs you have that opportunity. And it's even less today when everything's done as an outpatient or you're moved on so quickly through the system (see Footnote 3).

A former FNS early nurse who witnessed the effects to the service during its most profound changes in regard to the Appalachian culture, FNS personnel and health care delivery in the 1960s–1970s went so far as to say that any nurse that was not at the FNS prior to 1960 did not have the right to call herself an FNS nurse.[22] The cultures of FNS and Appalachia ran squarely into the vested interests of the nation's social, economic, professional and political establishments that were expanding exponentially, institutionalising and brokering power. These sorts of cultural politics are inherent in any historically based ideology. Therefore, any self-conscious group of people have to recognize where its cultural leadership comes from and needs to work out its relationship with other cultural voices as well [7].

There was no 'typical' FNS nurse or staff member and many newly graduated nurses came for FNS midwifery training who were ambitious, adventuresome and idealistic [8]. Other nurses who were older also came, attracted by the challenging job or simply because they liked horses and dogs. Most who stayed did so because they enjoyed the independence and responsibility of the work and because they fell in love with the mountains and its people, some so much so that they retired in Leslie County. However, changing societal values and trends do affect career choice. Understanding the factors that influence persons to choose nursing as a career has important implications for recruitment of nursing students during a severe nursing shortage. A study done to describe both the factors associated with the choice of nursing as a career and to determine the differential sources of influence found that the most important reason for choosing nursing was the "inner satisfaction of working with and helping people." Personal self-beliefs and the experience of caring for someone who was ill were also important influences on the decision to become a nurse. Students with a nurse in the family were more influenced by other people in their decision to become a nurse and other job characteristics that were important were flexibility, variety and ease of obtaining a job [9].

Most former FNS nurses who were in Appalachia in the late 1950s through the early 1960s said that they had heard about the FNS via 'word of mouth' from those nurses who had actually been at the FNS or who knew someone who had been there. They also heard about the service from nursing instructors in England and through advertisement literature designed for those wishing to travel abroad. The QNI had a unique relationship with the FNS. Many of the nurses who came to the service were recruited from the QNI in the 1950s, as they were uniquely qualified as public health and district nurse-midwives. Nurse-Midwives coming to the FNS from overseas had to sign on for at least 2 years of service in order for the FNS to provide travel expenses to and from the region. Potential students and employees generally sent letters of inquiry to the FNS upon hearing of it by promotional materials placed in nursing text books being used in the UK and US; advertisements placed in newspapers, nursing journals and popular Christian, business and secular magazines; or by hearing Mrs. Breckinridge speak at meetings set-up throughout the US at various locations by her committees. Later, Breckinridge's book on the

---

[22] Alice Herman. American former FNS Nurse (1956–1978).

FNS also served as a recruitment tool.[23] Information was then sent to prospective students or employees on what to expect from the FNS as well as what would be expected from them by the Service. In 1954 less than 1% of the FNS budget was being spent on promotion.[24]

One former American FNS nurse stated that she heard about the FNS from the 'face sheet' of her 'Obstetrics text book in (nurses) training' back in 1957. She stated that she had considered going to the FNS each time she thought of 'leaving nursing.' This nurse had entered the US Air Force Nurse Corp. a year post graduation, worked in a Veteran's Administration Hospital and was unhappy with nursing in an institutional setting. By 1963 she had determined to leave nursing and pursue a career in 'engineering' when she contacted the FNS indicating that she had 3 months before entering school and 'could they use her.' She arrived at the FNS in June of 1963, explaining:

> I don't remember that I filled out an application and certainly didn't have a physical. Once I arrived given the various experiences I had (they) put me right to work and even sent me out to Beech Fork (outpost) to fill in for a midwife that had to return home and then to Bullskin (outpost) for the same reason. Instead of going back to Seattle to start school (engineering program) I stayed 2½ years and the rest of my nursing career was based on the various experiences with the FNS (see Footnote 3).

This nurse expressed that the 'people we cared for and worked with,' with whom she still had contact with today, and the 'ability to use the education I had' were the best things she recalled about working for the Service. The experience also kept her in practice, which was provocative as she left a position that paid a much greater salary, benefits and provided an environment that was physically much less demanding in comparison. This would tend to support the notion that incorporation of the humanitarian piece of the nursing equation coupled with an increase in the moral inhabitability of the work environment served to keep this nurse in practice. Further, it would seem to have empowered her to do more within that practice. This nurse's career post FNS included, school nurse, visiting nurse supervisor and coordinator, assistant manager of a health and rehabilitation service, medical services consultant and eventually a position as a partner in a senior rehabilitation consultancy firm that bears her name as an associate today. She accomplished this never having gone any further in her education beyond that of a diploma graduate. She credited her professional achievements and decision to stay in practice entirely to her tenure at the FNS, stating:

> I have always thought because of the experience (at the FNS) that each job after was better-working there with the people made me aware of what life was really about and that has stayed with me.

---

[23] Schupp WE. The Good Neighbour of "Wide Neighbourhoods", In Kentucky, The official publication of the Commonwealth of Kentucky. (Summer Edition 1953). A feature on Breckinridge and the work of the FNS. 85M1: FNS, Box 36, Fol. 12. University of Kentucky in Lexington, USA.

[24] FNS Promotional & Fiscal Budget Material 1954. 85M1: FNS, Box 29, Fol. 17. University of Kentucky in Lexington, USA.

8.2   Retention Issues: Socio-Economic Versus Humanitarian Realities

Statements made by both American and British FNS nurses interviewed or surveyed, all of whom graduated from hospital nurse training (diploma) schools in the 1950s–1960s in either the US or the UK mirrored the cultural realities of the career choices for women that existed at this time. An American FNS nurse who was a 1957 Diploma graduate from a Hospital School of Nursing in Saginaw, Michigan when asked, "why nursing" summed it up nicely stating, 'it was either that, secretary, teacher or wife and mother in my day' (see Footnote 3). As late as the 1960s nursing was still viewed as one of the few professions open to single women outside of teaching and secretarial work, which provided a means of independence and self-sufficiency outside of marriage. Nursing, particularly district nursing at this time had the added incentive of offering more in the way of adventure and travel than other options. For young, single women with narrow employment prospects and even narrower prospects of working at all once married the opportunity to travel coupled with the adventurous experiences offered with this option could prove irresistible as evidenced by the following comment made by a former FNS nurse:

> I went to help out on my Uncle's farm in New Zealand back in 1957 for 1 year. I was unhappy there and on my return trip I met two nurses on the ship who told such lovely gory stories, I had to be a nurse![25]

All of the former American and British FNS nurses had relatives or acquaintances in nursing (or the medical field) which served as a positive recruitment influence and the dynamic, challenging or 'adventuresome' aspects of the work were cited as most appealing to all of those either interviewed or surveyed. The socio-economic advantages, nurses 'in the family' and the 'working with people' elements of nursing were strong motivators in the recruitment and retention of more recent nurse graduates as well.

Of the group of 19 US nurses and one Canadian nurse surveyed who are presently in practice, five reported the reason they chose nursing as a career was that they also had one or more close relative who was a nurse, had wanted to be a nurse or were in the medical field. One of these three nurses also added that she always said, 'she would never be a nurse' but when she became pregnant while going to college for a bachelors degree in biology she realized that she could make more money in less time with nursing and switched her major.[26] This 'never say never' reality was mirrored in a statement made by a former British FNS nurse who said that she 'was never, ever, ever going to be a midwife' (see Footnote 1). This nurse got into midwifery training only planning on doing the first 6 months and then quitting but found that she was surprised by how much she enjoyed it and ended-up not only finishing the course of study but practicing as a midwife, midwife-educator

---

[25] Judie Pridie-Halse. British former FNS Nurse-Midwife (1960–1961).

[26] Scarfe B. Hospital staff nurse for 6 years, critical care 2 years.

and FNS administrator from November of 1955 through March of 1967. One nurse in practice today also used the following language to further describe her career choice:

> I always wanted to be a nurse, and saw how my loved ones were treated by nurses when they were ill. I also had a few shining examples of what NOT to become![27]

This suggested identification with a human reward value system that was learned through observation. A former American FNS nurse also made a similar observation regarding what not to become while in training in 1957 when she made the following comment about a supervisor who was particularly harsh, "She was what you didn't want to be when you became what she was" (see Footnote 3). Another nurse presently in practice cited her being on the receiving end of 'good nursing care' that was the most 'significant' factor in her choice of a career in nursing.[28] Indeed, most of the nurses cited a desire to 'help others' and 'make an impact' or described their choice as 'a calling,' something they'd 'always wanted to be' or that had 'chosen them.' Only two of the 20 nurses presently in practice did not include identification with a human reward value system as a reason for entering nursing. Instead, both of these nurses cited a desire to 'work in health care,' one of them stating that they had their sights set on 'medicine.' Of these two nurses, one valued highly her ability to empower others, stated that she 'loved people' and was optimistic regarding the future of nursing while the other, though supportive of nursing was far less optimistic and admitted to feeling 'trapped' by her choice.

Apparently, the inner satisfaction associated with the humanitarian aspects of the work has been and continues to be a major draw into the profession, and can be sparked by an innate desire, observation or personal experience. Unfortunately, this has not been perceived by nurses as being valued within either their professional discipline or practice cultures. When British and American FNS nurses were asked if they would 'choose nursing' if they had it to do over again, they overwhelmingly responded 'no.' The rest of the British and FNS nurses felt that the opportunity to develop 'relationship' with your patients were, regrettably, a thing of the past largely due to the fact that the patient care which allowed nurses to make that connection had been given to non-licensed personnel and that patients are moved on so quickly through the system. The biggest impact to midwives cited by the nurses was the change from home to hospital births, which required less time to get to a patient and allowed midwives to care for more than one patient at a time but also inevitably decreased the 'one-on-one' care and interrupted students following a labour from front (pre-natal) to (post-natal) finish.[29]

When asked if these nurses would work for the FNS today, they also said 'no.' The reasons cited were that they had been back or had heard from some of the

---

[27] Onster V. Hospital staff nurse for 1 year, telemetry 3.5 years, critical care 2 years, dialysis 1 year, research 2 years.

[28] Smarr F. Hospital obstetrics nurse for 5 years.

[29] Phyllis Long. American former FNS Nurse (1964–1967; 1973–1976; 1993–1996).

Appalachian families they kept in contact with exactly what had happened to the Service since their departure. They felt they had been there at a time when they 'made a difference' to the families, that the district nursing clinic model that made the Service comprehensive and innovative no longer existed there and that, unfortunately, the FNS is not that different from hospitals and clinics elsewhere in the US today. One former FNS nurse said that at the time in history and time in her life that she was there it allowed her to grow as a person, specialist and caregiver.[30]

All of these narratives reveal a love and respect for the independence and importance of the practice, what this practice environment offered both personally and professionally, the administrative style they worked under or a combination of all of the above. These 'rewards' had less to do with salaries, public image or even a 'favourable' work environment but had much more to do with the people and the work done with and for the people, which often took precedence over personal comfort. Indeed, most stated that if they had it to do over again today, they would not choose to be nurses in what is now an obviously better paying and much less difficult work environment because of what has been lost within this contemporary practice environment. They are not alone. Job dissatisfaction continues to be a key issue contributing to the crisis related to recruiting and retaining nurses. In addition to the most commonly cited issues of inadequate staffing, heavy workloads and increased mandatory overtime inherent within the institutional setting, current research now supports what nurses have always known–lower RN to client ratios create adverse client outcomes [10]. What research has thus far neglected but is now beginning to explore is the fact that the lack of a 'culture of care' within purported institutions established for that purpose creates adverse nursing outcomes [11].

Outside of Appalachia, at the time that Breckinridge was beginning her Service, graduate nurses from US hospital schools of nursing diploma programs generally worked in a private duty capacity if they could find such work upon graduation and during the depression this was no easy feat. A former Chippewa County Graduate of 1934 stated in an interview that one of the reasons she went into training was that the work afforded a place to stay and food to eat and that in this way she could be a help to her parents by being one less mouth to feed at home [12]. This reality existed in the UK as well. During the 1930s there was a stream of young recruits because the only three choices for women was "domestic service, teaching or nursing" [13]. This nurse's reasons for entering the profession were contingent upon her socio-economic position. She also had an aptitude for the work and was a nurse throughout her marriage and at intervals between rearing her children until she retired. Socio-economic realities persist as a reason many women choose nursing as a career, albeit they are quite different than those which were presented during the Depression. Nurses today expect quite a bit more than a basic food and housing allotment while they train and the hope of work post training. Yet monetary incentives such as grants or scholarships to be used towards their education as well as

---

[30] Judy Haralson-Rafson. American former FNS Nurse (1971–1976; 1971 Graduate of FNS Family Nurse Practitioner Program).

expectations regarding salary, flexibility and professional opportunities post gradu-ation continue to be strong motivators for nurses to enter the profession [14].

Socio-economic motivators are not new, neither are they solely capable of keep-ing nurses in the profession once drawn into it. Although most of the nurses still in practice cited the economic advantages associated with nursing as a career choice as an incentive, only three of them said they were 'unsure' if they would make the same choice again and none of them cited 'economics' as the reason for their indecision. Of the three nurses who were 'unsure' if they would choose nursing again as a career, two had less than 5 years of experience and one had a little over 13 years of experience. All three went into nursing citing a strong human reward value system as their main reason for entering the profession, not salary, and all of these nurses worked in a hospital setting. In addition, all three of these nurses cited the lack of value, respect and autonomy afforded to the profession and the overall lack of concern for patients within the institutional setting as the main reason for their hesitancy in stating they would enter the field of nursing if they had it to do over again. Interestingly, of these three 'undecided' one expressed 'guilt' at the prospect of even contemplating having a nursing degree and not working in nurs-ing but stated that she would rather work in a field that 'feels more professional and respected'.[31] Another stipulated that this was a 'hard question' and that even though it had its problems nursing 'was really a good career' before admitting that she was not sure she would choose to do it again (see Footnote 28). Both of these nurses also stated that though they had thought about leaving nursing, they had also considered going on for an 'advanced degree' in 'teaching' or 'public health' or move into 'community health' where the environment was more conducive for both the patient and the nurse in lieu of leaving the profession altogether. This suggests that nurses today entering the profession still value humanitarian rewards highly, as well as professional autonomy, respect and recognition. It also suggests that if they cannot be found in institutional patient care environments nurses will seek them elsewhere. Unfortunately, these values may not exist elsewhere in nurs-ing as evidenced by the observations of this bachelor's prepared US nurse who had gone on for an advanced degree:

> I also find that my education is not honored. I have seen nurses with Masters and PhD's treated as if they were stupid. Their advanced degrees have not been held on par with others.[32]

A 2001 graduate from a bachelor of nursing degree program stated that she chose nursing as a career because it, 'provided flexibility and good financial opportunities' (see Footnote 32). She was in the midst of a divorce and needed to change careers. Nursing was a second degree for this nurse. Indeed, two other nurses, one a gradu-ate from an associate degree of nursing school and the other from a baccalaureate program also stated that after a divorce they were looking for a way to support themselves and their children and were attracted to the professions 'flexibility' and

---

[31] Jean A. Hospital oncology nurse <1 year.
[32] Sloan M. Hospital operating room staff nurse for 2.5 years, research. 5 years.

readily available job opportunities upon graduation due to how 'in-demand' nurses were. Divorce was also a factor for a nursing student who was reluctantly admitted to the Chippewa County Training School for Nursing in 1929. However, the following excerpt from her file demonstrates the stigma associated with being divorced at this time:

Very undesirable material. Tendency to prefer outside interests. Not a good example.[33]

This student was a transfer student from Grace Hospital in Detroit. This statement was on the student's transcript under 'remarks' from this school. She was recorded to have left training after 4 months at Grace Hospital's Nurse Training School. She also left War's training school with 'ill health' listed as the reason in April of 1930. Indeed, FNS founder, Mary Breckinridge was divorced at a time when such a state often precluded one from being trained in nursing at all. One would assume that it would be the nurses who cited socio-economic realities as one of the reasons or even the main reason that they chose nursing as a career to continue to be labelled the 'undesirable element' within the discipline by nurses who cited a more humanitarian motivation for entering practice but that has proven to be a more complex issue upon closer examination. Surprisingly, it was the divorced nurse who cited career flexibility and good financial opportunities as her main reason for entering the profession who expressed her displeasure in 'new' nurses coming into the profession for the same reason she did. She stated that though money and job security should be a reason to enter nursing, it should not be the "only" reason and that she felt that it was for many of the newer nurses entering practice (see Footnote 32).

A US nurse who graduated in 2006 admitted to choosing nursing as a career because it was "safe" as she came from a family of nurses, explaining, "I realized that I could make more money in less time with nursing. I didn't realize then that I would like my job and go on to further my education." This nurse also said that even though nurses do not have the "autonomy they should" and "are kept down with societal opinions of what they do," when asked if she had it to do over again would she choose nursing, she responded:

I think that I would have gone right to college and gotten my bachelors of Science degree in nursing earlier so that I would be making a real difference in nursing sooner (see Footnote 26).

This nurse was finishing a master's degree to become an Acute Care Nurse Practitioner. She also placed much of the blame for nursing's limitations on the fact that nurses do not demand to be treated as the educated professionals they are.

By the 1940s, hospital institutions began to see the necessity of decreasing work hours and providing incentives to entice nurses into employ that were being done in other businesses. At the same time, the FNS appealed not to nurses' socio-economic needs but rather to their humanitarian impulses to serve the health care needs of a community in a unique setting. The relational element inherent in her care model

---

[33]Chippewa County, et al., Sault Ste. Marie Hospital Training School of Nursing. Surviving Student Records for the Years 1926–1934.

made it not only culturally acceptable but extremely effective and fiscally efficient within the Appalachian community while simultaneously making it personally and professionally attractive to nurses, seeking a stimulating autonomous practice environment in which to grow professionally as well as personally. Breckinridge managed to keep her staff at a time when other organizations and institutions outside of Appalachia with less physically and emotionally demanding work environments could not. Importance was given at the FNS to ethical aspects, not just the physical or administrative aspects, of patient care and FNS personnel's morale, mental, physical and emotional well-being was also given priority in order to get the work done. Nurses today, though economically rewarded within the institutional setting lack the personal and professional respect and value that morally inhabitable environments such as Breckinridge's afforded her 'early nurses.' This disparity between the socio-economic and humanitarian needs of the nurse creates the moral distress associated with ineffective communication, fragmented care and a lack of advocacy on the part of the nurse, which in turn is associated with inadequate or inappropriate care as well as experiences of 'burnout.' Chapter 9 will further investigate how the professional and public image of nursing has been exploited and thus contributes to this crisis cycle.

References

1. Singleton K, Sun Z, Zell K, Vriezen K, Albert N. Multicenter study of nursing role complexity on environmental stressors and emotional exhaustion. Appl Nurs Res. 2016;30:52–7. https://doi.org/10.1016/j.apnr.2015.08.010.
2. Thierry P, Mitroff I. Transforming the crisis-prone organization: preventing individual, organizational and environmental tragedie. San Francisco. CA: Jossey-Bass. p. 182.
3. Martin J. Cultures in organizations: three perspectives. Oxford: Oxford University Press; 1992. p. 8.
4. Dammann N. A social history of the frontier nursing service. Sun City, AZ: Social Change Press; 1982. p. 123.
5. Breckinridge M. Wide neighborhoods: a story of the frontier nursing service. Lexington: University Press of Kentucky; 1981. p. 122–33.
6. Andrist C, Nicholas P, Wolf K. A history of nursing ideas. Burlington: Jones and Bartlett Publishers, Inc; 2006. p. 133.
7. Drake R. History of Appalachia. Lexington: University Press of Kentucky; 2003. p. 231.
8. Dammann N. A social history of the Frontier Nursing Service. Sun City: Social Change Press; 1982. p. 68.
9. Williamson M. Factors affecting the nursing career choice. Unpublished PhD dissertation, University of Texas Austin, USA; 1990. p. 179.
10. Hinno S, Partanen P, Vehvilainen-Julkunen K. Nursing activities, nurse staffing and adverse patient outcomes as perceived by hospital nurses. J Clin Nurs. 2012;11–12:1584–93. https://doi.org/10.1111/j.1365-2702.2011.03956.x. Epub 2011 Dec 15.
11. Tinsley C, France N. The trajectory of the registered nurse's exodus from the profession: a phenomenological study of the lived experience of oppression. Int J Hum Caring. 8.
12. West E. 'Wallis-Rye, A. Personal interview: war memorial hospital graduate recalls her training' featured in Sault Ste. Marie, Michigan Evening News, 29 August 2003.
13. Williams K. Nurse training in the Carnarfon and Anglesey hospital 1935–1949. N. Wales: University of Wales Bangor; 2000. p. 175.
14. Grant G, et al. Factors influencing job satisfaction among nurses. Br J Nurs. 1994;3(12):615–20.

Chapter 9
Cultural Identity, Public Image and Frontier Nursing

9.1 Cultural Identity, Public Image and the FNS

The special relationship that the Service had with the people was disrupted when the Appalachian culture began to erode in the advent of governmental interference on a much larger scale than ever before in the 1960s. The 'image' of nurses on horseback and babies in saddlebags, once highly esteemed by the people became suspect. After her death, Breckinridge was accused of using this image to garner funds for her Service while negatively depicting the people of the region.[1] The people also viewed the newer nurses with less respect because they wore jeans with their uniforms and the newer nurses demonstrated a lack of respect for what the uniform represented by opting to do so. The nurses also viewed the people differently than their predecessor's due in large part to the stereotypes being exported to them.[2]

Indeed, the Service along with every other influence from outside the region has been accused of being part of Appalachia's many economic, social and cultural problems ever since the publication of a book in 1963 by Harry M. Caudill entitled *Night Comes to the Cumberlands*. The book was an expose' against the coal industry, which Caudill believed exploited Eastern Kentucky and spawned many more publications of the same ilk. The book inspired many inside and outside of the area to look at the dynamics of regional politics and economic growth in Appalachia, which was certainly warranted. Unfortunately, it also created a lot of mud slinging by zealots in quarters where it was not justified though there were certainly individuals (including nurses) who came in from the outside that did take away and perpetuate a negative image of the people either intentionally or unintentionally. However, considering the Services long history, most coming to the FNS as staff, nurses or student nurses did not seek to tarnish its image. Perhaps the most notorious stereotype to come out of the hills was the publication of an

---

[1] Interview#78OH150FNS10 1982. Mary & Clyde Brewer.

[2] Interview #82OH05FNS148 1982. Dr. Mary Weiss & Dr. Pauline Fox.

© Springer Nature Switzerland AG 2019
E. West, *Frontier Nursing in Appalachia: History, Organization and the Changing Culture of Care*, https://doi.org/10.1007/978-3-030-20027-5_9

article in *Life Magazine* on 24 December 1949, by T.S. Hyland. It is one that neither the FNS nor Leslie County had forgotten or forgiven. Hylan was a former
science and medicine editor for *Time Magazine* whose apparent purpose was to
alert *Life* readers to the dangers of high birth rates in Central Appalachia while
simultaneously pointing out that the 'semi-illiterate surplus was over-running the
industrial Midwest' in post-war America. This infuriated Breckinridge, who had
tried to make certain that Hyland had accurate facts and figures. The birth rates he
published were blatantly inaccurate. He had said she could 'blue pencil' the story
and when he would not send her what he was planning to publish, she in turn
refused to give the magazine any of the photos they requested until she was permitted to do so. Unfortunately, the story she eventually proof-read was not the
story that ran alongside the photographs she submitted. Every fact she had given
the publication had been disregarded [1]. She ostensibly spent the rest of her life
attempting strategic public relations counterattacks against the backlash that the
Service received after this story ran with only marginal success. When asked by
Harper and Brother's publishers to write the story of the FNS she felt this would
be one way to set the record straight. It was published in 1952 with the title, *Wide
Neighbourhoods: A Story of the Frontier Nursing Service* and presented nary a
poor, ignorant, barefoot hillbilly from front to finish [2].

9.2   'Mission' Versus 'Medical Service': FNS as Image Broker

In a book entitled, *The History of Appalachia*, there is a very small paragraph, sand-
wiched in between two larger ones on Lexington's prominent physicians, that men-
tions a 'famous multi-county mission,' begun by Mary Breckinridge that 'specialized
in modern child bearing services' [3]. Only a small part of the service dealt with
child bearing. This service, a nursing service, not a 'mission,' treated the people of
the community from cradle to grave, promoted wellness when most other health
care organizations were not doing so, treated illnesses, provided public health and
district nursing as well as midwifery services to a community that spanned 1000
square miles when there were no roads to speak of. This same book goes on to herald the accomplishments of 'for profit' practices that had 'active political careers'
that included fighting for the causes of rights of miners suffering from black lung
disease which served to raise one general practitioner to prominence in West
Virginia reform politics, thus becoming protected by health insurance and government policy [4].

   This heralding of fine medical services and dedication on the part of doctors are
intimately connected with industry, politics, health insurance and governmental
policy, all of which are institutionalised entities within American society. The fact
that the causes of the rights of miners with black lung would warrant praise is not
surprising, what is surprising is that the achievements of an organization that
between 1925 and 1975 boasted a record of 17,000 deliveries (almost all of which

were in women's homes, often in primitive conditions) with only 11 maternal deaths was not even mentioned, let alone praised [5]. This omission conveyed a great deal in regard to which of these two health care endeavours and providers garnered the most value in society; direct, individual, personal patient advocacy versus politicised, institutionalised, publicized client (or consumer) advocacy. To add insult to injury, this book also reported that National Health Service Corps Scholarships had been offered to new medical school graduates as opportunities for service in the region and to pay off costs of medical school for these recipients. This was cited as helping to 'partly fill the region's physician gap' [4]. Apparently, the fact that the FNS had been offering scholarships for nurses to become midwives through their own organization since 1939 because the nation had no such offerings for nurses and have been filling that 'physician gap' quite nicely since 1925 also did not warrant mention.

In the early twenty-first century, Drake also commended the 'aggressive networking' of health services tied to the medical centres of the University of Kentucky, the University of Tennessee and the University of North Carolina. It is interesting to note that two of these institutions' medical centres were approached by FNS Physician, Rogers Beasley over 30 years before to aggressively network with the existing nursing service (FNS), the sole health care provider in Eastern Kentucky, for support and assistance in setting-up a nurse practitioner program in the late 1960s to better meet the needs of the people but declined doing so because of concerns regarding the expansion of these nurses' role. Perhaps another FNS doctor summed up nicely what these physicians were really concerned about when he made the following comment regarding the role of these nurses in an article for the Harvard Medical Alumni Bulletin:

> I learned too what 75 years of dedication by the nurse-midwives had meant to the people of Eastern Kentucky. One day, I fielded a call over the short-wave radio from a nurse-midwife who announced, "I'm bringing in a patient with a ruptured ectopic pregnancy!" The nurse soon appeared in her Land Rover, her patient attached to an intravenous and securely bedded on the floor of the vehicle. The woman's husband was offering her comfort. My interview and exam turned out to be superfluous because the nurse had coolly brought the situation under control. When I operated, I evacuated considerable blood from the patient's abdomen, clamped and removed the bleeding fallopian tube, closed the abdomen, and reported to the husband. He listened politely, but directed most of his questions to the nurse, as was proper. She was the person he knew, and the one who had intervened immediately to save his wife's life. To him, I was just another pair of hands [6].

The debate over the value and use of nurse-midwives amongst physicians included not only the actual benefit to the patient but also the economic advantage to the doctor. One physician stated that the nurse-midwife would allow 'time for reading, attendance at medical meetings' and an increase in the number of clients a practice could potentially take on, all of which would make the doctor 'financially better off' [7]. Arguments by physicians in favour of the use of nurse-midwives always included those less altruistic motives while arguments against their use tended to focus either on their educational lack, role limitations or either denying or ignoring entirely the mountain of evidence in existence proving their benefit to patient outcomes.

Breckinridge's publications, photographs and films of the Service and the region do not depict the Appalachian people as backward, anti-progressive or lazy. She was instrumental in making only one of the three films ever prepared for promotional use on the work of the Service. The first one, which was made in 1925 by her Cousin Marvin Breckinridge and was a black and white, silent film entitled 'Forgotten Frontier.' She did not appear in the film but rather solicited local people and real FNS Nurses to re-enact actual events portrayed in the film where the nurses had been called upon for help. The locals were aware of what the film was to be used for and the actual people who were helped agreed and appeared in the film.[3] Breckinridge used this film when she went outside of the region to solicit funds or personnel for the work of the Service at her speaking engagements. The second was entitled 'The Road' and was made in 1967, after her death but her successor, Helen E. Browne chose to follow her mentor's example. This film received several awards and was sold to numerous libraries. By spring of 1969 it had been shown on over 56 television stations in 51 cities. The US Information Agency distributed it in 70 countries and some ex-staff saw it in Africa, Asia and Latin America [8]. The third was created in 1974 and entitled, 'Cherish the Children.' In these latter two films, actual FNS nurses, doctors, employees and local people appear and re-enact the day-to-day operations of the FNS and select 'real events' that had occurred.

The most that can be construed from these latter promotional films is that music germane to the area is used (and played upon a dulcimer in the 1967 film) to give the viewer a feel for the culture being depicted. The latter films show jeeps being used not horses and depict the new hospital, people and more clinic than home visits by the FNS, which is again accurate for the changing times. The latter two films are narrated and stressed that in addition to giving all they know as 'nurses,' the FNS Nurse also gives all she is 'as a person,' which reflects the 'people orientation' of both the culture and Service.[4] One nurse who appeared in the 1974 film, 'Cherish the Children,' said that the roles portrayed in the film were not altogether accurate as physicians were depicted educating the patients when it was the nurses who did this in actual practice but in all other ways, the film depicted the people, work and area accurately.[5] This statement reflected the changes which occurred for the nurses there as their role became marginalized by the influx of medical doctors into the service area.

Images in all of these promotional materials depict the move from cabins to more modern homes that nurses visited on horseback and then in jeeps. The move to the hospital and modern equipment are also depicted alongside fuller curriculum out-

---

[3] FNS Audio Visual Series. Forgotten Frontier (1927). This is a silent, black and white film, the first made of the FNS. It was filmed by Breckinridge's cousin, Marvin Breckinridge. Factual stories were re-enacted by the FNS nurses and the families they served in the actual homes of the local people, depicting the work of the service. University of Kentucky in Lexington, USA.

[4] FNS Audio Visual Series. The Road (1967). This film is in colour and narrated. It also uses real nurses, patients and places at the FNS to depict the work of the service. University of Kentucky in Lexington, USA.

[5] Judy Haralson-Rafson. American former FNS Nurse (1971–1976; 1971 Graduate of FNS Family Nurse Practitioner Program).

lines and eventually included an outline on the Family Nurse Practitioner Program. Though it was certainly true that Breckinridge used the positive images associated with the FNS's long history and traditions in Appalachia to aid in recruitment, it cannot be said that she abused the use of the Service's earlier images of the community in order to get finances or staff. She always used her staff and local people who wanted to participate in all of her promotional materials, including the films. The films always portrayed the people to whom the events transpired when stories were being related regarding treatment received or the camera was merely brought into the clinic or home where the work was actually being done by real nurses; actors were never used nor were the peoples' stories dramatized or elaborated upon in any way.[6] Any 'staging' that occurred in promotional materials in the Service's latter years tended towards the inclusion of babies in saddlebags in the photographs. This alluded to the FNS's long, unique and respected history of delivering babies and doing home visits on horseback and it was the only 'staged' element within these photographs **(Photographs 2, 6)**. Breckinridge herself often appeared in promotional photographs with the locals and both they and she appeared in clothing and surroundings that were completely usual and natural **(Photograph 3)**. The same could not be said for promotional material outside of nursing's control in mainstream America. A large number of promotional materials for the armed services and American Red Cross did not always adequately reflect the nurse's role and tended to tie it to the more traditional, socially acceptable and restricted female role of 'mother.' When nursing was used in commercial advertisements they tended to reinforce the role of mother and caregiver, while often subliminally suggesting that these 'virtues' were merely a product of female genetics [9]. In addition, the promotional material for the Graduate Midwifery School reflected the changes that occurred at the Service by utilizing photographs of the newer clinics, hospital and use of jeeps, while also retaining a few of the historic photos of the nurses on horseback and 'exterior' cabin shots of the nurses with families or with saddlebags, the symbol associated with the organization. These photographs stressed the long history of unique, quality nursing care that the Service became known for while also stating emphatically that it had grown as times had changed and was now meeting the needs of the population using the latest techniques and treatments.[7] By 1971 the

---

[6] FNS Audio Visual Series, et al., 1927, 1967 & 1974, FNS Audio Visual Series, Cherish the Children (1974). This film is in colour and narrated. It also uses real nurses, patients and places at the FNS to depict the work of the Service but depicts physicians educating patients when the nurses had been the ones doing this. University of Kentucky in Lexington, USA.

[7] FNS Graduate Midwifery School Promotional Brochures 1925–1968. 85M1: FNS, Box 323, Fol. 1 & 2., Brochures from 1940s depict a car outside of the hospital, comfortable, rustic quarters, lectures by medical staff and hospital deliveries. There are shots of cabins and nurses on horseback as well. 1950s brochures depict jeeps and travel by jeep and horseback by nurses. 1960s brochures have updated photos of the hospital and newer equipment. 1960s–1970s materials include updated photographs of jeeps, nurses, clinics and the hospital with one 'baby in a saddlebag' shot on the back cover. 'FNS Family Nurse & Nurse Midwife Brochures (1971–1979)' have no photographs at all. University of Kentucky in Lexington, USA.

brochures included the Nurse Practitioner Program and had no photographs at all within the brochures.[8]

The nurses who came into the region from the rest of the nation as well as Great Britain said that they had been well informed as to what to expect via personal communication from the FNS as well as the brochures and promotional literature or publications that were generated by the Service. None said that they were 'surprised' in any way by the work or the people once they arrived as the promotional material was accurate and that the personal interviews with the director were straightforward in regard to what they would be expected to do there. Many also stated that they had learned a great deal about their own cultures as well as Appalachian culture and gleaned much in the way of professional growth from their experiences that they had no expectation of acquiring as well. Breckinridge has been described as an impassioned speaker by those who heard her speak and it is true that she 'played-up' the more exciting or adventurous elements of the work but this could hardly be viewed as deceptive if what was being expounded upon was true. She also stressed the best of Appalachian character, the people's family orientation, good-neighbour credo, trustworthiness, civility and reliability [10].

Breckinridge was shrewd and prolific in advancing her Service and in her desire to protect it and the community from caricatures. She did so in a variety of publications including Christian publications, popular secular magazines, nursing publications and even business, medical, physician and international publications.[9] In addition, the FNS has also generated its own *Quarterly Bulletin* since 1926. Various former FNS personnel have also published their experiences at the Service and by and large have been accurate and fair representations of the work, organization and local people; all of them recounted fondly by the nurses who spoke highly of the work and people in Eastern Appalachia [11].

FNS nurses in practice at the organization were often encouraged by Breckinridge to publish; articles on the work and her nurses even won the Harmon Prize and were published in the *Survey-Graphic*.[10] It should also be mentioned that one former British FNS nurse shared a slide presentation she had put together from photographs she had taken while she was there for a year in 1960 and an article that was published in Britain that also ran the photographs. Among them was an elderly woman, poorly attired and barefoot with a pipe in her mouth. The language used to

---

[8]FNS Family Nurse & Nurse Midwife Brochures 1971–1979. 85M1: FNS, Box 323, Fol. 1 & 2.

[9]Colliers Magazine 1946, Courier Journal Magazine 1953, Hi-Power News 1948, Life Magazine 1969, Nursing Mirror & Midwives Journal 1955, Scope Weekly 1958, The Progressive Farmer 1954. 85M1: FNS, Box 36, Fol.s 4–14.

[10]Breckinridge's Personal Correspondence, 14 September 1926. 85M1: FNS, Box 2, Fol. 20., Breckinridge writes, "A number of magazines have asked for articles on the work and the nurses are preparing them. An article entitled 'An Adventure in Midwifery' has won the Harmon Prize and was published in the October issue of the Survey-Graphic." University of Kentucky in Lexington, USA.

describe the people by both the nurse and within the publication was 'hillbilly'.[11] These images and descriptions were shared by this nurse in Britain after she left the service but the same images and disparaging language was also used by other American non-native Appalachian visitors and hurt the local community's image, and by default that of the FNS as collaborators in the perpetration of this image to the world.

A former American FNS nurse who was only at the Service for 8 months related the following memory of her drive to begin her work at the FNS:

> We (my mother and I) were driving up to Lexington and my mother was talking about when I'd come down and I suddenly said, "I'm not going." She says, "What do you mean?" I say, "No, it's not what I expected." I said one thing I couldn't tolerate was trash along the road or to see tipped over out-houses and my mother said, "Oh, for heavens sakes, go ahead, at least go for a year but whatever you do, don't bring home a hillbilly".[12]

The language and attitude expressed by this nurse suggested that she either did not have or did not share as deeply the values, beliefs and norms rooted within FNS culture as those of its earlier nurses. These comments could also have been due to her age and the fact that she came from an urban environment where this stereotype had been propagated. She was the youngest nurse to be hired by the FNS at this time, at 22 years of age. In any event she went and after 8 months with the Service her mother's worst fears were realized as she married a 'hillbilly,' to whom she is still married today. Therefore, the argument could be made that this nurse's latter action duly nullified her earlier prejudice toward the people and that she came away from the mountains with a very different view than she had going in with of its people.

Some interviews done in the late 1970s and early 1980s for the University of Kentucky Oral History Project made little attempt to hide their bias in framing questions such as, 'did the FNS do too much for the local people' thus 'robbing them of their independence,' to which the locals responded, 'no,' some appearing stunned by the suggestion.[13] In response to a statement made by an interviewer suggesting that the FNS portrayed the people to others in a manner that would continue donations, a local man said that when Breckinridge and the FNS first became involved in Leslie, Clay and Perry Counties they provided a "great service to the people who obviously appreciated it" and that conditions were "not far from the way she presented 'em".[14]

---

[11] Judie Pridie-Halse. British former FNS Nurse-Midwife (1960–1961).

[12] Roberta Stidham. American former FNS Nurse (1960–1961).

[13] Georgia Ledford, former Secretary for FNS Community Committee & long-time resident of Appalachia.

[14] Mary & Clyde Brewer. Long time residents of Appalachia who wrote a book on it called "Of Bolder Me" and later called "Rugged Trails of Appalachia."

9.3   Uniforms: Professional Identity or Symbol of Oppression?

Breckinridge's influence gave nurses the incentive to give their best. She expected her nurses to be in full uniform and look like FNS nurses who were proud of the uniform.[15]

There is another account of an FNS Nurse being asked why she did not wear her uniform cap, which she kept in her belt purportedly because she preferred the wind in her hair while horseback riding. This nurse responded that she thought the world of her little cap, just not upon her head [12]. Breckinridge never reprimanded her for this lapse in uniform protocol whereas a breach in protocol of this magnitude would have been severely sanctioned in the more common institutional settings outside of Appalachia. It is well documented in a variety of sources, and among nurses and student nurses at the FNS who have been interviewed that the FNS uniform was well respected and worn with a certain amount of humble recognition of the fact that the reason it was so esteemed was due entirely to the work of the early nurses who had worn it before them and had earned that respect from the community. In other words, it was not the uniform as object that garnered respect but rather the people (women) who had earned it from the local population. The uniform later symbolized, embodied, the entire organization. As one FNS nurse who joined the service in the 1960s aptly stated, they had influence with the people and were accepted just by virtue of being in an FNS uniform as a direct result of the respect those early nurses had earned within the community. She stated, 'the men would listen and follow through' and this in a culture where women did not instruct men.[16]

Another former FNS nurse recalled her interview with Breckinridge's successor, Helen E. Browne, remembering that Browne was wearing "denim jeans" and "hoeing in the garden" when she arrived and that she thought at the time that this was "not proper attire for an interview" (see Footnote 12). Indeed, proper attire, or 'dressing for success' are concepts relevant to the business world and institutions have long controlled both its employees and image to the general public by its dress code [13]. Perhaps this is also why the uniform question remains a curious phenomenon germane to nursing and serves as point of conflict among nurses [14]. Historically, it crops up, unsolicited in dialogues concerning professionalism in both positive and negative connotations and has been used by nurses and non-nurses alike to categorize nurses and nursing. Surviving records from nurse training schools in both the US and UK contain descriptors associated with the uniform and student 'appearance' in said uniform within student evaluations. Very similar language was used to describe students in uniform and included, 'smart,' 'neat,' 'tidy,' 'untidy,' and 'healthy looking.' A nurse who wore her uniform well gave the 'appearance of confidence' and was apparently highly valued by the gate-keepers of the discipline. This should not be surprising as societal grounding within a particular culture is

---

[15] Betty Lester, former long-time FNS Nurse (English).
[16] Anne Lorentzen. American former FNS Nurse (1963–1965).

identified via adherence to a particular selection of clothing and observable in the form of personal behaviour attributed to the social group to which one belongs [15].

Both the British and American former FNS nurses as well as nurses presently in practice broached the topic of uniforms in their discourse while answering very disparate questions surrounding personal as well as professional motivation and image. FNS nurses who came to Appalachia either alluded to or stated outright in their discourse that a desire to wear the uniform was a motivating factor in their decision to become FNS nurses but generally suggested this in connection with the reputation that the uniform inspired. This suggests that the FNS uniform was not in and of itself the determinant of professional identity or image but rather a symbol of it and for FNS nurses this symbol held no negative or controversial connotations as the identity of the organization, as well as the discipline of nursing within the organization was well established and accepted by the community they served in the organization's early years. Indeed, there were two FNS uniforms worn by the nurses, a summer and winter uniform that were either blue or grey respectively; the winter uniform was wool because of the harsh Appalachian winters. The uniforms were certainly unique, for any era as they included knee high boots, riding pants and cap, and a riding crop. The nurses carried supplies in saddlebags. The respect, admiration and value that this uniform came to represent not only to nursing but also to the nation was evident by the fact that a winter uniform and saddlebag is displayed at the Smithsonian Institute's National Museum of American History in Washington DC. The uniforms designed by Breckinridge were practical to the extreme with a passing reference to the organization via a patch on the sleeve. The district nurses wore these uniforms and the hospital staff wore the more traditional white uniforms that were worn elsewhere in the US prior to the 1960s.

In a twenty-first century article entitled, *In My Opinion... What is Uniform about the Nursing Uniform*, a male nurse attributed the change in nursing uniforms with "science," citing that the nursing cap was jettisoned because it was suspected of harbouring bacteria as well as becoming incompatible with burgeoning technology, which made it a hazard to wear, and the sweeping changes of the 1960s wrought by feminism and social change that saw the white uniform as a "symbol of oppression" [14]. In the turbulent 1960s the nursing uniform was not immune to the immense transformations taking place in society. Feminism was a catalyst for all women to examine their place and role, and not surprisingly, a perfectly white uniform worn by a mostly female workforce within institutional hierarchies where doctors (mostly men) were in control was seen not as a symbol of power but of oppression. He connected the image of Florence Nightingale with her lamp to that of a "uniformed nurse" reasoning that the lay public (and often nurses themselves) found these familiar, albeit outdated, images as nostalgic, compelling and understood them to represent nursing. Pinard concluded that the nursing uniform was a relic from the past and not practical in the modern hospital setting despite the controversy surrounding professionalism amongst nurses in relation to the uniform and the pleas made by the general public to "know who the nurses are" amongst the cornucopia of health professionals within the institutional setting [14]. What were particularly compelling about these statements were the obvious cultural references to science, technology and popular culture and their impact on shaping the professional attire of nurses. The problem with Pinard's interpretation was that it did not take into account the role that this culture also had in shaping this image as well as his own opinions. Assumptions about gender have historically been branded as the cause for many of nursing's woes and science and technology, which are more highly valued by society than care and service values, as attributes to be sought by the discipline in the hope of raising its status within the culture. In response to his arguments, a senior nurse with 27 years of experience stated that her patients routinely commented that they appreciated knowing who she was and that the strong argument being made by nurses for a professional look and 'dressing for success' instead of in white in order to be "respected and compensated" was undermined and not abetted by modern V-neck scrub uniforms that exposed midriffs and underwear when hanging intravenous solution bags or bending over to administer patient care [16]. A 2005 bachelor's degree nurse in practice today agreed and stated in her discourse, "I don't like the lack of professionalism I feel when wearing pyjama-like scrubs and a ponytail".[17] In addition, many of the older former FNS nurses who had been hospitalized recently commented on the fact that you never knew if the person who entered your room was a nurse or housekeeping staff.[18] Oddly enough, discourse surrounding the uniform question invariably led to the negative changes associated with new nurses as well as the hospital. One former FNS nurse who is still practicing as a Senior Rehabilitation Consultant in a firm at which she is a partner discoursed on all of these issues in answer to the question, 'Would you choose to be a nurse or nurse-midwife today?

> The majority of people that I know today that have gone into nursing, they have no want of taking care of people. They see themselves as pseudo-physicians, and you know, nothing was closer to being a physician or a practitioner than us (FNS nurses). You know, we had the first Peace Corps Nurses spending time with us. We taught them… and I have difficulty when I go into a hospital in my job, I'm in most hospitals in the state of Michigan, and I have difficulty when I can't find the nurse, or don't know who the nurse is… (see Footnote 16)

All of the older former FNS nurses also tended to connect the uniform change with the obvious negative care changes within the hospital setting and many of them also saw 'younger' nurses as lacking in humanitarian impulses. One former British FNS nurse strongly implied that the appalling care she had experienced herself when recently hospitalized was due to the fact that much of the care had been "taken out of the professional nurses' hands and given to untrained people".[19]

Age or gender does not appear to be the driving force behind the uniform controversy. Both the young and older female nurses found scrubs 'unprofessional,' while a male nurse found uniformed nurses 'outdated.' A nurse with 26 years of experience presently in practice perhaps best mirrored the ambiguity inherent when evaluating change, uniform or otherwise, within the discipline of nursing. In answer to

---

[17] Jean A. Hospital oncology nurse < 1 year.

[18] Molly Lee. British former FNS Nurse-Midwife (1950–1970s).

[19] Margaret (Maggie) Willson. British former FNS Nurse-Midwife (1955–1967).

the question how nursing had changed, she shared that though she certainly felt it was a positive thing that the "old school" ways of strict hierarchy and restrictive nursing practice norms had given way to far more scope and opportunity within nursing, there were also many things that had been lost. She observed that nurses 'knew who they were' though she thought the 'handmaiden image' was inappropriate. She did not advocate for the return of nursing caps but at the same time felt that the profession had lost tremendously in the image department as a direct result of the "sloppy" uniforms, which were often ill fitting 'scrubs and mismatched items that gave an extremely poor image, as does "hair unrestrained and jewellery everywhere" (especially in this day of major infection control issues). She saw the change as a "generally unkempt appearance" that hurt nursing. She also stated that you could not tell the nurses from anyone else. She goes on to say, "Sometime an area (hospital unit) will have nicely coordinated name tags, but too often the name and credential of the staff member is far smaller than the unit name. As a clinical instructor, I can't even tell who's who half the time".[20]

It is ironic that the cap was abandoned according to one nurse due to its possible infection risk only to have been replaced with jewellery and unkempt hair as potential risks for infection by another nurse; neither hypothesis having been proved. Perhaps the question should not focus on the symbol but rather the cultural identity that the symbol is supposed to represent. Indeed, could the change associated with the symbol of nursing (the uniform) so drastically and completely obliterate the cultural identity of the discipline or is it not perhaps more reasonable to assume that the current ambiguity concerning the uniform question has more to do with the lack of cohesion within the discipline regarding what that identity was, is and should be for nurses? Name tags that identify people to a particular hospital unit and uniforms that do not define a particular identity save that of 'staff' suggests a desire on the part of the institution to foster a solely institutional identity among its employees and a desire to perpetuate this identity to its customers. The institution may even be either intentionally or inadvertently obliterating nursing's professional identity through marginalization by confusing it with untrained personnel while physicians continue to be easily identified as the "Captain of the ship" wearing only a white lab coat with their title and name either embossed or pinned upon it over what ever attire they choose to don beneath it.

Nurses who argued for the return of the white nursing uniform sought neither a romanticized or oppressive professional *image* but rather a return of professional *identity* the uniform symbolized to the world, regardless of practice environment, which had been lost when retired from public view. The public also preferred this symbol, despite the negative baggage that the image obviously carried for some nurses because of the trustworthiness it had earned. A 2018 Gallup Poll found nurses to be "the most trusted profession" amongst the general populous. Nurses topped the 2018 Gallup Poll ranking of how Americans view 20 major professions, with 84% of the public, four in five Americans, rating their honesty and ethical

---

[20] Morrison S. Hospital staff nurse for 1 year, critical care for 10 years, pain management for 13 years.

standards as "high" or "very high." Nurses have ranked first for 17 consecutive years and every year except for one in the 20 years that Gallup has surveyed public opinion on the honesty and ethical standards of various occupations.as it has done for the past 17 years [17]. It stands to reason that if nurses are most trusted by the general public it would be in the disciplines best interest to make sure the public knew who they were.

Recent studies have found that nursing uniforms reflect the profession in a positive light and were preferred by patients and nurses alike [18]. Furthermore, the language used, regardless of gender or age, to identify the image projected by the standard white uniform when compared to the cacophony of print uniforms amongst the general populous was "professional" [19]. Feminist perspective may well have viewed the standard, white nursing uniform as a symbol of oppression but the general public and many nurses, feminist or otherwise, do not. The discipline's decision to separate itself from the 'handmaiden' image associated with its symbol, which had also garnered some very compelling and powerful positive images, instead of combating the perpetuation of the servant role within institutional hierarchies has served to do the exact opposite of what it was intended to do. In addition, it has served to weaken the discipline's recognizable, established position amongst those from whom it had always garnered its greatest support, the general public.

This reality was verified at the FNS when the same forces identified by Pinard, technology, modern feminism and social change, created an identity crisis at the Service in its latter years. A former FNS nurse recounted that you had an "automatic in" with the locals as a direct result of the uniform by the time she was there. She said you still had to "pass mustard," that is prove you were caring and honest with them but if you did you became "part of the family, were respected, appreciated and cared for deeply." The respect they had for nurses held for many years. They (the people) would say, "My granddad was delivered by Helen Browne!" (see Footnote 5). When FNS nurses began to wear blue jeans with their uniform tops in the 1960s, the community at large did not know quite what to make of it. They tended to view the change negatively and described the nurses as looking 'sloppy' a term also used by a nurse in practice today to describe ill-fitting scrubs.

There was unquestionably a culture clash at the FNS on many levels that occurred at the same time the uniform standards were relaxed. This created interpersonal conflicts between nurses and administration as well as patient dissatisfaction that went far beyond the question of what nurses should wear. At the time that younger nurses began wearing blue jean bottoms with their uniforms, institutional bureaucracy and government overregulation was also reducing the Service's ability to accomplish its primary function, which was to provide quality patient care to the local community. Cooperman's (1978) thoughts regarding the damaging effect of bureaucratic overregulation on the teaching profession, a profession that was also female dominated and categorized as within the 'vocational sector,' can be paralleled with the nursing profession [20]. Cooperman argued that to burden an organization with secondary functions is to reduce its ability to accompany its primary function. He calls this axiomatic to management science. The fact that this same argument is still being made in the twenty-first century in regard to "bridging professional and organizational quality" in health care is indeed telling [21]. For nursing, the most damaging effect continues to be that bureaucratic overregulation is not just escalating costs of health care or even driving nurses from the health care system, although both are considerable, but rather the reduction in the autonomy and authority of health care providers, namely nurses that *create* this mass exodus from practice. Government regulations are merely mechanisms by which society ensures that our health care institutions and the nurses within them carry out these certain specific secondary functions.

The problem of overregulation of nursing is really part of a much larger problem in wider-society, namely prizing technological skill and advancement to the exclusion of humanitarian endeavours. One nurse in practice today stated that she had witness the role of nursing "reduced to a technician" and that she was in some ways sad to see the creation of the nursing assistant role as they seemed to handle all of the tasks that can connect the nurse most to the patient while reducing the nurse to "pill pusher and recording secretary".[21] This was a significant observation as former FNS nurses also equated the advent of institutionalized care in Eastern Appalachia with the curtailment of professional autonomy, an increase in interpersonal conflict between older and younger staff and administration, and a loss of connectedness with the local community (see Footnote 18). Yet these realities have somehow become embodied within nursing discourse about generation or gender disparity and domination, uniforms and image when perhaps these issues are merely symptoms of a much larger, more complex and deeper problem of identity confusion.

9.4 'Angels of Mercy': Image, Identity, Myth or Marketing Ploy?

Like the nursing uniform, the most popular image of nurses in the twentieth century, that of 'Angels of Mercy,' has also been perceived by some as akin to the 'handmaiden' label and decidedly a negative one [22]. Unfortunately, it is an image that persists today [23]. A Canadian nurse in practice since 2002 answered an open ended-question about what she didn't like about nursing thus:

> I do not like the culture that nurses have created for themselves. We are seen as health care angels and I think it is time that we use our professional voice to create change. I think at times as nurses because we have the label of "angel" we assume the role, we often don't see our own faults as a profession. I think we really need to look more critically at the way we work to initiate and create change.[22]

This nurse felt that the 'angel' image was created and perpetuated by nurses who assumed the role to the detriment of positive change within the profession when in

---

[21] Sloan M. Hospital operating room staff nurse for 2.5 years, research. 5 years.

[22] Tipper N. Hospital telemetry nurse for 3 years. Date surveyed: 05/11/2007.

fact the image was more of a non-collaborative effort on the part of mass media, the government and other institutional regulators as well as the discipline of nursing who presented fictional and factual; popular and official representations of nursing and nursing's work in publications, on film, television and in recruitment literature [22].

In a publication on the FNS describing the work of the nurses in *Colliers Magazine* (1946) the nurses were referred to as "Heroines on Horseback".[23] In 1953, another publication began an article on the work of the FNS with "Mercy Hits the Trail" and was followed by a statement that boldly heralded that the FNS sent out "Florence Nightingales on Horseback".[24] Frontier nurses were identified from time to time as "Angels on Horseback" as well, due in large part to the various publications that described the nurses in a way so as to extrapolate on the existing image nurses had garnered as 'angels' of 'mercy' during war time. Indeed, many of the publications had advertisements for nurses that sought nurses with the same qualities as those of our "army and Navy Nurses".[25]

Breckinridge used these existing images to foster public relations and recruit nurses. A former American FNS nurse amusedly related that with the absence of horses and advent of motorcycles, some of the nurses chose to ride. They came to be known by the locals as "Hills Angels," this being a play on words for the well-known American motorcycle gangs known as "Hells Angels" (see Footnote 5). All of these images were embraced by the FNS nurses as well as the local community and were viewed as positive images. A book that was first published in 1972 and is still in publication today entitled, 'Angel Coming' by Heather Henson was a children's book about a little girl waiting for the "Angel on Horseback" to bring her a new baby brother or sister [24]. This book included a section at the back which briefly described the woman who had inspired the book, Mary Breckinridge and the Frontier Nursing Service. A more recent publication by well known children's author Rosemary Wells entitled 'Mary on Horseback: Three Mountain Stories' was written after the author read about Breckinridge and the FNS. The book began with a very brief depiction of life in Kentucky's Appalachian Mountains during the early 1920s and was followed by three stories gleaned from the 1930 film 'The Forgotten Frontier' and Breckinridge's autobiography 'Wide Neighbourhoods' [25].

The FNS was uniquely positioned in society with a nurse as its founder, administrator, financier and public relations officer. Breckinridge played an active role in how both she and her Service were portrayed in the print and film media, which was something that most nurses had very little control of outside of Appalachia. Indeed, it was due to this diligence that the image that has been extrapolated upon in recent publications has not been unduly distorted, and if so, has been distorted in

[23] Heroines on Horseback by Dorothy Miles. 85M1: FNS, Box 36, Fol. 5. Colliers Magazine (3 August 1946). University of Kentucky in Lexington, USA. p. 275.

[24] Courier Journal Magazine. 85M1: FNS, Box 36, Fol. 13. Mercy Hits the Trail: The FNS Sends Out Florence Nightingales on Horseback. (29 November 1953) University of Kentucky in Lexington, USA. p. 7.

[25] Trained Nurse. 85M1: FNS, Box 36, Fol. 11. May 1930 (3rd. Edition, 1946). Magazine features FNS nurse on horseback and another in a jeep on the cover with a story on the FNS inside. University of Kentucky in Lexington, USA. p. 275.

an optimistic and affirmative way by the media. The resources utilized by Wells were publications and films about the FNS and its founder that were generated *by* the FNS and its founder. Those journalists, filmmakers and writers that Breckinridge did not know or thoroughly trust to give an honest accounting of the nurses, work or people who petitioned her to come out, view the FNS first-hand and write about it, she procured final draft approval from prior to publication or they were not permitted to come [1].

The FNS's perception by the general public was singular when compared with the images that were being presented in the print, film and visual media about nurses and the work of nursing outside of Eastern Appalachia. In articles written on the founder, organization's work or nurses in the Service's early years may have been considered 'romanticized' due to the sometimes vivid and flowery wording used by some in praise of the more altruistic aspects of the work. This was evident in a reference made in a Christian publication that stated that 'Christianity was first place in her (Breckinridge's) life and work, permeating and shining through all of her activities, which was the secret of her success in developing the FNS'.[26] The use of this language never excluded the more practical and professional aspects of either the woman or the work in a majority of publications. This same article stated that though childbirth was observed by the author to be "beautiful," the removal of "fear" and "pain" in childbirth with anaesthetics or episiotomy incisions made to prevent tears during labour was something the midwives had learned to do to control delivery while also eliciting the full and conscious cooperation of the patient thus allowing mothers to express their joy at the precise moment their child was born. She goes on to stay that in "modern medicine, the mother was anesthetized for the episiotomy" and missed this experience entirely. She concluded that "Midwifery as it is practiced by the FNS Graduate Nurse-Midwife was indeed an art which modern obstetricians might well envy."

When articles about the FNS included references to the local population, it may have included imagery to describe the work as a "three-pronged weapon against suffering" but it also included vital statistics about the hospital, outpost clinics and Graduate Midwifery program and "how it compared with today's practice of obstetrics and gynaecology" [26]. References also included the realities of life there that the nurses encountered; paper on the cabin walls, the quaint earthy language, the below per capita income and sanitation issues but also mention the freeways being built, supermarkets and slow steady "progress" being made to the areas economic, social and health care problems. What was certainly always mentioned about the organization's founder and nurses were their titles and educational achievements, something that does not always happen when nurses are being written about or interviewed today.

The Pittsburgh, PA *Tribune-Review* ran an article entitled 'Nurse at Children's Hospital gives Strength to Kids, Families' that used the word 'nurse' once in the six-page feature and never mentioned the nurses' credentials, title or educational background at all except to say, "Armed with advanced degrees and hospital street

---

[26] The Frontier Nursing Service by Adelaide Mueller. In: The Walther League Messenger (April 1968). 85M1: FNS, Box 36, Fol. 7. University of Kentucky in Lexington, USA. p. 16.

smarts, (she) keeps tabs on patients whose doctors don't know if they will survive."
She was described by one physician in the article as, "compassionate and kind."
Many physicians are mentioned in the article and each time, their titles and credentials are mentioned and role clearly defined. Though the article does a good job of
describing the nurses' compassion and the emotional support she provided to dying
patients and their families it also does a dismal job of highlighting exactly what it
was this nurse did in her capacity of advocate, educator, and care manager for them.
The hospital's program and physician's role within it, however, was clearly identified, whereas the nurse was described in the article as the "most paged *employee*"
[27]. It was also of interest to note that the many photographs used in the article that
depicted the nurse show her in street clothes at the patients' bedside and no visible
means of identification. Conversely, FNS nurses and its founder were more frequently than not depicted in uniform and on horseback or in a jeep, which left little
doubt as to their role.

Indeed, it was as rare to see disparaging images of the mountaineers as it was
to see vague references to the FNS in print. It was even rarer to see negative
images of the people generated by former FNS staff. It was for this reason that the
local population was far more reluctant to attribute its negative image and ultimate cultural devastation at the hands of corporate America to either Breckinridge
or her Service. Perhaps the single most important action on the part of
Breckinridge's long-time secretary, which helped to keep her memory and by
default her Service from becoming a casualty in the 'blame game' for Appalachia's
cultural upheaval and ruination after her death was the burning of her personal
diary and correspondence.[27]

When asked why she did this, Breckinridge's secretary said, because they were:

> Highly emotional and sentimental things she wrote in her day book and would have been
> grabbed up, published, would have made a lot (of money). That was her own inner young
> life and she didn't want it to be seen and I'm glad she didn't. I was delighted to burn it after
> she died. (I also) Burned Breckie's (Breckinridge's deceased son's) shoes and her hus-
> band's shirts.

It would appear that Breckinridge had a sentimental side that she was wise
enough to see could also be used after her death to romanticize her or besmirch the
integrity of her organization. An interviewer with the Oral History Project at the
University of Kentucky managed to unearth that Breckinridge harboured latent
'spiritualist' tendencies and 'communicated' with her dead son from another former
FNS secretary who was also privy to her personal correspondence.[28] But considering the era to which Breckinridge was born and raised, this was hardly surprising.
Spiritualism flourished in the US from 1840s to the 1920s as it did in most English-
speaking countries and was prominent amongst the social class from which she
sprang [28]. The cultural and political upheaval, which occurred roughly during the
years 1958–1974, are evident in the oral history transcripts of the same time frame.
Many of this particular interviewer's questions were designed to elicit negative

---

[27] Interview #82OH03FNS146 1982. Agnes Lewis.
[28] Interview#82OH11FNS154 1982. Wilma Duvall Whittlesey.

responses toward the FNS and its founder insinuating that Breckinridge thought her self superior to the locals because she discouraged too much socialization of her staff with them, she didn't encourage them to call her "Mary" and asking if they thought she treated them like "slaves." Yet even so, the only negative response this particular interviewer could get was that Breckinridge frowned on her nurses "mixing" with the local men.[29] It should also be mentioned that a former FNS nurse from New England who married a local man in 1958 received a congratulatory note from Breckinridge which read, "My affectionate good wishes go out to this young descendent of some of the best families I know" (see Footnote 12).

So, how did the FNS, an organization that had successfully improved the health care of Eastern Appalachia and who had earned the trust and respect of the community it served become a target of social activists as being part of the problem in Appalachia in its latter years? In the same way that the once positive images associated with heroism and humanitarian service such as 'Angels of Mercy (or on horseback)' in nursing became images to be reviled by nurses. The uniform, once a symbol of empowerment, the only one available for women for a very long time in history, became a "symbol of oppression" to so many nurses. These symbols were overtaken by institutions and the nurses within them who perpetuated an image that corporate culture could manipulate. In much the same way, iconic figures such as Florence Nightingale and Mary Breckinridge have been viewed through a lens largely outside of historical context, politicized and then judged with an eye toward furthering a particular ideology by nurses and non-nurses alike. In Breckinridge's case, it was to bolster the cause against colonialism and the rising corporate culture in Appalachia. In Nightingale's, it was to discard the 'handmaiden' image associated with her. The problem with such an approach was that it also meant discarding the tremendous advances made in sanitation even before the advent of germ theory in patient care and the advancement of professional nursing as both an art and science, which required intellect and training wrought by Nightingale at a time when the discipline was thought by most in Victorian society to be unsuitable for women who were supposed to know only the things necessary to bring up children and keep house. Such an approach also ignored the tremendous contributions made by Breckinridge in US nurse-midwifery and public health as well as the decline in infant mortality rates and overall improvement in the quality of life of the people of Appalachia. It would appear that Appalachia was not alone in its corporate colonization; Breckinridge and her Service shared the cultural upheaval experienced by the local community via Federal Government intervention and in so doing came to be viewed as the oppressor.

Nurses who fought in world wars and were volunteers with the Red Cross embraced the label 'Angel' and wore it proudly. A book entitled, "We Band of Angels" gave an accounting of the untold story of American nurses trapped on Batann and incarcerated in a Japanese internment camp during World War Two [29]. The title of the book was a deliberate play on a well-known phrase in literature and history, which denoted military groups and depicted the dedication and loyalty

---

[29] Interview#82OH34FNS177 1982. Mary Stewart.

amongst these groups. First use of the term, "Band of Brothers" was by perhaps the greatest of English playwrights, William Shakespeare, in his famous history play, *Henry V*. In it a military group spills their blood, mixes it together in desperate battles and this makes them a family as close as any blood tie can make them. In their desperation, their comradeship, their shared struggle they become a "band of brothers" [30]. This phrase has since been used to express group solidarity of the kind wrought by shared hardships and triumphs. How the discipline hopes to emancipate itself while simultaneously obliterating its foundational roots, ignoring its epic historical achievements and blatantly disregarding its shared desperation, comradeship, struggles and solidarity is unclear. What is clear is that nursing has exhibited oppressed group behaviour similar to that of Appalachia and its people [31]. The root of this cycle of oppression is a learned belief by dominated people that they are inferior. Although this belief is not accurate, the belief occurs because the dominant group crates norms and values for the culture in its own image, and the group initially has the power to enforce it and subordinate groups learn to hate their own attributes [32]. Furthermore, nursing has successfully identified many of the norms and values of the dominant culture from without the discipline, which has fostered its disempowerment. However, it has been much less successful in recognizing, identifying and addressing how these 'inferiority complexes' persist and why there is such a lack of pride and respect of its own culture, cultural attributes and each other within the profession.

Perhaps the conclusions drawn from a study on nurse recruitment in 1947 emphasize the complexity of the problem. In it the statement was made that "successful" recruitment required "*selling*" [italics added] the applicant not only on the kind of school but far more importantly on "nursing." It was not conducive to stress the fact that so few are in the profession now as this would raise questions as to "why," "what is wrong with the endeavour" or "why are so few interested?" [33] Instead, the discipline should emphasize not the need but rather the "opportunities" that nursing has to offer, use the slogans used in 1947, "Nursing is a Proud Profession," not stress the "shortage" and endeavour instead to explain the reasons for "increased demand." Note the use of business language imbedded within these statements. We should 'Sell' the applicant, use 'slogans' and endeavour to explain the increase in 'demand' to the recognized 'supply' needs. This approach mirrors those used by corporations in their consumer marketing strategies. The discipline does not want prospective applicants to ask the very questions that we have been reluctant to explore the complexities of too closely, 'why are there so few in nursing,' 'what is wrong with the endeavour,' 'Why are so few interested?' Instead, we confuse "image" with "character." Daniel Boorstin's book, *The Image* detailed how mass media created an image often devoid of substance by replacing character with an *image* [Italics added] of it [34]. Indeed, in the Service's later years, nurses who read about the FNS who were inspired by its achievements stated that they came in order to 'wear that uniform' (see Footnote 12). Older FNS nurses commented that many of these young nurses began coming out to Appalachia for reasons other than the primary one, which was humanitarian service. One nurse commented that the FNS's couriers, volunteer assistants who were often daughters of the Service's wealthy financial supporters in cities outside of Appalachia, also began coming out for the personal experience or prestige associated with the organization and that those who did so were 'not really interested in the people or the actual work with them' (see Footnote 18).

The FNS's public image as well as the professional nurse's identity changed in the Service's latter years. This was due in large part to the cultural changes imposed upon both the community and organization. For the community, the shift from people to object focus that the corporate/business model caused created a lack of trust and disruption of relationship between the organization and the local population. For the FNS, the medical model (centralized power structure) displaced its nursing model (decentralized power structure). Publications and promotional material was controlled by Breckinridge which placed her in a unique position regarding the image presented to the outside world of nursing, her organization and the local community. This was a reality not fully realized by nurse leaders outside of Appalachia as they were never in complete control of nursing's image elsewhere. Image brokering on the part of the FNS prior to Breckinridge's demise in the 1960s strove to depict the people, the work and the school of Midwifery realistically, while stressing the best of Appalachian character, the people's family orientation, good-neighbour credo, trustworthiness, civility and reliability. Despite this fact, her organization was scrutinized after her death and blamed by some as a cause of image distortion of the people as gun toting, illiterate, prolifically breeding, barefoot hillbillies. In addition, publications outside of Appalachia described the FNS as a "mission," whereas physician run services were viewed as "medical services" and connected with industry, politics, health insurance (of which they were the sole point of access to) and governmental policy, all of which are institutionalized entities of value within American society.

The traditional nursing uniform, a powerful symbol of nursing, has been manipulated by sources both within as well as without the profession and has thus shaped the opinions nurses as well as non-nurses as representative of 'oppression' or 'professionalism.' The popular images of nurses as 'angels of mercy' or 'Nightingales' has also been embraced and viewed by nurses as sources of pride; representative of what is best about nursing while simultaneously being used as "slogans" to "sell" an image to the general public. These images have been accused by nurses of not honestly representing the character or cultural identity of nurses but rather depicting an *image* devoid of substance and non-existent within the culture of modern organizational life.

References

1. Dammann N. A social history of the Frontier Nursing Service. Sun City: Social Change Press; 1982. p. 80.
2. Dammann N. A social history of the Frontier Nursing Service, vol. 81. Sun City: Social Change Press; 1982.
3. Drake R. History of Appalachia. Lexington: University Press of Kentucky; 2003. p. 192.
4. Drake R. History of Appalachia. Lexington: University Press of Kentucky; 2003. p. 193.
5. Lepreau F. Babies in saddlebags. Harv Med Alumni Bull. 2000;28:51.

6. Lepreau F. Babies in saddlebags. Harv Med Alumni Bull. 2000;28:53.
7. Criss B. Culture and the provision of care: FNS, 1925–1940. Utah: University of Utah; 1988. p. 10.
8. Dammann N. A social history of the Frontier Nursing Service. Sun City: Social Change Press; 1982. p. 126.
9. Hudson-Jones A. Images of nurses: perspectives from history, art and literature. Philadelphia: University of Pennsylvania Press; 1988.
10. Breckinridge M. Wide neighborhoods: a story of the frontier nursing service. Lexington: University Press of Kentucky; 1981.
11. Reid D. Saddlebags full of memories. USA: Burt Lake Michigan.
12. Gardner C. Cleaver country: Kentucky mountain trails, vol. 27. New York: Fleming H. Revell Company; 1931.
13. Martin J. Cultures in organizations: three perspectives. USA: Oxford University Press; 1992. p. 90.
14. Pinard B. In my opinion … what is uniform about the nursing uniform? New Hampshire Nurs News. 2006;30(2):19.
15. Bates D, Plog F. Cultural anthropology. p. 10.
16. Chambers M. In response to "In my opinion… what is uniform about the nursing uniform?" by Brandond T. Pinard, RN in May 2006. New Hampshire Nurs News. 2006;30(4):23.
17. National Nurses United. Press Release. Once again nurses top gallup poll as most trusted profession 17 years running, December 20, 2018. https://www.nationalnursesunited.org/press/once-again-nurses-top-gallup-poll-most-trusted-profession-17-years-running. Accessed 16 Feb 2019.
18. Spragley F. Nursing uniforms: professional symbol or outdated relic? Nurs Manag. 2006;37(10):55–8.
19. Skorupski VJ. Patients' perceptions of today's nursing attire: exploring dual images. J Nurs Adm. 2006;36(9):393–401.
20. Cooperman P. The literacy hoax: the decline of reading, writing and learning in the public schools and what we can do about it. New York: William Morrow & Company; 1978. p. 174.
21. Berg M, Schellekens W, Bergen C. Bridging the quality chasm: integrating professional and organizational approaches to quality. Int J Qual Health Care. 2005;17(1):75–82. https://doi.org/10.1093/intqhc/mzi008.
22. Hallam J. From angels to handmaidens: changing constructions of nursing's public image in post war Britain. Nurs Inq. 1998;5:32–42.
23. Daly J, Speedy S, Jackson D. Context of nursing, Chapter 4: heroines, hookers and harridans: exploring popular images of nurses and nursing, by Darbyshire, P. Churchill Livingstone: Elsevier; 2014. p. 53–7.
24. Henson H. Angel coming. USA: Simon & Schuster; 2005.
25. Wells R. Mary on horseback: three mountain stories. USA: Puffin Books; 2000.
26. Clem A, Hardenbrook H. Edge of a dark land. Abbottempo. 1964:15–21.
27. Fabregas L. Nurse at children's gives strength to kids, families. Tribune Review, Greensburg, Pennsylvania (2 December 2007), 1–6.
28. Brandon R. The spiritualists: the passion for the occult in the nineteenth and twentieth centuries. New York: Alfred A. Knopf, Inc; 1983.
29. Norman E. We band of angels: the untold story of American nurses trapped on Bataan by the Japanese. New York: Random House; 2000. p. 2013.
30. Band of brothers in history and literature. indepthinfo.com. http://www.indepthinfo.com/band-of-brothers/index.shtml. Accessed 16 Feb 2019.
31. Billings DB, Norman G, Ledford I. Confronting Appalachian stereotypes: back talk from an American region. Lexington: University Press of Kentucky; 2000.
32. Feire P. Pedagogy of the oppressed. 50th anniversary ed. New York: Bloomsbury Academic; 2018.
33. Carrington M. Looking through the years: 1947, a National Student Nurse Recruitment Program. Creat Nurs. 2000;7(7):16.
34. Boorstin DJ. The image: a guide to pseudo-events in America. 50th anniversary ed. USA: Vintage Books; 1992. p. 45.

Chapter 10
Conclusions

The American economy exploited the Appalachian people more on their mountain farms than it did later when it had to pay them fully family-supported wages (welfare). Both the Appalachian regional economy and America's national economy benefited more from these people when they were subsistence farmers and supplied subsidized workers to industry than it has benefited from them since they have joined more fully in the money economy and are no longer self-sufficient [1]. The same can certainly be said of nurses prior to the country's shift from community-based to the institutionalised provision of health care. While nurses continue to call for increased salaries, reduced nurse-patient ratios, greater professional autonomy and safer working conditions they are simultaneously continuing to leave the profession in droves citing their frustration with a system that continually curtails their ability to provide the type of humane, meaningful, quality care they feel obligated to provide to the people they serve [2]. For both Appalachia and the nursing profession it was not the 'enterprise' system itself that weakened the culture; it was the form that it took. For Appalachia, it was working for currency instead of people and for the FNS and in a larger sense for the profession of nursing as well, it was working for institutions instead of patients.

In much the same way that researchers have examined Appalachia's socio-economic woes; the profession of nursing has also been ruminated upon by those both within and without the culture. Remarkably, similar causes for the profession's troubles have also been identified as reasons for Appalachia's afflictions, namely, gender role biases, government intervention (lack of substantial or consistent financial assistance) or government interference (institution of regulatory measures), image distortion by outsiders and a loss of autonomy brought about by an influx of the socio-cultural and economic changes that occurred nationally over the last two centuries that created a rise in corporate culture (objective pursuits and rewards) and an accompanying decline in people focus and reward systems [3]. As a result, the culture of institutionalized nursing has been described by nurses as 'oppressive' due primarily to the lack of power and control within the existing health care delivery system [4]. In addition, nurses have often felt ineffectual and trapped in a national

© Springer Nature Switzerland AG 2019
E. West, *Frontier Nursing in Appalachia: History, Organization and the Changing Culture of Care*, https://doi.org/10.1007/978-3-030-20027-5_10

culture that does not value their unique contributions as humanitarians or as skilled health professionals due to gender or role assignations and the value placed upon them by society as well as the differing agendas of the medical, institutional and governmental establishments with whom the discipline brokers power on a decidedly inequitable playing field. As a result, they are unable to meet the needs of their patients and often feel like cogs in the wheel of the health care industry, trapped by structural and bureaucratic rigidity that exist within their own professional organizations as well as the governmental organizations and institutional care environments in which they are forced to work [5]. Nurses within these care environments are not able to reconcile the care culture they envision for their practice with the care culture that actually exists within their practice. This was clearly demonstrated by the changes that occurred at the FNS in its latter years.

FNS founder, Mary Breckinridge founded and ran her organization for over 40 years on the philosophy of generalist nursing care, working through rather than for people, having standards 'without standardization,' 'unity' while 'avoiding uniformity,' and 'experimentation' instead of 'rigidity'.[1] The focus on technological and scientific advancement, and economic developments at the expense of the socio-cultural needs of the people, which occurred after Breckinridge's death, fell far short in meeting both the professional needs of the nurses, as well as the health care needs of the population her organization served.

Historically, nursing like many other disciplines has attempted to emulate those corporate entities that have risen to power in order to attain the respect, political clout, organizational power structure and professional autonomy that these bodies have attained. However, the profession has also inherited a culture that has proven to be self-defeating as it has also perpetuated many of the corporate cultural traits that have proven to be incongruent with its professional identity and goals [6]. Nursing's attempts to offer an explanation for inter-disciplinary conflict have nearly always been influenced by oppression and feminist theories and although these theories can be insightful they are also limiting as they omit the finer grained-analysis necessary for a fuller understanding of these conflicts. The focus thus far tended to be on the alleged disempowerment of nursing in relation to other perceived dominant groups, especially male doctors and the denial of power, control and access to rewards, material or otherwise that are a result of this disempowerment [7].

Analysis of the FNS exposed a stark contrast between the relationships that existed between community, staff nurse, physician and administration, as well as the moral inhabitability of the work environment, in its 'early years' (pre-corporate-consumer culture) versus its 'latter years' (corporate-consumer culture assimilation). Moreover, these relationships defied the conventional causes of disenfranchisement cited by nurses outside of Eastern Appalachia while the organization was nurse-run, decentralized and relatively free from outside interference. Narratives of nurses in practice today not only supported many of the issues raised by former British and American FNS nurses who experienced the crisis changes

---

[1]Reprint from the FNS Quarterly Bulletin 1948. 85M1: FNS, Box 25, Fol. 21.

imposed upon the adoption of the national health system but also reflected how deeply imbedded within institutional cultures these crisis issues have become and remain. Yet in most cases liberation from oppression is said to come from unveiling the cycle of oppression and the myth developed within the system and not from the leadership or even the dominant group within it [8].

Erikson suggested that people experience an identity crisis when they lose "a sense of personal sameness and historical continuity" and only those individuals who succeed in resolving the crisis will be ready to face future challenges in life [9]. This was evidenced by nurses in this study who volunteered unsolicited confirmation of the profession's dialogue in the literature, which centred on questioning the credibility of icons and distancing itself from history in an effort to reconcile its professional identity to that of the prevailing institutional culture. Further, identity crisis may also be a recurring phenomenon, as the changing world demands us to constantly redefine ourselves and given today's rapid development in technology, global economy, dynamics in local and world politics, identity crises are expected to be more common than they were 30 years ago, when Erikson formed his theory [9]. Much of nursing's supposed resistance to change can be traced to these rapid developments within an equally rigid practice environment.

Perhaps a first step in getting nurses to become culture change ready is to identify the true nature of our problems. Indeed, Lafer argues that *there has never really been a 'nursing shortage,' but there has always been cyclical "shortages of nurses willing to work under the current conditions created by hospital managers"* [Italics added] [10]. The nurse interview and survey data presented here have also indicated a strong consensus regarding both the cause and potential solution to this problem and until their voices are heeded, the cycle will continue. Therefore, the question emerging from analysis of the FNS, which needs to be posed to the profession as a whole is, "Has the embracing of institutional identity (namely, the business and medical models) within the nursing profession, its higher education and practice settings impeded the discipline's ability to impact more successfully for sustained, positive change within these environments?" In order to answer this question, nurses must first be aware that the continual recruitment, retention, work environment and image concerns that nursing faces are not caused solely by those barriers which exist external to the profession, such as a lack of political power, funding or even the institutionalization of health care. They also are being created by the inability to deal with the barriers within the profession that have been either caused or created by the profession's inability to deal with them inside the existing institutional culture.

In an article entitled, *From Tall Poppies to Squashed Weeds: Why Don't Nurses Pull Together More,* Farrell concluded that it was not only the alleged misogyny intrinsic to oppression or feminist theory that shackled and impeded nurses, but nurses themselves who in their everyday work and interpersonal interactions, act as insidious gatekeepers to an iniquitous status quo [7]. Nursing shortages are created by both of these barriers and cannot be stopped by either viewing them as merely 'endemic to modern organizational life' or by blaming all of the discipline's schisms upon its outside forces.

A poll of 5679 senior leaders from 77 US based companies revealed that the reason they determined to join, stay with or leave a company was: *values and culture* [Italics added] (58%), freedom and autonomy (56%), exciting job challenges (51%), well managed (50%) and career advancement (39%) [11]. For nurses in practice today, as well as FNS nurses who witnessed the changes within the organization in its latter years, the major reason cited for dissatisfaction was a lack of autonomy and poor management. *Oddly enough, culture and values often were either not identified as a factor or not addressed.* The responses generated from both older as well as younger nurses presented here validate what is happening nationwide. According to the US Department of Health and Human Services, nurses may constitute the most dissatisfied profession in the US today. Slightly more than 23 of registered nurses 69.5% reported being even "moderately satisfied" with their jobs in 2000. In 2010 that level of satisfaction dropped to 51.8% [12]. Reporting recent changes in the *industry* [italics added], a survey done by the Nursing Executive Centre reported in 1999 that 51% of all registered nurses stated that they were less satisfied with their jobs than they had been just 2 years earlier [13]. Hospital staff nurses had the lowest satisfaction at 66% than any other type of nurse when analyzed by place of work. Numerous studies by those within as well as without the profession have focused on the multiple frustrations facing nurses such as, "feeling exhausted and discouraged, powerless to affect the change necessary for safe, quality patient care and feeling frightened for themselves or their patients" since even before the twentieth century with much the same or worse results [14].

Yet while nurse dissatisfaction is endemic, survey after survey also reports that nurses would like to continue working as nurses if job conditions were improved, many stating that they would stay, and many others who have left nursing altogether stating that they would consider returning if certain conditions were met. As a group, nurses have among the lowest engagement levels of any category of workers Gallup has studied. Nearly one in four nurses (25%) are currently actively disengaged, compared to only 16% of the U.S. working population. Gallup defines actively disengaged staff as "physically present but psychologically absent." They are unhappy with their work situations and insist on sharing their unhappiness with their colleagues. So, even nurses with no plans to leave the profession also echo many of these same sentiments [15]. What is perhaps most telling about this condition is that the business issues of compensation and better work hours have been repeatedly cited and addressed since 1948, to positive effect, at least in the short term. However, though the 'humanization' of the institutional setting has also been cited since before 1948, little or no sustained positive change has been forthcoming in regard to the cultural issues of respect and a morally inhabitable work environment [16].

Nursing's crisis issues cannot be halted solely by gaining political knowledge, socio-economic clout or by embracing science and technology over humanitarian aims. Unfortunately, some nurse administrators within the system have bought into the ethos of the existing 'crisis-prone' management style of the establishment. They manage in the belief that a crisis can be handled by increasing power or technology, denying the possibility of a crisis or involving fate as an excuse to do nothing about it. Trapped by the same structural and bureaucratic rigidity as their employees or students within these organizations, they often end-up trying to survive within the system instead of serving as leaders, movers and shakers for constructive transformation [17]. Further, the profession's attempts at change, which focus on issues surrounding 'Nightingalism,' men in nursing, uniforms, public image and attempts at professional recognition that solely focus on salary increases or hours of work decreases are really just treatment of the symptoms and not the root causes of the profession's main problem; namely, its cultural identity crisis and need for core belief clarification.

Friss noted that as early as 1915, leaders in the nursing profession were concerned with the "image problem of nurses," which they saw as needing improvement. She stated that since then, countless studies, reports, and commissions have attempted to explain and solve perceived shortages of registered nurses, which have always occurred regularly after brief periods of quiescence or oversupply. Usually their recommendations have not dealt with the real issues of nursing work but rather on the 'image' of the profession [18]. These studies and commissions do little more than recycle data and obscure the profession's fundamental problems which in turn create role and identity confusion within its ranks. Their ineffectiveness to bring about sustained positive change suggests the need for less "image enhancement" and more actual leadership and effort to garner support from physicians, hospital administrators, the government and the public to bring about health care system reform instead of continuing the cycle of investing in recruitment in times of perceived 'shortage' while simultaneously doing nothing to foster retention within the institutional setting. The reality is that only top organizational managers have the power to bring about major cultural change and these managers must also be professional leaders. Leaders like Nightingale and Breckinridge, who set an excellent ethical example and removed or reprimanded those lax in monitoring ethical compliance; encouraged fresh ideas and suggestions; tolerated mavericks with creative ideas, giving them room to operate; and who were willing to tolerate failures and reward success, while encouraging people who championed unsuccessful ideas to try again.

Nurse leaders can be a catalyst for change but this can only be achieved by impacting a society or organization's core beliefs. Values, fears, behaviours and infrastructure all flow from core beliefs. Therefore, attempts at changing culture by changing these elements are doomed to failure until the core beliefs are changed [19]. Historically, the discipline of nursing has always had to change and evolve while maintaining commitment to its 'care' roots. Adaptive cultures are also said to have a strong commitment to timeless principles; a sense of confidence among all employees to do what is needed to ensure long-term success and to be proactive in implementing workable solutions. In addition, adaptive cultures are supportive of people proposing useful change, adept at changing the right things in the right way and genuinely concerned about the well-being of others [20]. These traits are all hallmarks of nursing and decidedly stem from a 'people focused' perspective. Indeed, Breckinridge's philosophy regarding the importance of managers and employees being receptive to risk-taking, experimentation, innovation and changing strategies are also values indicative of an adaptive, people focused culture. All of the traits associated with strong and high-performance cultures are people oriented, emphasizing achievement and excellence and producing extraordinary results with ordinary people [21]. These are all values that made the FNS successful for so long and which, even after Breckinridge's death helped the organization to survive. Further, these traits were perpetuated within the FNS via stories/history; rituals; material symbols and language [22].

What is necessary to heal nursing's identity crisis is for the profession to embrace the changes wrought by science, technology and global economics while simultaneously recommitting itself to the community-based and service (or people) oriented vision of its founders. These are not mutually exclusive concepts and either concept should not be embraced as of superior value to the other. What can be gained from this historical analysis is the needed for nursing to rediscover its core values and beliefs and begin to use them to shape the social context of our times, instead of vice versa. Though this has been happening as evidenced by the rise of nurse led clinics, services and in consulting and advanced practice roles, it is of particular interest to note that of the six former FNS nurses interviewed who were at the Service during the end of Breckinridge's tenure, and who stayed well beyond their 2-year commitment, all had careers beyond Appalachia that included furthering their education and becoming nurse leaders' them-selves. All of these nurses credited Breckinridge's leadership and organizational environment as their inspiration, in much the same way that Breckinridge herself credited Nightingale as her muse. The far-reaching and empowering value inherent within a morally inhabitable environment made so by strong nurse leaders, who embrace, value and seek to perpetuate their profession's identity in the marketplace; who are ready, willing and able to take a seat at the negotiating table with institutional administrators and physicians to push for sustained positive change for nurses and their patients cannot be underestimated.

References

1. Salstrom P. Appalachia's path to dependency: rethinking a region's economic history, 1730–1940. Lexington: University Press of Kentucky; 2015, 133, 34.
2. Lu H, Zhao Y, While A. Job satisfaction among hospital nurses: a literature review. Int J Nurs Stud. 2019;94:21–31. https://doi.org/10.1016/j.ijnurstu.2019.01.011.
3. Abramson R, Haskell J. Encyclopaedia of Appalachia. Knoxville: University of Tennessee Press; 2006. p. 1563.
4. Cleland V. Sex discrimination: nursing's most pervasive problem. Am J Nurs. 1971;71:1542–7.
5. Thierry P, Mitroff I. Transforming the crisis-prone organization: preventing individual, organizational and environmental tragedies. San Francisco: Jossey-Bass Inc.; 1992. p. 6.
6. Lipset S. American intellectuals: their politics and status. In: Political man: the social basis of politics. p. 12.
7. Farrell G. From tall poppies to squashed weeds: why don't nurses pull together more? J Adv Nurs. 2001;35(1):26–33.
8. Feire P. Pedagogy of the oppressed. New York: Bloomsbury Academic; 2018.

9. Cote J. Fifty years since "identity: youth and crisis": a renewed look at Erikson's writings on identity. Int J Theory Res. 2018;18(4):251–63. https://doi.org/10.1080/15283488.2018.1524328.
10. Lafer G. Hospital speedups and the fiction of a nursing shortage. Labour Stud J. 2005;30(1):27–46.
11. Chambers EG, Foulon M, Handfield-Jones H, Hankin SM, Michaels EG. The war for talent. McKinsey Q. 1998;1(3):44–57.
12. The registered nurse populations 2008: findings from the National Sample Survey of Registered Nurses. Washington DC: Division of Nursing, Bureau of Health Professions, US Department of Health & Human Services, Health Resources & Services Administration; 2010. p. 31. https://bhw.hrsa.gov/sites/default/files/bhw/nchwa/rnsurveyfinal.pdf.
13. American Federation of State, County & Municipal Employees (AFSCME). Listening to nurses: dissatisfaction and burnout on the job. https://www.afscme.org/news/publications/health-care/solving-the-nursing-shortage/listening-to-nurses-dissatisfaction-and-burnout-on-the-job. Accessed 16 Feb 2019.
14. Tovey EJ, Adams AE. The changing nature of nurses' job satisfaction: an exploration of sources of satisfaction in the 1990s. J Adv Nurs. 1999;30(1):150–8.
15. Blizzard R. Nurses may be satisfied but are they engaged? Gallup poll. 2002. https://news.gallup.com/poll/6004/nurses-may-satisfied-they-engaged.aspx. Accessed 16 Feb 2019.
16. Cohen J. Minority report: working party on the recruitment and training of nurses. London: Metropolitan Library Archives; 1948.
17. Thierry P, Mitroff I. Transforming the crisis-prone organization: preventing individual, organizational and environmental tragedies. San Francisco: Jossey-Bass Inc.; 1992.
18. Friss L. Nursing studies laid end to end form a circle. J Health Polit Policy Law. 1994;19(3):597–631.
19. Van den Steen E. On the origin of shared beliefs (and corporate culture). Rand J Econ. 2010;41(4):617–48.
20. Thompson A, Strickland A. Strategic management: concepts and cases. New York: Irwin/McGraw-Hill; 2001.
21. Kotter J, Heskett J. Corporate culture and performance. New York: Simon & Schuster; 2011.
22. Johnson G. Rethinking incrementalism. Strateg Manag J. 1988;9(1):76.

Illustration(s) (Photographs)

Illustration(s) (Photographs) 2

Judy Halse Posing
For FNS Bulletin
(1960s)

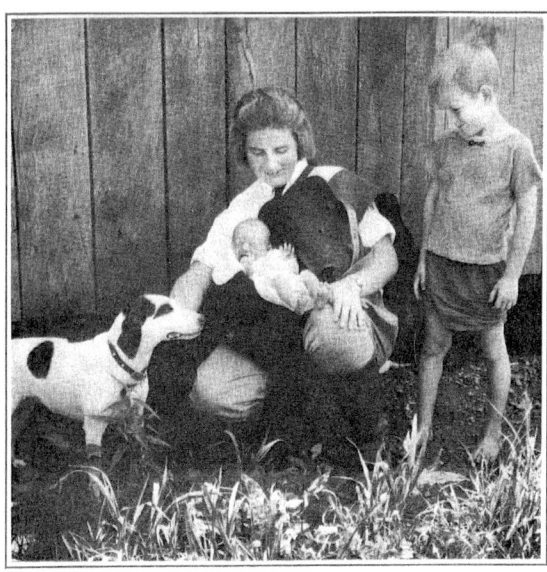

FRONTIER NURSING SERVICE
QUARTERLY BULLETIN

VOLUME 40   SUMMER, 1964   NUMBER 1

THIRTY-NINTH ANNUAL REPORT

SADDLEBAG BABY

© Springer Nature Switzerland AG 2019
E. West, *Frontier Nursing in Appalachia: History, Organization and the Changing Culture of Care*, https://doi.org/10.1007/978-3-030-20027-5

Illustration(s) (Photographs) 3

Mary Breckinridge with "Third Generation" FNS 'Baby' outside of her home and administrative offices, 'The Big House' (Circa 1960s) .... Note both Breckinridge's and the child's attire and surroundings…

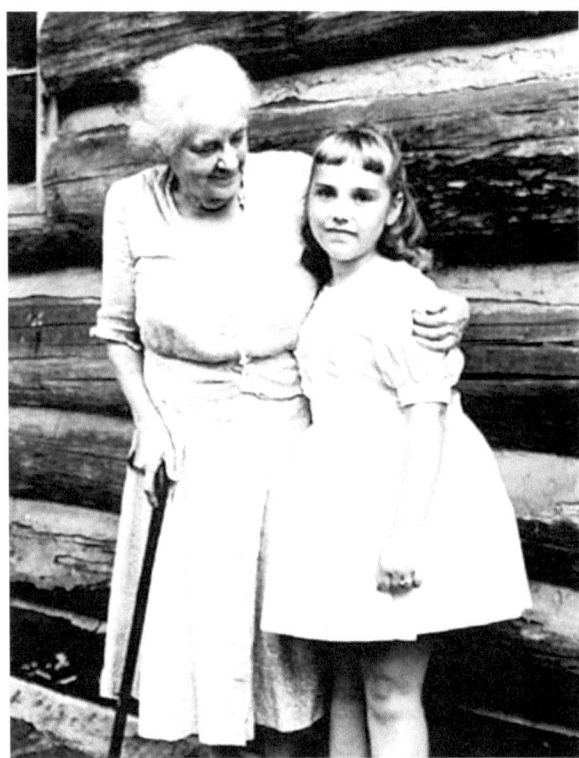

Illustration(s) (Photographs) 4

'Big House' interior, then and now, with Molly Lee at Thanksgiving Dinner in 'then' photo (circa 1960s).

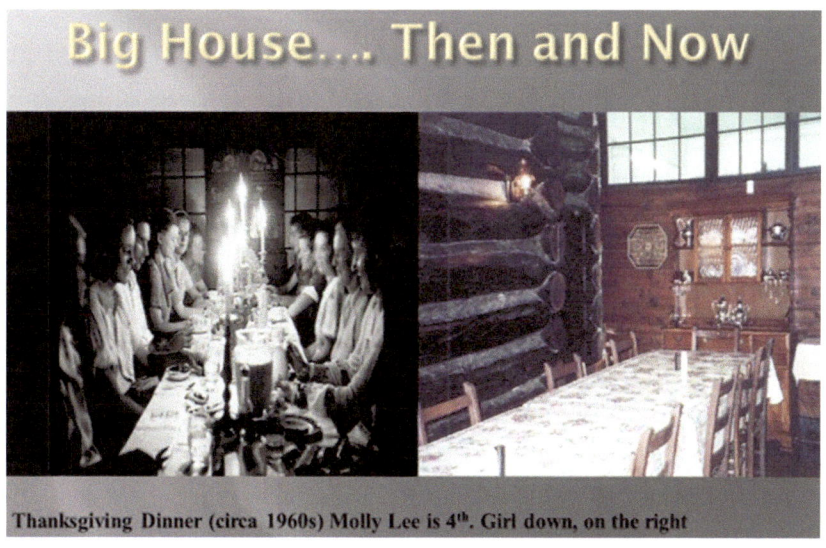

Thanksgiving Dinner (circa 1960s) Molly Lee is 4th. Girl down, on the right

Illustration(s) (Photographs) 5

Former British FNS Nurse Maggie Willson (standing) with (left to right): Helen Browne, FNS Founder, Mary Breckinridge and her Cousin, Marvin Breckinridge.

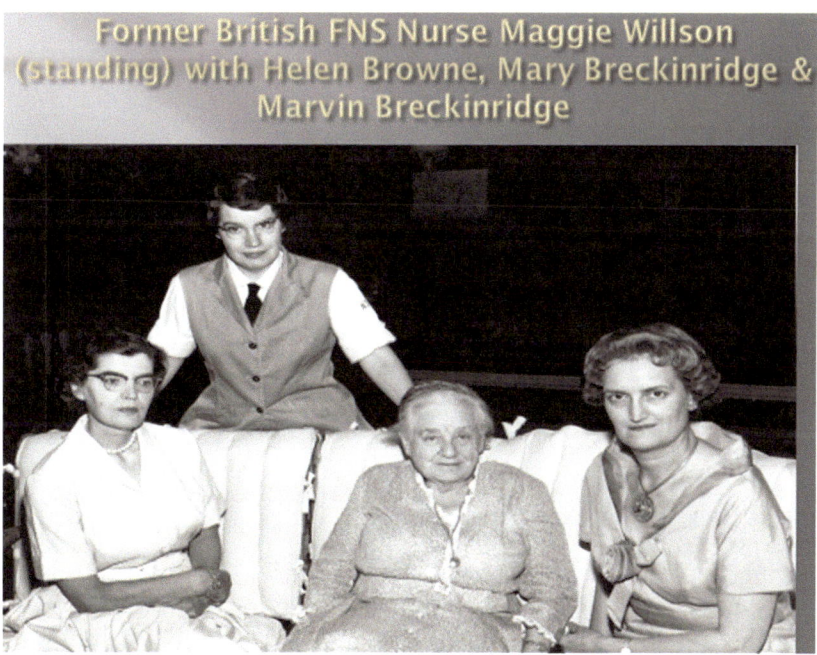

Illustration(s) (Photographs) 6

Former British FNS Nurse, Maggie Willson with 'Baby in her Saddlebag' promotional photograph.

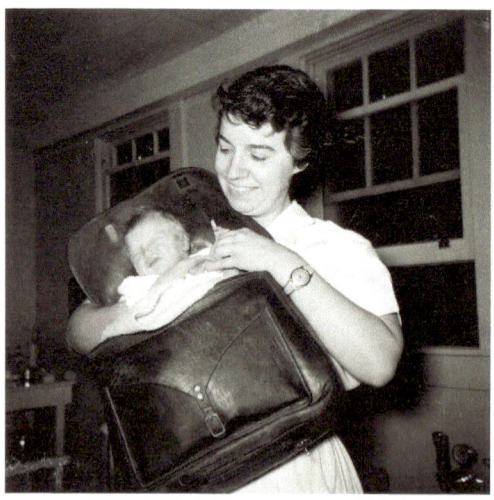

Illustration(s) (Photographs) 7

Author, Dr. Edie West, with former British FNS Nurses Judy Halse and Maggie WIllson, then and now…

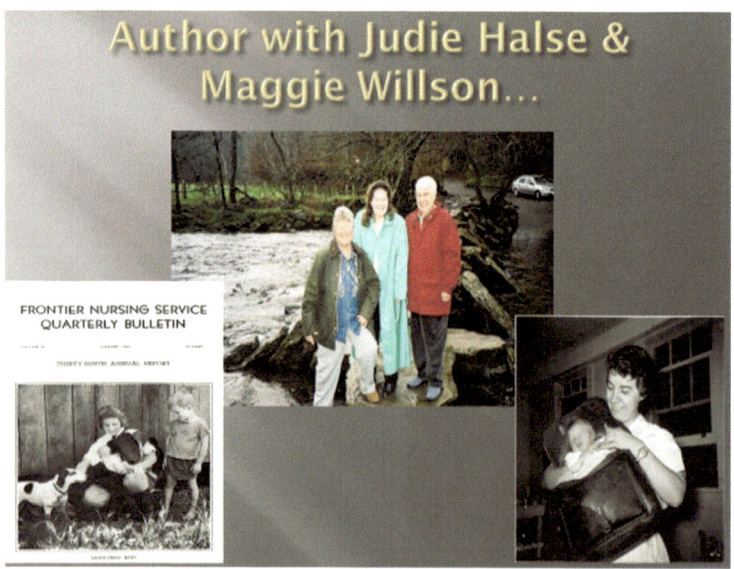

Illustration(s) (Photographs) 8

Former British FNS Nurse, Molly Lee, with Appalachian mother and twins she delivered.

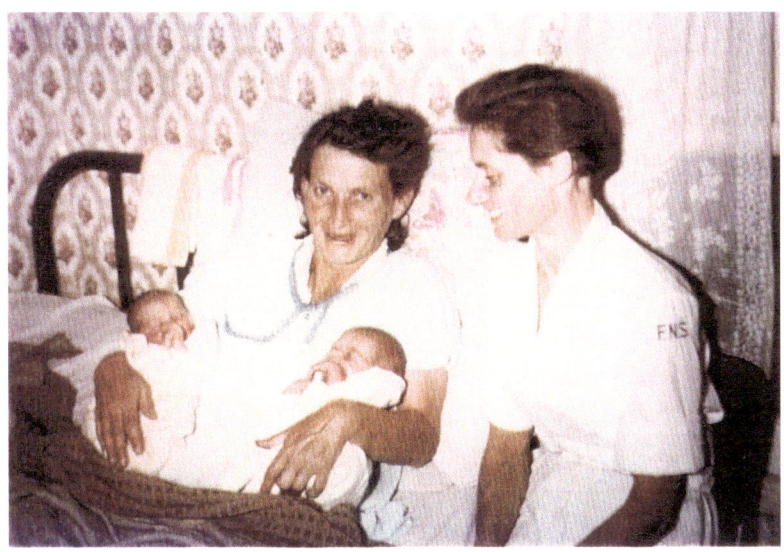

Illustration(s) (Photographs) 9

Former British FNS Nurses: Molly Lee & Betty "Hilly" Hillman… then and now.

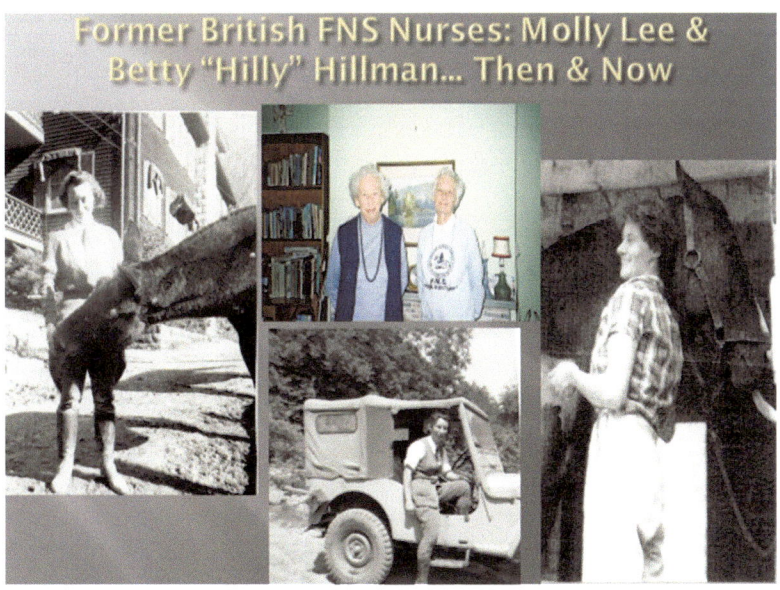

Illustration(s) (Photographs) 10

Former British FNS Nurse, Betty "Hilly" Hillman on an Appalachian home visit.

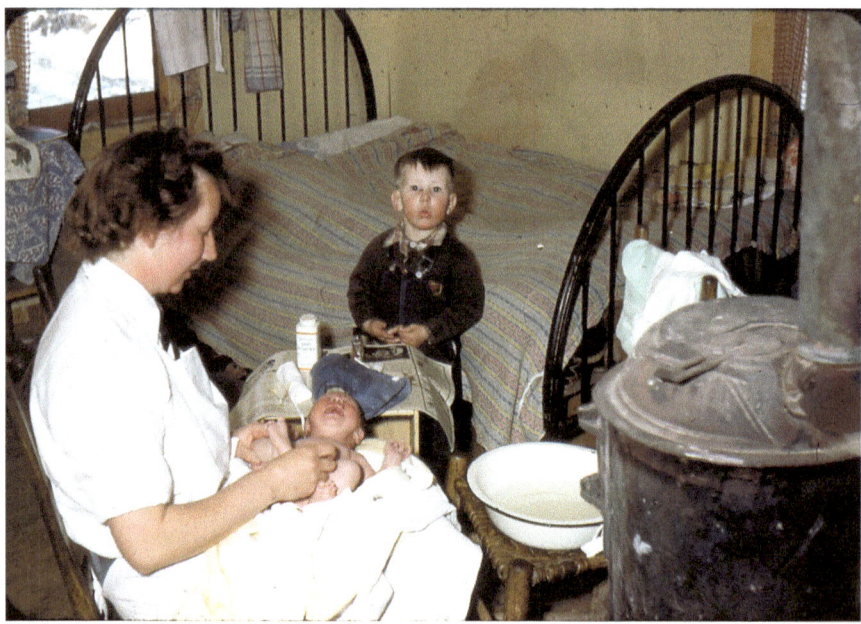

Illustration(s) (Photographs) 11

British FNS Nurse Betty Lester (on white horse), FNS Founder, Mary Breckinridge, former British FNS Nurse Molly Lee (far right) and one other FNS Nurse on horseback preparing to ride on "Mary Breckinridge Day."

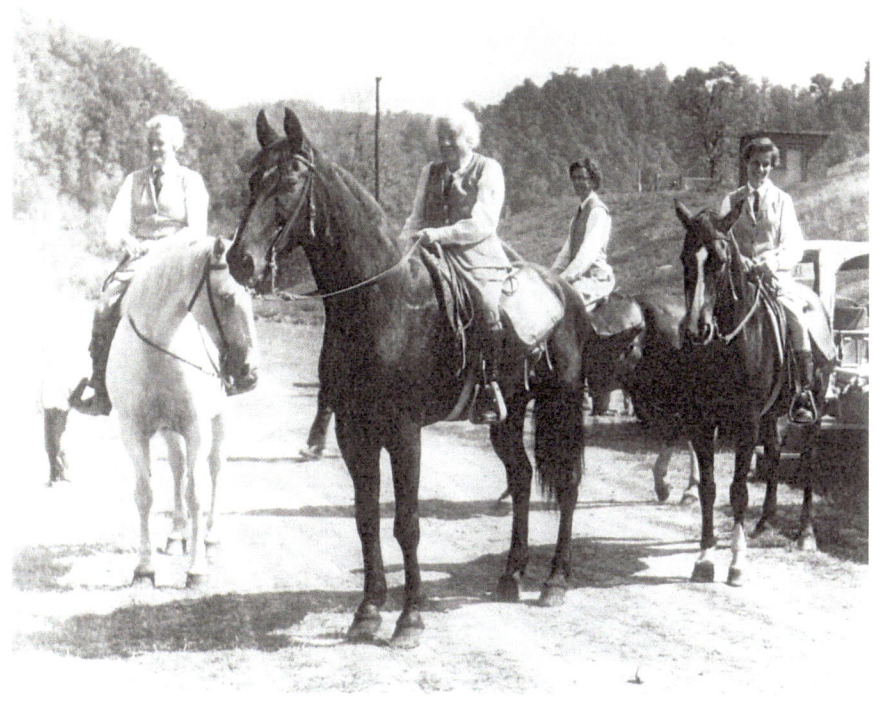

Illustration(s) (Photographs) 12

Unidentified FNS Nurse, her dog and jeep (circa 1960s).

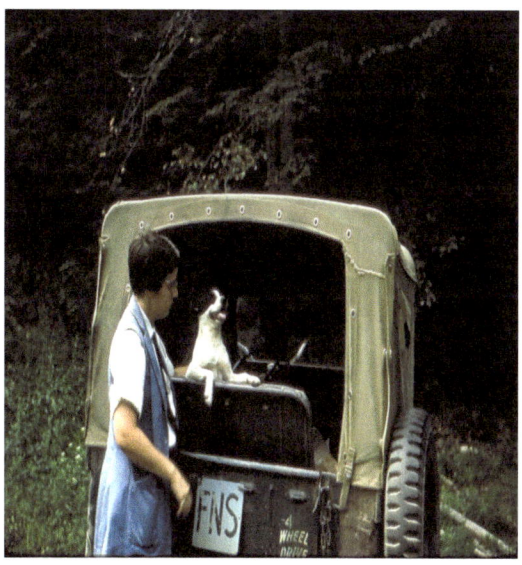

Illustration(s) (Photographs) 13

Former American FNS Nurse and one of the first graduates of the Frontier Graduate School of Midwifery, Doris E. Reid and her dog on horseback.

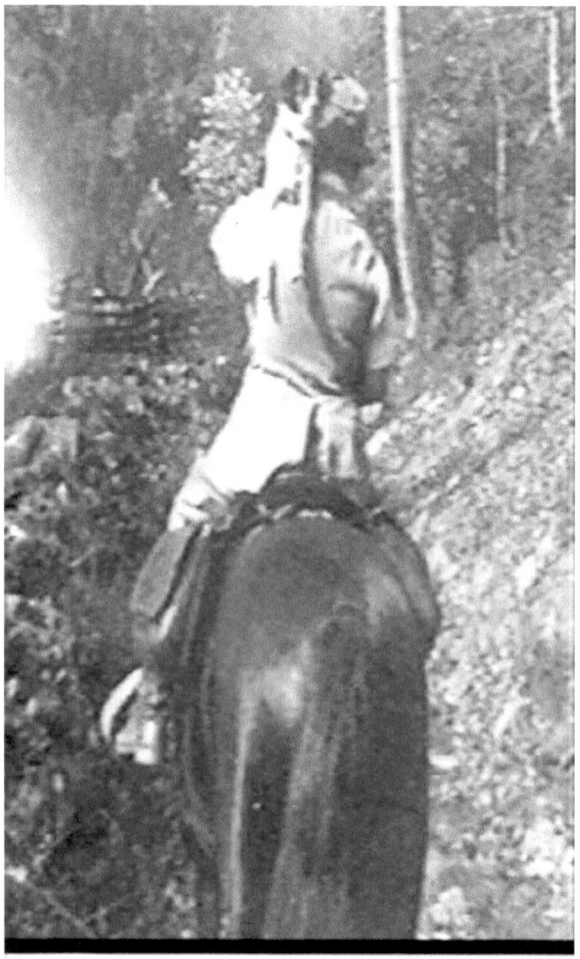

Good Bye

Illustration (Maps) 14: The Appalachian Region as Defined by The Appalachian Regional Commission (ARC)

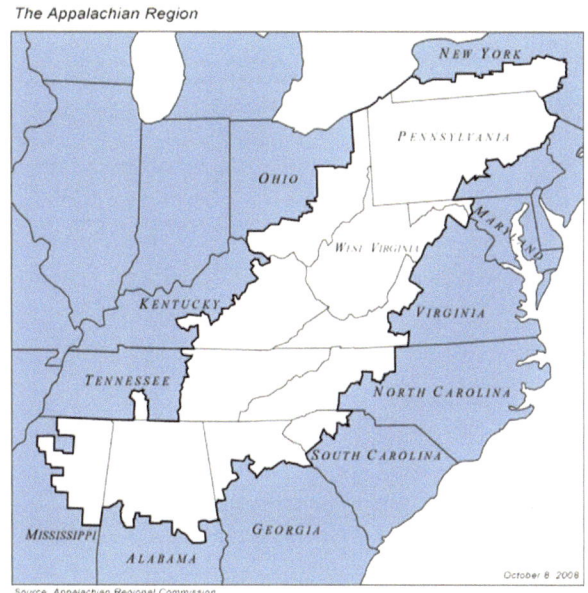

Counties or county-equivalents 420
States 13
Population (2010)
Total 25 million

Appendix A: Interview Questions

1. Demographic data (education level, nationality, background, practice history/area, "Tell me a bit about yourself")
2. What did you know about nursing before you went into training?
3. Why did you choose to become a nurse? (**In addition for FNS nurses: "How did you learn about the FNS and why did you choose to go there?"**)
4. Was nursing all you thought it would be? (**In addition for FNS nurses: "Was working for the FNS all you thought it would be?"**)
5. What do you like best about nursing? (**In addition for FNS nurses: "What did you like best about nursing at the FNS?"**)
6. What do you like least about nursing? (**In addition for FNS nurses: "What did you like least about nursing at the FNS?"**)
7. How long have you been a nurse? Would you consider leaving nursing and if so, why? (**In addition for FNS nurses: "How long were you at the FNS? When did you leave, and why?"**)
8. Would you choose nursing as a career now if you had it to do over again? (**In addition for FNS nurses: "Would you choose to go work for the FNS today if you had it to do over again? How did your work at the FNS compare with nursing you did elsewhere?"**)
9. Have nurses changed? (**In addition for FNS nurses: "Did you notice a change in nurses at the FNS during your tenure there?"**)
10. Has the profession changed? (**In addition for FNS nurses: "How did the FNS change during your tenure there?"**)
11. What do you see the future of nursing as being?
12. How do you think the public views nurses and nursing? (**In addition for FNS nurses: "Did the people in Appalachia view nurses differently than people outside of that area?"**)

© Springer Nature Switzerland AG 2019
E. West, *Frontier Nursing in Appalachia: History, Organization and the Changing Culture of Care*, https://doi.org/10.1007/978-3-030-20027-5

Prompt Questions

Can you give an example…?
Can you elaborate…?
Can you explain…?
What makes you think that…?

Appendix B: FNS 'Early Years' Organizational Chart (Undated)

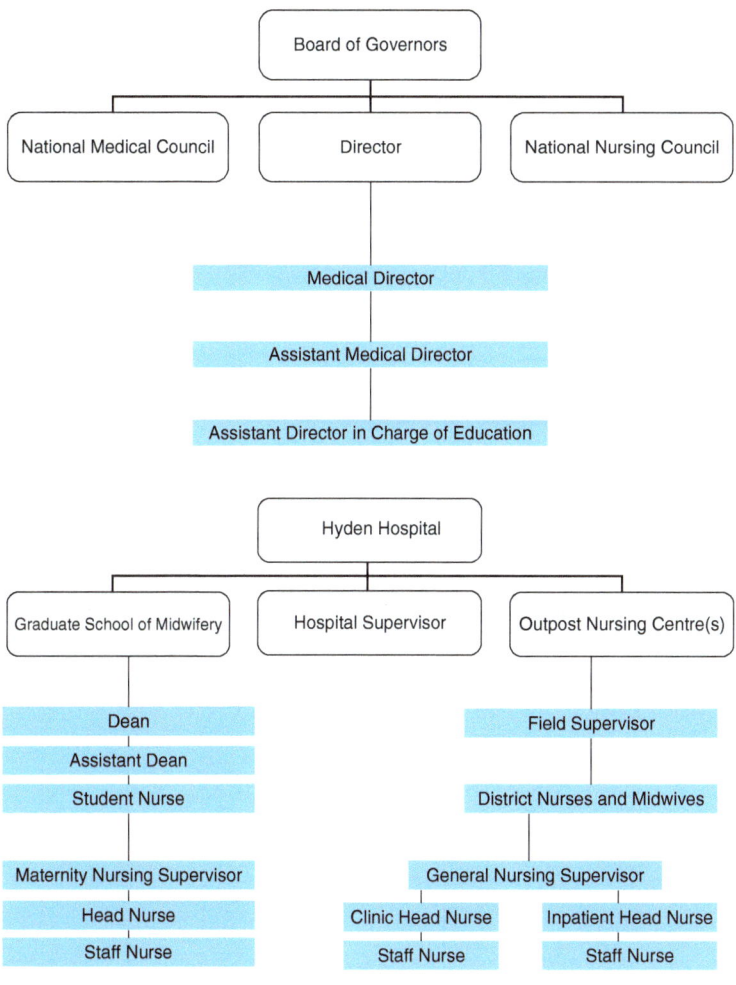

© Springer Nature Switzerland AG 2019
E. West, *Frontier Nursing in Appalachia: History, Organization and the Changing Culture of Care*, https://doi.org/10.1007/978-3-030-20027-5

Appendix C: FNS Organizational Chart, 2007

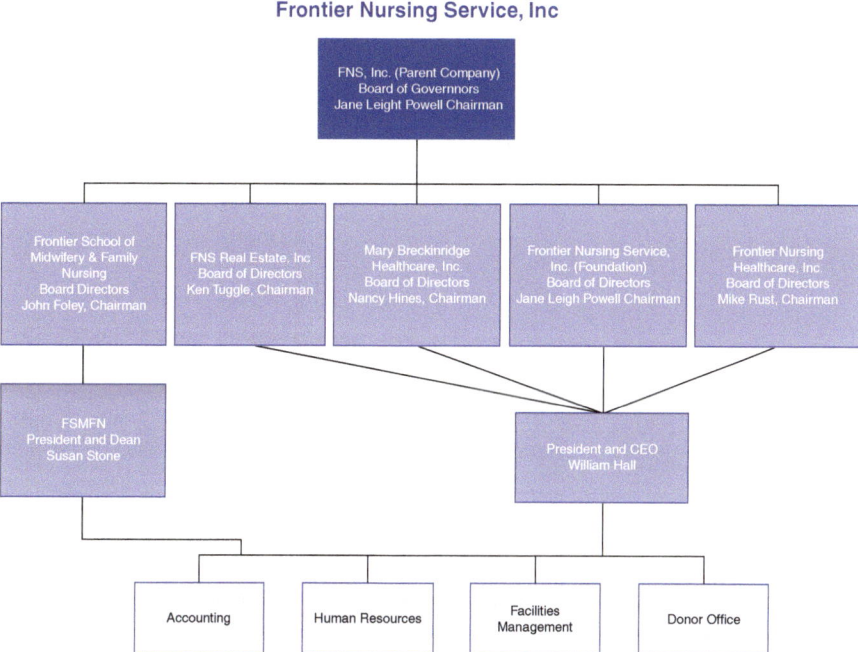

© Springer Nature Switzerland AG 2019
E. West, *Frontier Nursing in Appalachia: History, Organization and the Changing Culture of Care*, https://doi.org/10.1007/978-3-030-20027-5

Appendix D: FNS Philosophy, 2007

Philosophy

FNS Object

To safeguard the lives and health of mothers and children by providing and preparing trained nurse-midwives and nurse-practitioners for rural areas where there is inadequate medical service;

To give skilled care to women in childbirth;

To give nursing care to the sick of both sexes and all ages;

To establish, own, maintain and operate hospitals, clinics, nursing centers and educational programs for nurse-midwives and nurse-practitioners;

To carry out preventive public health measures to educate the rural population in the laws of health, and parents in baby hygiene and child care;

To provide expert social service;

To obtain medical, dental and surgical services for those who need them, at a price they can afford to pay;

To promote the general welfare of the elderly and handicapped;

To ameliorate economic conditions inimical to health and growth and to conduct research toward that end;

To do any and all other things in any way incident to or connected with these objects, and, in pursuit of them to cooperate with individual and with organizations, private, state or federal;

And thought the fulfillment of these aims to advance the cause of health, social welfare and economic independence in rural districts with the help of their own leading citizens.

From the Articles of Incorporations of the Frontier Nursing Service. Article III as amended June 8, 1984.

© Springer Nature Switzerland AG 2019
E. West, *Frontier Nursing in Appalachia: History, Organization and the Changing Culture of Care*, https://doi.org/10.1007/978-3-030-20027-5

Appendix E: American Nurses Association (ANA) Code of Ethics with Interpretive Statements

1. The nurse will handle professional relationships with compassion and respect for inherent worth, dignity, uniqueness of every individual.
2. The nurse's primary commitment is to the patient (individual, family, group or community)
3. The nurse promotes, advocates for and strives to protect health, safety and the rights of patients.
4. The nurse is responsible and accountable for individual nursing practice and determines appropriate delegation of tasks consistent with the nurses obligation to provide optimum patient care.
5. The nurse oversees the same duties to self as to others, including integrity, safety, and competence, personal and professional growth.
6. The nurse participates in establishing, maintaining, and improving health care that are consistent with the values of the profession through individual and collective action.
7. The nurse participates in advancement of the profession through continued practice, education, administration and knowledge development.
8. The nurse collaborates with other health professionals and the public in promoting community, national and international efforts to meet health needs.
9. The professional nurse as represented by the association and their members is responsible for articulating nursing values, for maintaining the integrity of the profession and its practice, and for shaping social policy.

© Springer Nature Switzerland AG 2019
E. West, *Frontier Nursing in Appalachia: History, Organization and the Changing Culture of Care*, https://doi.org/10.1007/978-3-030-20027-5

.

Glossary

Adaptive culture The effectiveness or degree with which members within a culture meet the standards of personal independence and social responsibility expected of them when acclimatizing to a new culture.

Business model A framework for creating economic, social, and/or other forms of value. The term is used for a broad range of informal and formal descriptions to represent core aspects of a business, including purpose, offerings, strategies, infrastructure, organizational structures, trading practices, and operational processes and policies. In the most basic sense, a business model is the method of doing business by which a company can sustain itself—that is, generate revenue. The business model spells-out how a company makes money by specifying where it is positioned in the value chain.

Centralized power structure The organization, that is the governing authority of a political unit, the ruling power in a political society and/or the apparatus through which a governing body functions and exercises authority. It is the central authority to which local governments are subject. Centralization occurs both geographically and politically.

Control systems The processes in place to monitor what is going on. Role cultures would have vast rulebooks. There would be more reliance on individualism in a power culture.

Corporate-consumer culture The combined beliefs, values, ethics, procedures, and atmosphere of an organization devoted to the equation of personal fulfilment or happiness with the purchase of goods and services or material possessions. This culture is often expressed as "the way we do things around here" and consists of largely unspoken values, norms, and behaviours that become the natural way of doing things.

Culture Generally refers to patterns of human activity and the symbolic structures that give such activities significance and importance. Cultures can be understood as systems of symbols and meanings that even their creators contest, that lack fixed boundaries, that are constantly in flux, and that interact and compete with one another. Culture can be defined as all the ways of life including arts, beliefs

© Springer Nature Switzerland AG 2019   231
E. West, *Frontier Nursing in Appalachia: History, Organization and the Changing Culture of Care*, https://doi.org/10.1007/978-3-030-20027-5

and institutions of a population that is passed down from generation to generation. Culture has been called 'the way of life for an entire society', including codes of manners, dress, language, religion, rituals, games, norms of behaviour such as law and morality, and systems of belief as well as art.

Cultural assimilation When an individual or individuals adopts some or all aspects of a dominant culture (such as its religion, language, norms, values etc.). Cultural assimilation is a process of socialization. It is mostly a voluntary or "natural" process, but can sometimes be the result of involuntary political decisions.

Decentralized power structure The distribution of administrative functions or powers of a central authority among local authorities.

Enculturation The process whereby an individual learns the accepted norms and value emphases of an established culture through repetition, so that the individual can become an accepted member of the society and find his or her suitable role. Most importantly, it establishes a context of boundaries and correctness that dictates what is and is not permissible within that society's collective framework.

Feeder culture The cultures or environments external to a particular culture that permeates the boundaries of said culture. Some of the cultural elements within that boundary will be truly distinctive to the organization, while other elements, some of which may well be erroneously believed to be unique, will reflect cultural influences external to the organization.

Fragmentation perspective Views culture as a loosely structured and incompletely shared system that emerges dynamically as cultural members experience each other's events and the organisation's contextual features. This perspective acknowledges the integration perspectives search for consistency and the differentiation perspective's search for inconsistency within organizational cultures but goes further, deeper, on to complexity.

High performance culture Companies that emphasize achievement and excellence have a 'results-oriented' culture, pursue policies and practices inspiring people to do their best and produce extraordinary results with ordinary people.

Humanitarian rewards Personal and moral satisfaction generated within an individual as well as social standing or status placed upon an individual by society for their civil, charitable, compassionate and just undertakings with and for others in addition to any professional skill or expertise.

Institutional identity Individuals within an organization embrace and assume the character and persona of the establishment, whatever that ethos may be, in order to survive within that environment.

Low performance culture Characterized by a politicized internal environment (that is autonomous fiefdoms operated by influential managers who resist change and in which issues are resolved on the basis of turf or coalitions), where a hostility toward change exists (i.e., experimentation discouraged, status quo maintained at all costs, and managers promoted who understand structures, systems and controls better than vision, strategies and culture building), and where an aversion exists toward looking outside the organization for superior practices.

Medical model Describes the approach to illness that is dominant in Western medicine. It aims to find medical treatments for diagnosed symptoms and syndromes and treats the human body as a very complex mechanism.

Moral distress When one knows the right thing to do, but institutional constraints make it nearly impossible to pursue the right course of action; the painful psychological disequilibrium that results from recognizing the ethically appropriate action, yet not taking it, because of such obstacles as lack of time, supervisory reluctance, an inhibiting medical power structure, institution policy, or legal considerations; the physical or emotional suffering that is experienced when constraints (internal or external) prevent one from following the course of action that one believes is right.

Moral inhabitability The degree to which a work environment is fit for human habitation, that is without oppressive regulatory components that chafe and containing the rewards inherent in 'a way of doing things' that is not devoid of human interaction, connectedness and the sense of belonging and purpose that give meaning to life.

Nurse-midwife An individual who holds a diploma (or degree) in nursing who has also completed the further educational (degree) requirements and accompanying licensure to practice nursing and midwifery (as a specialty) in the US.

Object-focused 'Bottom-line' centred dealings with others. The end-product is more important than the person or the method used to reach the desired object, or result.

Organizational (or institutional) culture The attitudes, experiences, beliefs and views of an organization, the elements of which describe or influence its paradigm, control system, organization and power structures, symbols, rituals, routines, stories and myths.

Organizational structures Reporting lines, hierarchies, and the way that work flows through the business.

Paradigm What the organization is about; what it does; its mission; its values.

People-focused Relationship-centred dealings with others. The person involved as well as the process used toward achieving a desired result is as important as the end-product or objective of said result.

Power structures Configuration regarding who makes the decisions, how widely power is spread, and on what the power is based.

Professional A person in a specialized occupation or vocation that requires certain types of skilled work requiring formal training or education. In western nations, the term commonly describes highly educated, mostly salaried workers, who enjoy considerable work autonomy, economic security, a comfortable salary, and are commonly engaged in creative and intellectually challenging work.

Professional identity An individual in a specialized occupation or vocation that has embraced the profession's ethos, taken on that culture's characteristics and persona, and is perpetuating it within their existing practice and education environments.

Socio-economic rewards Social standing or status and financial remuneration or wealth bestowed upon an individual for a technical skill or intellectual trait valued within the culture.

Spirituality In a narrow sense, concerns itself with matters of the spirit, a concept closely tied to religious belief and faith, a transcendent reality. Spiritual matters are thus those matters regarding humankind's ultimate nature and meaning, not only as material biological organisms, but as beings with a unique relationship to that which is perceived to be beyond the bodily senses, time and the material world.

Stories and myths A build-up about people and events that conveys a message about what is valued within the organization.

Strong culture Is said to exist where staff respond to stimulus because of their alignment to organizational values. In such environments, strong cultures help firms operate like well-oiled machines, cruising along with outstanding execution and perhaps minor tweaking of existing procedures here and there.

Sub-culture A group of people with a culture (whether distinct or hidden) which differentiates them from the larger culture to which they belong.

Values The principles, standards, or quality which guides human actions; a property of objects, including physical objects as well as abstract objects (e.g. actions), representing their degree of importance that is independent of subjective valuations by any individual.

Weak culture Where there is little alignment with organizational values and control must be exercised through extensive procedures and bureaucracy.

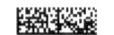